IMMUNOTHERAPY OF HUMAN CANCER

The University of Texas System Cancer Center
M. D. Anderson Hospital and Tumor Institute
22nd Annual Clinical Conference on Cancer

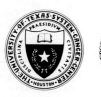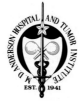

Published for
The University of Texas System Cancer Center
M. D. Anderson Hospital and Tumor Institute
Houston, Texas, by Raven Press, New York

The University of Texas System Cancer Center
M. D. Anderson Hospital and Tumor Institute
22nd Annual Clinical Conference on Cancer

Immunotherapy
of
Human Cancer

Raven Press ■ New York

Raven Press, 1140 Avenue of the Americas, New York, New York 10036

Library of Congress Cataloging in Publication Data

Clinical Conference on Cancer, 22nd, Anderson Hospital
    and Tumor Institute, 1978.
    Immunotherapy of human cancer.

    Includes bibliographical references and indexes.
    1. Cancer--Immunological aspects--Congresses.
2. Immunotherapy--Congresses. I. Anderson Hospital
and Tumor Institute, Houston, Tex. II. Title.
RC271.I45C55   1978   616.9'94'079   77-17701
ISBN 0-89004-263-2

The material contained in this volume was submitted as previously unpublished material, except in the instances in which credit has been given to the source from which some of the illustrative material was derived.

Great care has been taken to maintain the accuracy of the information contained in the volume. However, the Editorial Staff and The University of Texas System Cancer Center cannot be held responsible for errors or for any consequences arising from the use of the information contained herein.

Contents

ix   Introduction
     R. Lee Clark, Robert C. Hickey, and Evan M. Hersh

Heath Memorial Award Lecture

3   Introduction of Heath Memorial Award Recipient
     Robert C. Hickey

5   Active Immunotherapy: Experimental and Rational Basis
     Georges Mathé

Immunologic and Clinical Basis of Immunotherapy

31   Principles of Immunology with Relevance to Immunotherapy
     J. L. Fahey

41   Host Mechanisms for Control of Tumor Growth That Can Be Modulated by Nonspecific Immunotherapy
     David W. Weiss

63   Experimental Basis of Immunotherapy for Metastatic Disease
     Isaiah J. Fidler

83   Clinical Rationale for Immunotherapy and Its Role in Cancer Treatment
     Evan M. Hersh, Jordan U. Gutterman, Giora M. Mavligit, Christine H. Granatek, Roger D. Rossen, Adan Rios, Allan L. Goldstein, Yehuda Z. Patt, Ernesto Rivera, Stephen P. Richman, Joseph C. Bottino, David Farquhar, Dexter Morris, and Khoji Ezaki

Approaches to Immunotherapy

101   Chairman's Introduction—Animal Models of Cancer Immunotherapy: Some Considerations
     David W. Weiss

111   BCG Immunotherapy: Efficacy of BCG-Induced Tumor Immunity in Guinea Pigs with Regional Tumor and/or Visceral Micrometastases
     M. G. Hanna, Jr. and Leona C. Peters

131   Immunotherapy for Tumors with Microbial Constituents or Their Synthetic Analogues. A Review
     Edgar Ribi, Charles A. McLaughlin, John L. Cantrell, Werner Brehmer, Ichiro Azuma, Yuichi Yamamura, S. Michael Strain, Kou M. Hwang, and Raoul Toubiana

155   Actions and Interactions of *Corynebacterium parvum* in Experimental
       Tumor Systems
       Lester J. Peters

173   Thymosin Therapy: Approach to Immunoreconstitution in Immunodefi-
       ciency Diseases and Cancer
       Allan L. Goldstein, Gailen D. Marshall, Jr., and Jeffrey L. Rossio

181   Combined Levamisole Therapy: An Overview of Its Protective Effects
       Michael A. Chirigos and William K. Amery

197   Transfer Factor and Immunotherapy for Cancer
       H. Sherwood Lawrence

213   Active-Specific Immunotherapy
       Ariel C. Hollinshead

Clinical Immunotherapy

237   Chemoimmunotherapy for Acute Myelocytic Leukemia
       James F. Holland, J. George Bekesi, and Janet Cuttner

245   Preliminary Results of Three Chemotherapy-Immunotherapy Protocols
       for Treatment of Acute Lymphoid Leukemia in Children
       *Georges Mathé, Francoise de Vassal, Léon Schwarzenberg, Miguel Del-
       gado, Roy Weiner, Marianne Gil, Juan Pena-Angulo, Dominique Bel-
       pomme, Pierre Pouillart, David Machover, Jean-Louis Misset, José-
       Luis Pico, Claude Jasmin, Maurice Hayat, Maurice Schneider, Albert
       Cattan, Jean-Louis Amiel, Marina Musset, Claude Rosenfeld, and Pa-
       tricia Ribaud*

257   Immunotherapy for Malignant Melanoma
       *Jordan U. Gutterman, Giora M. Mavligit, Stephen P. Richman, Robert
       S. Benjamin, Anne Kennedy, Charles M. McBride, Michael A. Burgess,
       Shelley L. Bartold, Edmund A. Gehan, and Evan M. Hersh*

267   Immunology and Immunotherapy of Human Sarcomas
       *Joseph G. Sinkovics, Carl Plager, Nicholas Papadopoulos, Marion J.
       McMurtrey, Jimmy J. Romero, Ruth Waldinger, and Marvin M.
       Romsdahl*

289   Immunotherapy for Genitourinary Cancer
       David Eidinger

303   Immunotherapy for Gynecologic Malignancies
       Stanley A. Gall

321   Immunotherapy and Chemoimmunotherapy for Human Breast Cancer
       *G. N. Hortobagyi, J. U. Gutterman, G. R. Blumenschein, A. U. Buzdar,
       S. P. Richman, C. Wiseman, and E. M. Hersh*

347   Nonspecific Immunotherapy for Lung Cancer
      Martin F. McKneally

355   Adjuvant Immunotherapy for Colorectal Cancer
      *Giora M. Mavligit, Mary Anne Malahy, Nancy Zatopek, and Evan M.
      Hersh*

Principles and Prospects for Immunotherapy

363   Some New Approaches to Cancer Immunotherapy in Man
      Lucien Israël, Richard Edelstein, and Raymond Samak

375   Limitations, Obstacles, and Controversies in the Optimal Development
      of Immunotherapy
      Michael J. Mastrangelo, David Berd, and Robert E. Bellet

395   Prospects for the Future of Immunotherapy: The Need for Individualism
      Jordan U. Gutterman

407   *Author Index*

409   *Subject Index*

Introduction

R. Lee Clark, M.D., D.Sc. (Hon.),* Robert C. Hickey, M.D.,†
and Evan M. Hersh, M.D.‡

*President, The University of Texas System Cancer Center, and Professor of Surgery,
M. D. Anderson Hospital and Tumor Institute; †Executive Vice President, The University
of Texas System Cancer Center, and Director and Professor of Surgery, M. D. Anderson
Hospital and Tumor Institute; ‡Professor of Medicine, Chief, Section of Immunology,
and Deputy Head, Department of Developmental Therapeutics, M. D. Anderson Hospital
and Tumor Institute, Houston, Texas

The concepts that human tumors are antigenically distinct from the host and might be subject to attack by host defense mechanisms, and that therapeutic manipulations might alter or augment these host defense mechanisms go back to the turn of the century and to the writings of Paul Ehrlich. These concepts remained highly controversial until the 1950s, when Ludwik Gross unequivocally demonstrated the presence of tumor antigens and tumor immunity in mouse tumor systems. During the last two decades, many studies have demonstrated that tumor-associated antigens and tumor-associated immune responses are present in many, if not all, experimental animal and human tumors. These responses include classic cell-mediated and humoral immunity as well as nonspecific host defense mechanisms involving the reticuloendothelial system and macrophages.

Slightly less than 20 years ago, it was demonstrated in mice that immunologic manipulation of the host, namely, administration of bacillus Calmette-Guérin (BCG), protects animals from the subsequent development of tumors induced by chemical carcinogens or oncogenic viruses. During the last decade, expansion of this experimental basis has laid the foundation for the gradually emerging clinical discipline of immunotherapy. Also during the last decade, development of techniques through which the human immune response can be critically evaluated, demonstration of the immunosuppressive effects of the tumor-bearing state, characterization of the immunosuppressive effects of conventional cancer treatment, and documentation of the relationship between immunocompetence and prognosis in cancer have added a strong, rational, scientific basis to this field.

During the first half of the 20th century, a number of empirical clinical trials of immunotherapy appeared positive. However, several subsequent clinical experiments, which now can be considered classic, have established the clinical foundations of immunotherapy. These include the demonstration by Professor Georges Mathé that remission duration in childhood acute leukemia can be prolonged by the administration of BCG, irradiated allogeneic tumor cells, or both. Also important were the demonstration by Dr. Donald Morton that cutaneous, metastatic melanoma nodules can be induced to regress in immunocompetent patients through the intralesional injection of BCG, and the demonstration by Edmund Klein that a variety of primary cutaneous tumors can be caused to regress by the topical application of DNCB after sensitization of the subject to that hapten. In the latter study, it was most important that in patients with multiple, recurrent, primary skin tumors, the rate of new tumor formation was retarded after intralesional or topical therapy for a few primary tumors.

Tumor immunobiology and experimental and clinical immunotherapy have been prominent in the program at M. D. Anderson Hospital and Tumor Institute of The University of Texas System Cancer Center for some time. This is evidenced by the prominence of these topics in several of our annual basic science symposia and the presentation of the annual Ernst W. Bertner Memorial Award to Dr. Ludwik Gross in 1963 and to Dr. George Klein in 1973 for their preeminent work in tumor immunobiology and virology. Furthermore, our staff has developed a major program for both animal model work and clinical immunotherapy trials during the last seven years. Currently, there are more than 20 active clinical immunotherapy protocols at M. D. Anderson Hospital, and several thousand patients are receiving immunotherapy as an adjunct to conventional therapy.

As the science of modern immunobiology has developed, the various approaches to immunotherapy have become well defined; these include active-nonspecific immunotherapy with adjuvants such as BCG, active-specific immunotherapy by immunization with tumor cells or tumor antigen, adoptive immunotherapy with host defense cells or subcellular components such as transfer factor, immunorestorative immunotherapy with such agents as thymic hormones and levamisole, and possibly, passive immunotherapy with specific antitumor antibody.

Immunotherapy, now in its earliest stages of development, should be considered the fourth major modality of cancer treatment. The immunotherapeutic agents and approaches currently available for clinical application are, in general, crude and poorly defined. The mechanism of action of many of the immunotherapeutic agents is poorly or incompletely understood. The optimal timing of immunotherapy in relationship to conventional therapy has not been worked out. Highly purified and specific immunotherapeutic agents are yet to be developed. Despite these obstacles, there is evidence that immunotherapy of various types has activity in terms of increasing the remission rate or prolonging remission duration and survival for patients with such diverse malignancies as acute leukemia, soft tissue and osteogenic sarcoma, and malignant melanoma, as well as the more common malignancies, such as gynecologic and genitourinary cancer, and carcinoma of the breast, colon, and lung. In addition, several newer and unique approaches, such as the use of thymic hormones or the immunorestorative agent levamisole, and specific immunologic maneuvers, such as plasmapheresis to remove blocking factors, offer considerable promise for the future. It is our feeling that the proceedings of this conference adequately summarize the past development, current status, and future prospects for immunotherapy and will represent a landmark in its development.

Acknowledgments

To all whose knowledge and support made possible the 22nd Clinical Conference we extend our gratitude and give special thanks to the National Cancer Institute and the American Cancer Society, Texas Division, Inc., for their continued support. We also thank the Division of Continuing Education of The University of Texas Health Science Center at Houston for their assistance.

We wish to thank especially the members of the Program Committee, Evan M. Hersh and Joseph G. Sinkovics (cochairmen), Richard Ford, Jordan U. Gutterman, Giora M. Mavligit, Charles M. McBride, Marion J. McMurtrey, Samuel G. Murphy, Ellen S. Richie, and Max Schlamowitz, who arranged and organized the conference.

We are grateful for the excellent editorial work of the Publications Office of the Department of Information and Publications, M. D. Anderson Hospital, and especially the professional assistance of Linda Higgins, Editor, in compiling this volume.

Contributors

William K. Amery, M.D.
Janssen Pharmaceutica
Beerse, Belgium

Jean-Louis Amiel, M.D.
Institut de Cancérologie et
  d'Immunogénétique
Hôpital Paul-Brousse
Dèpartement d'Hématologie
Institut Gustave-Roussy
94800 Villejuif, France

Ichiro Azuma, Ph.D.
The Third Department of Internal
  Medicine
Osaka University Hospital
Osaka, Japan

Shelley L. Bartold, Ph.D.
Department of Biomathematics
The University of Texas System Cancer
  Center
M. D. Anderson Hospital and Tumor
  Institute
Houston, Texas 77030

J. George Bekesi, Ph.D.
Department of Neoplastic Diseases
Mount Sinai School of Medicine
New York, New York 10029

Robert E. Bellet, M.D.
Melanoma Unit
Fox Chase Cancer Center
Philadelphia, Pennsylvania 19111

Dominique Belpomme, M.D.
Institut de Cancérologie et
  d'Immunogénétique
Hôpital Paul-Brousse
Dèpartement d'Hématologie
Institut Gustave-Roussy
94800 Villejuif, France

Robert S. Benjamin, M.D.
Department of Developmental
  Therapeutics
The University of Texas System Cancer
  Center
M. D. Anderson Hospital and Tumor
  Institute
Houston, Texas 77030

David Berd, M.D.
Melanoma Unit
Fox Chase Cancer Center
Philadelphia, Pennsylvania 19111

G. R. Blumenschein, M.D.
Department of Medicine
The University of Texas System Cancer
  Center
M. D. Anderson Hospital and Tumor
  Institute
Houston, Texas 77030

Joseph C. Bottino, M.D.
Department of Developmental
  Therapeutics
The University of Texas System Cancer
  Center
M. D. Anderson Hospital and Tumor
  Institute
Houston, Texas 77030

Werner Brehmer, M.D.
Robert Koch Institute
Berlin, West Germany

Michael A. Burgess, M.B.B.S.
Department of Developmental
  Therapeutics
The University of Texas System Cancer
  Center
M. D. Anderson Hospital and Tumor
  Institute
Houston, Texas 77030

A. U. Buzdar, M.D.
Department of Medicine
The University of Texas System Cancer
Center
M. D. Anderson Hospital and Tumor
Institute
Houston, Texas 77030

John L. Cantrell, Ph.D.
Rocky Mountain Laboratory
National Institute of Allergy and Infec-
tious Diseases
National Institutes of Health
Hamilton, Montana 59840

Albert Cattan, M.D.
Institut de Cancérologie et
d'Immunogénétique
Hôpital Paul-Brousse
Dèpartement d'Hématologie
Institut Gustave-Roussy
94800 Villejuif, France

Michael A. Chirigos, Ph.D., D.Sc.
Virus and Disease Modification Section
Laboratory of RNA Tumor Viruses
Division of Cancer Cause and Prevention
National Cancer Institute
National Institutes of Health
Bethesda, Maryland 20014

R. Lee Clark, M.D., D.Sc. (Hon.)
President
The University of Texas System Cancer
Center
Professor of Surgery
M. D. Anderson Hospital and Tumor
Institute
Houston, Texas 77030

Janet Cuttner, M.D.
Department of Neoplastic Diseases
Mount Sinai School of Medicine
New York, New York 10029

Miguel Delgado, M.D.
Institut de Cancérologie et
d'Immunogénétique
Hôpital Paul-Brousse
Dèpartement d'Hématologie
Institut Gustave-Roussy
94800 Villejuif, France

Francoise de Vassal, M.D.
Institut de Cancérologie et
d'Immunogénétique
Hôpital Paul-Brousse
Dèpartement d'Hématologie
Institut Gustave-Roussy
94800 Villejuif, France

Richard Edelstein, M.D.
Chemotherapy and Immunotherapy Unit
University of Paris XIII
Centre Hospitalier Universitaire de
Bobigny
93000 Bobigny, France

David Eidinger, M.D., Ph.D.
Department of Microbiology
Faculty of Medicine
University of Saskatchewan
Saskatoon, Saskatchewan S7N 0W0

Khoji Ezaki, M.D.
Department of Developmental
Therapeutics
The University of Texas System Cancer
Center
M. D. Anderson Hospital and Tumor
Institute
Houston, Texas 77030

J. L. Fahey, M.D.
Department of Microbiology and
Immunology
UCLA School of Medicine
Los Angeles, California 90024

David Farquhar, Ph.D.
Department of Developmental
Therapeutics
The University of Texas System Cancer
Center
M. D. Anderson Hospital and Tumor
Institute
Houston, Texas 77030

Isaiah J. Fidler, D.V.M., Ph.D.
Biology of Metastasis Section
Cancer Biology Program
Frederick Cancer Research Center
Frederick, Maryland 21701

Stanley A. Gall, M.D.
Department of Obstetrics and Gynecology
Duke University Medical Center
Durham, North Carolina 27710

Edmund A. Gehan, Ph.D.
Department of Biomathematics
The University of Texas System Cancer
  Center
M. D. Anderson Hospital and Tumor
  Institute
Houston, Texas 77030

Marianne Gil, M.D.
Institut de Cancérologie et
  d'Immunogénétique
Hôpital Paul-Brousse
Dèpartement d'Hématologie
Institut Gustave-Roussy
94800 Villejuif, France

Allan L. Goldstein, Ph.D.
Department of Biochemistry
The George Washington University Medi-
  cal Center
Washington, D.C. 20037

Christine H. Granatek, Ph.D.
Department of Developmental
  Therapeutics
The University of Texas System Cancer
  Center
M. D. Anderson Hospital and Tumor
  Institute
Houston, Texas 77030

Jordan U. Gutterman, M.D.
Department of Developmental
  Therapeutics
The University of Texas System Cancer
  Center
M. D. Anderson Hospital and Tumor
  Institute
Houston, Texas 77030

M. G. Hanna, Jr., Ph.D.
Cancer Biology Program
Frederick Cancer Research Center
Frederick, Maryland 21701

Maurice Hayat, M.D.
Institut de Cancérologie et
  d'Immunogénétique
Hôpital Paul-Brousse
Dèpartement d'Hématologie
Institut Gustave-Roussy
94800 Villejuif, France

Evan M. Hersh, M.D.
Department of Developmental
  Therapeutics
The University of Texas System Cancer
  Center
M. D. Anderson Hospital and Tumor
  Institute
Houston, Texas 77030

Robert C. Hickey, M.D.
Executive Vice President
The University of Texas System Cancer
  Center
Director
M. D. Anderson Hospital and Tumor
  Institute
Houston, Texas 77030

James F. Holland, M.D.
Department of Neoplastic Diseases
Mount Sinai School of Medicine
New York, New York 10029

Ariel C. Hollinshead, Ph.D.
Department of Medicine
The George Washington University Medi-
  cal Center
Washington, D.C. 20037

G. N. Hortobagyi, M.D.
Department of Medicine
The University of Texas System Cancer
  Center
M. D. Anderson Hospital and Tumor
  Institute
Houston, Texas 77030

Kou M. Hwang, Ph.D.
Department of Developmental
  Therapeutics
The University of Texas System Cancer
  Center
M. D. Anderson Hospital and Tumor
  Institute
Houston, Texas 77030

Lucien Israël, M.D.
Chemotherapy and Immunotherapy Unit
University of Paris XIII
Centre Hospitalier Universitaire de
  Bobigny
93000 Bobigny, France

Claude Jasmin, M.D.
Institut de Cancérologie et
  d'Immunogénétique
Hôpital Paul-Brousse
Dèpartement d'Hématologie
Institut Gustave-Roussy
94800 Villejuif, France

Anne Kennedy, B.A.
Department of Biomathematics
The University of Texas System Cancer
  Center
M. D. Anderson Hospital and Tumor
  Institute
Houston, Texas 77030

H. Sherwood Lawrence, M.D.
Infectious Disease and Immunology
  Division
Department of Medicine
New York University School of Medicine
New York, New York 10016

David Machover, M.D.
Institut de Cancérologie et
  d'Immunogénétique
Hôpital Paul-Brousse
Dèpartement d'Hématologie
Institut Gustave-Roussy
94800 Villejuif, France

Mary Anne Malahy, Ph.D.
National Large Bowel Cancer Project
The University of Texas System Cancer
  Center
M. D. Anderson Hospital and Tumor
  Institute
Houston, Texas 77030

Gailen D. Marshall, Jr., M.S.
Department of Biochemistry
The George Washington University Medi-
  cal Center
Washington, D.C. 20037

Michael J. Mastrangelo, M.D.
Melanoma Unit
Fox Chase Cancer Center
Philadelphia, Pennsylvania 19111

Georges Mathé, M.D.
Institut de Cancérologie et
  d'Immunogénétique
Hôpital Paul-Brousse
Dèpartement d'Hématologie
Institut Gustave-Roussy
94800 Villejuif, France

Giora M. Mavligit, M.D.
Department of Developmental
  Therapeutics
The University of Texas System Cancer
  Center
M. D. Anderson Hospital and Tumor
  Institute
Houston, Texas 77030

Charles M. McBride, M.D.
Department of Surgery
The University of Texas System Cancer
  Center
M. D. Anderson Hospital and Tumor
  Institute
Houston, Texas 77030

Martin F. McKneally, M.D., Ph.D.
Department of Surgery
Albany Medical College
Albany, New York 12208

Charles A. McLaughlin, D.V.M., Ph.D.
Rocky Mountain Laboratory
National Institute of Allergy and Infec-
  tious Diseases
National Institutes of Health
Hamilton, Montana 59840

Marion J. McMurtrey, M.D.
Department of Surgery
The University of Texas System Cancer
  Center
M. D. Anderson Hospital and Tumor
  Institute
Houston, Texas 77030

Jean-Louis Misset, M.D.
*Institut de Cancérologie et
d'Immunogénétique
Hôpital Paul-Brousse
Dèpartement d'Hématologie
Institut Gustave-Roussy
94800 Villejuif, France*

Dexter Morris, B.A.
*Department of Developmental
Therapeutics
The University of Texas System Cancer
Center
M. D. Anderson Hospital and Tumor
Institute
Houston, Texas 77030*

Marina Musset, M.D.
*Institut de Cancérologie et
d'Immunogénétique
Hôpital Paul-Brousse
Dèpartement d'Hématologie
Institut Gustave-Roussy
94800 Villejuif, France*

Nicholas Papadopoulos, M.D.
*Department of Medicine
The University of Texas System Cancer
Center
M. D. Anderson Hospital and Tumor
Institute
Houston, Texas 77030*

Yehuda Z. Patt, M.D.
*Department of Developmental
Therapeutics
The University of Texas System Cancer
Center
M. D. Anderson Hospital and Tumor
Institute
Houston, Texas 77030*

Juan Pena-Angulo, M.D.
*Institut de Cancérologie et
d'Immunogénétique
Hôpital Paul-Brousse
Dèpartement d'Hématologie
Institut Gustave-Roussy
94800 Villejuif, France*

Leona C. Peters, B.S.
*Cancer Biology Program
Frederick Cancer Research Center
Frederick, Maryland 21701*

Lester J. Peters, M.D.
*Department of Radiotherapy
The University of Texas System Cancer
Center
M. D. Anderson Hospital and Tumor
Institute
Houston, Texas 77030*

José-Luis Pico, M.D.
*Institut de Cancérologie et
d'Immunogénétique
Hôpital Paul-Brousse
Dèpartement d'Hématologie
Institut Gustave-Roussy
94800 Villejuif, France*

Carl Plager, M.D.
*Department of Medicine
The University of Texas System Cancer
Center
M. D. Anderson Hospital and Tumor
Institute
Houston, Texas 77030*

Pierre Pouillart, M.D.
*Institut de Cancérologie et
d'Immunogénétique
Hôpital Paul-Brousse
Dèpartement d'Hématologie
Institut Gustave-Roussy
94800 Villejuif, France*

Patricia Ribaud, M.D.
*Institut de Cancérologie et
d'Immunogénétique
Hôpital Paul-Brousse
Dèpartement d'Hématologie
Institut Gustave-Roussy
94800 Villejuif, France*

Edgar Ribi, Ph.D.
*Rocky Mountain Laboratory
National Institute of Allergy and Infec-
tious Diseases
National Institutes of Health
Hamilton, Montana 59840*

Stephen P. Richman, M.D.
Department of Developmental
Therapeutics
The University of Texas System Cancer
Center
M. D. Anderson Hospital and Tumor
Institute
Houston, Texas 77030

Adan Rios, M.D.
Department of Developmental
Therapeutics
The University of Texas System Cancer
Center
M. D. Anderson Hospital and Tumor
Institute
Houston, Texas 77030

Ernesto Rivera, M.D.
Department of Developmental
Therapeutics
The University of Texas System Cancer
Center
M. D. Anderson Hospital and Tumor
Institute
Houston, Texas 77030

Jimmy J. Romero, B.S.
Department of Medicine
The University of Texas System Cancer
Center
M. D. Anderson Hospital and Tumor
Institute
Houston, Texas 77030

Marvin M. Romsdahl, M.D., Ph.D.
Department of Surgery
The University of Texas System Cancer
Center
M. D. Anderson Hospital and Tumor
Institute
Houston, Texas 77030

Claude Rosenfeld, M.D.
Institut de Cancérologie et
d'Immunogénétique
Hôpital Paul-Brousse
Dèpartement d'Hématologie
Institut Gustave-Roussy
94800 Villejuif, France

Roger D. Rossen, M.D.
Department of Microbiology and
Immunology
Baylor College of Medicine
Houston, Texas 77030

Jeffrey L. Rossio, Ph.D.
Department of Microbiology and
Immunology
Wright State University School of
Medicine
Dayton, Ohio 45431

Raymond Samak, M.D.
Chemotherapy and Immunotherapy Unit
University of Paris XIII
Centre Hospitalier Universitaire de
Bobigny
93000 Bobigny, France

Maurice Schneider, M.D.
Institut de Cancérologie et
d'Immunogénétique
Hôpital Paul-Brousse
Dèpartement d'Hématologie
Institut Gustave-Roussy
94800 Villejuif, France

Léon Schwarzenberg, M.D.
Institut de Cancérologie et
d'Immunogénétique
Hôpital Paul-Brousse
Dèpartement d'Hématologie
Institut Gustave-Roussy
94800 Villejuif, France

Joseph G. Sinkovics, M.D.
Department of Medicine
The University of Texas System Cancer
Center
M. D. Anderson Hospital and Tumor
Institute
Houston, Texas 77030

S. Michael Strain, B.S.
Hamilton Biochemical Research
Laboratory
Hamilton, Montana 59840

Raoul Toubiana, Ph.D.
CNRS Institute de Chimie des Substances
Naturelles
Gif sur Yvette, France

Ruth Waldinger, R.N.
Department of Nursing
The University of Texas System Cancer
 Center
M. D. Anderson Hospital and Tumor
 Institute
Houston, Texas 77030

Roy Weiner, M.D.
Institut de Cancérologie et
 d'Immunogénétique
Hôpital Paul-Brousse
Dèpartement d'Hématologie
Institut Gustave-Roussy
94800 Villejuif, France
Present address: Division of Medical
 Oncology
University of Florida
Gainesville, Florida 32611

David W. Weiss, Ph.D., D.Phil.Med.
Lautenberg Center for General and Tu-
 mor Immunology
Hebrew University—Hadassah Medical
 School
Jerusalem, Israel

C. Wiseman, M.D.
Department of Medicine
The University of Texas System Cancer
 Center
M. D. Anderson Hospital and Tumor
 Institute
Houston, Texas 77030

Yuichi Yamamura, M.D.
The Third Department of Internal
 Medicine
Osaka University Hospital
Osaka, Japan

Nancy Zatopek, B.A.
Department of Developmental
 Therapeutics
The University of Texas System Cancer
 Center
M. D. Anderson Hospital and Tumor
 Institute
Houston, Texas 77030

HEATH MEMORIAL AWARD LECTURE

Immunotherapy of Human Cancer,
The University of Texas System Cancer Center
M. D. Anderson Hospital and Tumor Institute.
Raven Press, New York © 1978.

Introduction of Heath Memorial Award Recipient

Robert C. Hickey, M.D.

Executive Vice President, The University of Texas System Cancer Center, and Director and Professor of Surgery, M. D. Anderson Hospital and Tumor Institute, Houston, Texas

It is my privilege to introduce the 1977 Heath Memorial Award recipient, Dr. Georges Mathé of France. His lecture is entitled "Active Immunotherapy: Experimental and Rational Basis."

The award, memorializing three brothers, Guy H., Dan C., and Gilford G. Heath, was made possible by the late William W. Heath, former chairman of The University of Texas System Board of Regents. The award honors, after careful selection, a person who has made "outstanding contributions to the care of patients with cancer." There is hardly a scientist in the world today whose contributions in immunology and immunotherapy can equal those of Dr. Mathé.

Dr. Mathé was born in France on July 9, 1922. He received his Doctor of Medicine degree from the University of Paris in 1948. He was Head of the Clinic from 1952 to 1953 and Professor of Cancer Research from 1956 to 1967 in the Faculty of Medicine at the University of Paris Medical School. Since 1961, he has been Head of the Hematology Service of Gustave-Roussy Institute; and from 1965 to the present, he has been the Director of the Institute of Cancerology and Immunogenetics in Villejuif, France. He is Editor-in-Chief of *Biomedicine,* and an editor of *Cancer Immunology and Immunotherapy* and *Cancer Chemotherapy and Pharmacology.*

Dr. Mathé has been a major contributor to clinical and basic cancer research since the early 1960s. He introduced bone marrow grafts in man in 1958 and the aseptic environment for bone marrow grafts and intensive chemotherapy at the same time, and described and characterized the effectiveness of immunotherapy in a mouse leukemia model. He demonstrated that BCG alone or BCG plus tumor cells was able to prolong survival of mice with leukemia.

In 1962, he designed a clinical trial, based on his animal model work, in which patients with acute leukemia treated with chemotherapy alone were compared with patients given immunotherapy with a leukemic cell vaccine, BCG, or the combination of tumor cells and BCG. In children with acute lymphocytic leukemia, he showed that immunotherapy definitely prolonged disease-free survival, and indeed, seven of the 20 patients in his original trial who received immunotherapy are still in remission some 16 years later. Dr. Mathé has done numerous studies that have been major contributions to cancer immunology and immunotherapy.

He was one of the pioneers in the treatment of malignant disease with combination chemotherapy. He was one of the early developers of leukocyte transfusion therapy and bone marrow transplantation in the management of leukemia. He has also been active in the development of chemotherapy and immunotherapy regimens for malignant lymphoma and more recently has been conducting important clinical trials of immunotherapy for lung cancer. Dr. Mathé's pioneering work with the use of BCG immunotherapy and active-specific immunotherapy with tumor cells has inspired a whole generation of studies of immunotherapy, not only for leukemia, but also for solid tumors.

Finally, Dr. Mathé may be considered a humanist in that he has repeatedly put forth concepts of the humanistic approach to clinical research in cancer. His concepts that each patient must receive the best available treatment, that clinical experiments are different from laboratory experiments in animals, and that ethical considerations are extremely important in clinical cancer research have made an important impact throughout the world.

These contributions, plus his organization of numerous scientific meetings and symposia, his publication and coordination of numerous books on cancer research, and his development of some important cancer research journals, make it entirely appropriate that he be the recipient of the Heath Memorial Award.

Immunotherapy of Human Cancer,
The University of Texas System Cancer Center
M. D. Anderson Hospital and Tumor Institute.
Raven Press, New York © 1978.

Active Immunotherapy: Experimental and Rational Basis

Georges Mathé, M.D.

Institut de Cancérologie et d'Immunogénétique, Hôpital Paul-Brousse, and Dèpartement d'Hématologie de l'Institut Gustave-Roussy, 94800 Villejuif, France

Active immunotherapy not only has a strong rational basis, but has been the object of many experimental studies, the conclusions of which are not known by enough clinicians who conduct clinical trials. A wider knowledge of experimental results could accelerate clinical progress in this new field of cancer treatment.

ACTIVE IMMUNOTHERAPY FOR MINIMAL RESIDUAL DISEASE LEFT BY OTHER CANCER TREATMENT(S)

The treatment of minimal residual disease was our objective when we embarked, 15 years ago, on the cancer immunotherapy adventure, for two reasons: (1) Many patients relapse after local tumor treatment(s), up to 90% in the case of breast cancer surgery (Brinkley and Haybittle, 1975) because of the growth of the few cells already emigrated at the time of operation, and up to 35% in the case of acute lymphoid leukemia remission maintenance (Bernard, 1975) because chemotherapy obeys first-order kinetics (Skipper *et al.,* 1964, 1965, 1967) and therefore often leaves a few cells alive. We predict, on the basis of results of our study on the murine L1210 leukemia mean inductive cell number, that surgery, radiotherapy, or chemotherapy—provided it is not immunosuppressive—must leave no more than ten cells to cure the disease (Mathé, 1976a). However, these treatment modalities are often immunosuppressive (Mathé and Kenis, 1976; Clarysse *et al.,* 1976). (2) Attempt at immunoprophylaxis with a specific vaccine made of irradiated tumor cells and a systemic immunity adjuvant, such as bacillus Calmette-Guérin (BCG), increases the mean inductive cell number of L1210 leukemia to 10^5 (Mathé, 1976a).

Hence, our first question was: Are similar immunointerventions that are efficient in prevention also efficient in therapy, after the tumor is established? We

Abbreviations used in this chapter: EORTC—European Organization for Research on Treatment of Cancer; ICIG—Institut de Cancérologie et d'Immunogénétique; RFCNU—[(chloro-2-ethyl)-1-(ribofuranosyl-isopropylidene-2′-3′-paranitrobenzoate-5′)-3-nitrosourea].

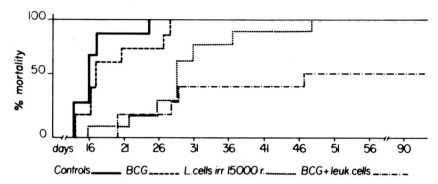

Figure 1. Cumulative survival times of mice grafted with 10³ L1210 leukemia cells and treated with either BCG 24 hours after graft (injection was repeated every four days), irradiated leukemic cells (one injection 14 hours after graft), or both. (Reproduced from Mathé *et al.,* 1969, with permission of H. K. Lewis & Co. Ltd.)

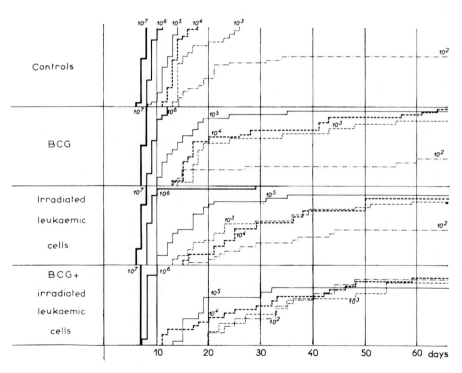

Figure 2. Cumulative survival times of mice grafted with 10² to 10⁷ L1210 leukemic cells and treated with either BCG 24 hours after graft (1 mg per mouse, injected intravenously every four days), 10⁷ irradiated leukemic cells (one subcutaneous injection), or both. (Reproduced from Mathé, 1968, with permission of Editions Mèdicales Flammarion.)

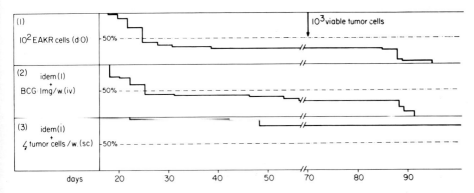

Figure 3. Results of active systemic immunotherapy with BCG alone and irradiated tumor cells alone for EAKR murine leukemia inoculated with 10^2 tumor cells.

conducted experiments with several tumors—L1210 leukemia (Mathé, 1968; Mathé *et al.,* 1969), RC-19 (Mathé *et al.,* 1971), and AKR (Mathé *et al.,* 1973a)— and demonstrated that immunotherapy, that is, the immunointervention applied after the tumor is established, eradicates such tumors, at least in certain conditions which we will define.

Some of the conditions of action concern the modality of active immunotherapy: The combination of irradiated tumor cells as the specific stimulus and BCG as a nonspecific immunity adjuvant is often more active than leukemic cells or BCG alone, for instance, in the case of L1210 leukemia (Fig. 1) (Mathé, 1968; Mathé *et al.,* 1969). This observation was confirmed by Parr (1972). Other conditions concern the size of the tumor cell population: Active immunotherapy is able to cure only mice that have received 10^5 leukemic cells or less (Fig. 2), and has no effect on those grafted with 10^6 or more cells (Mathé, 1968).

For some tumors, especially some leukemias (e.g., EAKR), if the number of inoculated tumor cells is small, 10^3 or 10^2, the specific stimulus induced by repeated injections of irradiated tumor cells may be sufficient by itself to cure animals, whereas BCG is ineffective (Fig. 3) (Olsson *et al.,* unpublished data). On the contrary, if the tumor cell number has been reduced by a previous treatment, the nonspecific immune application of a systemic adjuvant may be sufficient to cure animals: Figure 4 shows that BCG is highly effective after chemotherapy with cyclophosphamide for L1210 leukemia (Mathé *et al.,* 1974a); Figure 5, that it is slightly effective after radiotherapy for Lewis tumor (Martin *et al.,* 1975a); and Figure 6, that this mycobacterium applied intravenously after tumor and draining lymph-node surgery for melanoma B16 is able to cure animals for which surgery is unsuccessful (Economides *et al.,* 1977).

In all these experiments, BCG was injected intravenously at the dose of 1 mg per mouse, which we had shown to be the optimal dose to stimulate immune reactions in the hemolytic plaque-forming assay. Higher doses, such as 3 mg or 5 mg, induce immunosuppression (Mathé, 1976a,b) by stimulating suppressor

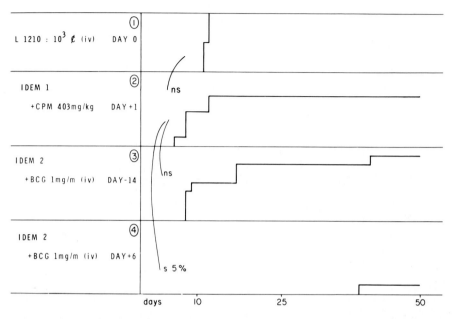

Figure 4. Immunotherapeutic effect of BCG (1 mg per mouse) administered intravenously five days after injection of 403 mg/kg cyclophosphamide (CPM). BCG treatment has protective effect against early bone marrow (and lymphoid?) toxicity. Mice were inoculated with 10^3 L1210 leukemia cells one day before chemotherapy. (Reproduced from Mathé *et al.*, 1974a, with permission of Pergamon Press Ltd.)

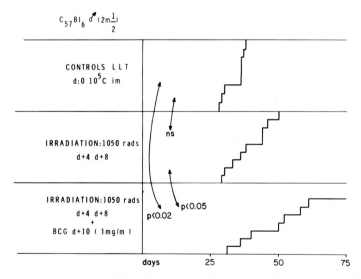

Figure 5. Results of radiotherapy followed by active systemic immunotherapy for Lewis tumor in C57BL/6 mice. (Reproduced from Martin *et al.*, 1975a, with permission of Masson.)

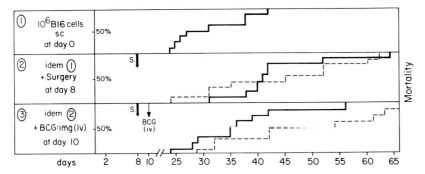

Figure 6. Effect of postsurgical systemic immunotherapy on B16 melanoma.

cells, as shown by Geffard and Orbach-Arbouys (1976) in our laboratory. Injected intravenously at a dose of 1 mg per mouse, BCG induces a septicemia (Fig. 7), the presence of which we have shown to be necessary for the antitumor effect (Khalil *et al.,* 1975). Among the other efficient modalities of administration is the application of BCG by scarification or via the Heaf gun (Fig. 8) (Martin *et al.,* 1975b). The subcutaneous route of administration, which does not induce such a septicemia, can not only cause tumor rejection, but may in fact produce enhancement of the Lewis tumor (Fig. 9) (Mathé *et al.,* 1973c).

Not all BCG preparations work. Submitting ten preparations to our experimental screening for systemic immunity adjuvants (Mathé *et al.,* 1973c, 1975b), we observed that only fresh Pasteur preparation is efficient in all tests (Mathé *et al.,* 1973b).

In conclusion, immune manipulation may eliminate some neoplasms, provided the tumor cell number is small, which is the condition of minimum residual disease left by the first treatment(s), and provided some conditions concerning the modalities of preparations used for specific and nonspecific stimuli and the methods of their application are respected. However, as illustrated by the dose-

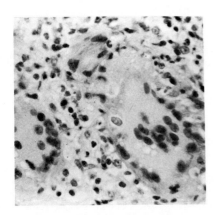

Figure 7. Granuloma in tissue of mouse induced by intravenous injection of 1 mg fresh BCG (Pasteur strain). (Reproduced from Khalil *et al.,* 1975, with permission of Masson.)

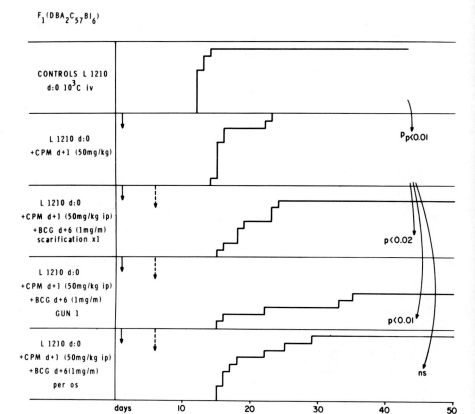

Figure 8. Effect of BCG by different routes of administration in active systemic immunotherapy following chemotherapy for murine L1210 leukemia. CPM, cyclophosphamide; C, cells; d, day; m, mice; ns, not significant. (Reproduced from Martin *et al.*, 1975b, with permission of Masson.)

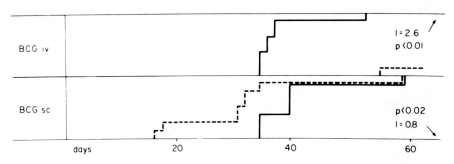

Figure 9. Immunoprophylactic effect of BCG injected intravenously and growth-accelerating effect of BCG injected subcutaneously at same dose (1 mg per mouse) on Lewis lung tumor. Animals were injected with 2×10^6 tumor cells on day 0; BCG was administered on day 14. ———, controls; ---------, treated animals; I, median survival time for experimental animals (days)/median survival time for controls (days). Statistical significance determined by nonparametric test of Wilcoxon. (Reproduced from Mathé, 1976a, with permission of Springer-Verlag.)

Table 1. *Tumor Characteristics in Relation to Tumor Cell Cytotoxic Potential of Antibodies and Lymphoid Cells in Mice Treated with BCG and Irradiated Tumor Cells**

| | Group† | | | | | |
| | 1 | | 2 | | | |
Parameter	A	B	A	B	3	4
Tumor size‡	<	=	<	=	−	...
Tumor cells (%) in peritoneal fluid‡	<	=	<	=	=	...
Lymphocytes (%) at days 13 & 18‡	>	=	>	=	=	...
Immunoblast-like cells (%) at days 13 & 18‡	>	=	>	=	=	...
Complement-dependent, antibody-mediated cytotoxicity (CDAC)	++	++	++	++	+(+)	0
Inhibitor of CDAC	++	++	++	++	++	−
Direct lymphocyte cytotoxicity						
Lymph nodes	0	0	0	0	0	0
Spleen	++	±	++	±	±	(+)
Antibody-dependent, cell-mediated cytotoxicity						
Spleen	++	(+)	++	(+)	(+)	(+)
Lymph nodes	++	0	++	0	0	0
Cells from peritoneal fluid	++	−	++	...	...	...

Symbols: ++, high cytotoxicity; +, mean cytotoxicity; (+), weak, but significant cytotoxicity; −, no significant cytotoxicity.
* Reproduced from Olsson *et al.*, 1977.
† Group 1, BCG alone; group 2, BCG plus irradiated tumor cells; group 3, irradiated tumor cells; group 4, tumor-bearing controls; subgroup A, tumor smaller than that of controls; subgroup B, tumor size equal to that of controls.
‡ Compared with that in control animals.

effect correlation of BCG, which is immunosuppressive at high doses (Mathé, 1976b), and by the enhancement of Lewis tumor growth after subcutaneous injection of BCG (Mathé *et al.*, 1973c), one must underline the importance of monitoring nonspecific immune reactions during any attempt at immunotherapy. We compared the effects of active immunotherapy with BCG and irradiated tumor cells in two groups of EAKR-carrying mice, one in which BCG was effective and one in which it was not, and we could correlate the antitumor efficiency only with an increase of antibody-dependent cell-mediated cytotoxicity (Table 1) (Olsson *et al.*, 1977).

INTERSPERSION OF INTERMITTENT CHEMOTHERAPY AND IMMUNOTHERAPY

Another approach that we have also studied experimentally was introduced by an M. D. Anderson Hospital group: the interspersion of chemotherapy and immunotherapy (Gutterman *et al.*, 1974). There are several reasons for the combination and interspersion of chemotherapy and immunotherapy.

In most of the experiments mentioned above, some mice were cured, but

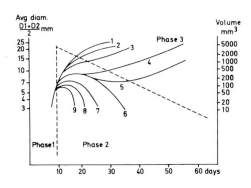

Figure 10. Growth curves for tumors obtained from mice treated with BCG and irradiated cells one day after injection of 10^4 L1210 cells. (Reproduced from Mathé, 1976a, with permission of Springer-Verlag.)

rarely 100%, even with the best conditions of active immunotherapy application. Figure 10 illustrates this phenomenon (Mathé, 1976a). After subjecting subcutaneously grafted L1210 leukemia to active immunotherapy, we observed three kinds of results: a decrease in the tumor volume, and cure; an absence of effect on the tumor volume, which increases until death; and a plateau in the tumor volume, which is followed by an increase until death, suggesting an initial effect followed by immunoresistance. Figure 10 also indicates that active immunotherapy has no effect on cells in the exponential phase (in which all the cells are in the cycle) but has effect only on cells in the saturation phase. Figure 11 shows the results of our studies of active immunotherapy with cells at the different phases of the cell cycle, and explains this phenomenon more basically: Active immunotherapy works only on cells in G_0 and/or G_1 phase (Olsson and Mathé, 1977). These two experiments suggest possible reasons for interspersing immunotherapy and chemotherapy: (1) to try to reduce the number of cells when the tumor volume curve has attained the plateau to the number accessible to immunotherapy, i.e., 10^5 or 10^3; and (2) to increase the number of target cells, as immunotherapy has effect only on cells in the G_0-G_1 phase (Olsson and Mathé, 1977) and chemotherapy, mainly on cells in the other phases of the cycle (Bruce *et al.,* 1966; van Putten, 1972).

Moreover, we have observed that a given chemotherapy regimen that does not cure leukemic mice immunosuppressed by antithymocyte serum may cure leukemic animals that are not immunosuppressed (Mathé, 1977; Mathé *et al.,* 1977c).

Another reason for interspersing active immunotherapy and chemotherapy is that immunity adjuvants, such as BCG, accelerate blood cell restoration after chemotherapy (Fig. 12) (Mathé, 1974). This suggests that such adjuvants act on stem cells. Using the techniques of determining the number of colony-forming units in the spleen and in agar culture and the tritiated thymidine suicide method, we observed that BCG increases the number of both types of stem cells in the S phase of the cell cycle (Table 2) (Mathé, 1974; Pouillart *et al.,* 1975, 1976).

Finally, there is another reason for the interspersion of carefully selected

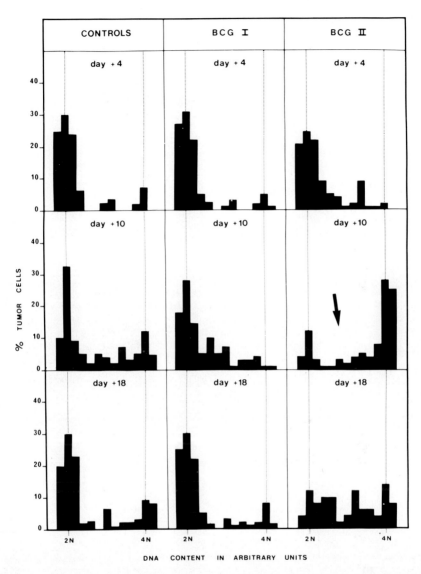

Figure 11. Percentage distribution of ascitic tumor cells as function of single-cell DNA content at various times after intraperitoneal inoculation of 10^5 tumor cells. 2N indicates mean DNA content of cells in G_1 phase, and 4N, mean DNA content of mitoses (cells in G_2 phase). Each value is mean for three to five mice. Group I, BCG-treated mice with tumor load and tumor-cell mitotic activity no different from that of control animals; group II, BCG-treated mice with lower tumor-cell number and higher tumor-cell mitotic activity than that of control animals. (Reproduced from Olsson and Mathé, 1977, with permission of Cancer Research, Inc.)

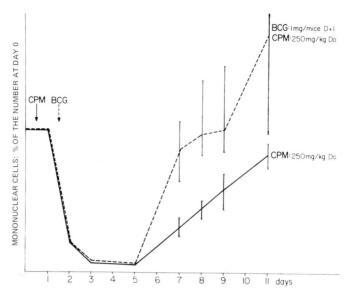

Figure 12. Effect of BCG on lymphoid stem cells. Restoration of blood lymphocyte number after cyclophosphamide (CPM) aplasia is faster when BCG is administered one day after cytostatics. (Reproduced from Mathé, 1976a, with permission of Springer-Verlag.)

chemotherapy and active immunotherapy: Systemic immunity adjuvants at high doses may induce immunosuppression (Mathé, 1976b) through the stimulation of suppressor cells (Geffard and Orbach-Arbouys, 1976). These cells may be sensitive to cytostatic drugs different from those active on cytotoxic T cells, helper T cells, B cells, K cells, and macrophages. Thus, selective chemotherapy is an important objective to work toward and necessitates the "interspersion" of the most qualified immunologists and chemotherapists.

Table 2. *Number of Colony-Forming Units per Femur After Intravenous Injections of 1 mg Fresh BCG to (DBA/2 × C57BL/6) Mice**

Hours After Injection	No. of CFUs†/Femur	After ³H-TdR Suicide Technique	No. of CFUa‡/ Femur	After ³H-TdR Suicide Technique
0	335	325	$1{,}090 \pm 40$	904 ± 54
12	630	560	$1{,}524 \pm 95$	$1{,}030 \pm 36$
24	410	260	$1{,}410 \pm 75$	$1{,}060 \pm 60$
36	. . .	. . .	$1{,}540 \pm 90$	$1{,}080 \pm 45$
48	350	280	$1{,}620 \pm 45$	$1{,}110 \pm 60$
72	470	310	$1{,}910 \pm 120$	$1{,}240 \pm 60$

* Reproduced from Mathé, 1976a, with permission of Springer-Verlag.

† CFUs (colony-forming units in the spleen) are more sensitive to ³H-TdR after two days, hence a higher fraction of them are in S phase.

‡ CFUa (colony-forming units in agar culture) increase after 12 hours; after this time, a third of them are sensitive to ³H-TdR, hence in S phase.

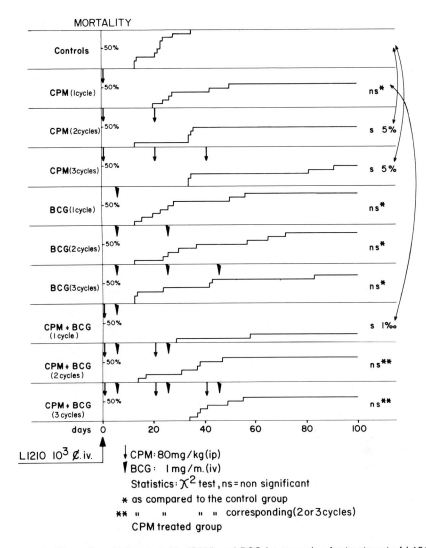

Figure 13. Effect of cyclophosphamide (CPM) and BCG interspersion for treatment of L1210 leukemia when sequential combination is given two to three times. Effect is poorer than that obtained by one injection of cyclophosphamide followed by one administration of BCG. (Reproduced from Mathé *et al.*, 1977d, with permission of Pergamon Press Ltd.)

We were encouraged, therefore, to conduct experiments with immunotherapy-chemotherapy interspersion. In our first experiments, we interspersed cyclophosphamide and BCG in the treatment of L1210 leukemia, for which we had seen previously that the sequence cyclophosphamide → BCG is much more efficient than cyclophosphamide alone (Mathé *et al.*, 1974a). We were unpleasantly surprised, however, to observe that two or three interspersion sequences of these two agents were no more efficient than cyclophosphamide alone and much less efficient that the single sequence of one cyclophosphamide and one BCG injection (Fig. 13) (Mathé *et al.*, 1977d). The same result was observed for the solid Lewis tumor (Mathé *et al.*, 1977d).

As the single sequence cyclophosphamide → BCG is more effective than cyclophosphamide alone (Mathé *et al.*, 1974a), we wondered if the reverse sequence, BCG → cyclophosphamide, was less effective. Figure 14 shows that this is the case: The sequence BCG → cyclophosphamide is significantly less efficient than cyclophosphamide alone (Mathé *et al.*, 1974a). As we had shown that the effect of cyclophosphamide is much poorer in immunosuppressed animals (Mathé, 1977; Mathé *et al.*, 1977c), we wondered if BCG followed by cyclophosphamide induced immunosuppression as BCG pushes the lymphocytes in the cycle, rendering them more sensitive to the lymphostatic action of cyclophosphamide, a cycle-dependent agent. An experiment with allogeneic skin grafting (Mathé *et al.*, 1974b) demonstrated the validity of this hypothesis: The sequence BCG → cyclophosphamide greatly prolongs allograft survival compared with cyclophosphamide alone (Fig. 15).

The problem was then to investigate whether this phenomenon was true for all chemotherapy agents, or only for those known to be immunosuppressive (Mathé and Kenis, 1976; Clarysse *et al.*, 1976). Hence, we performed a similar

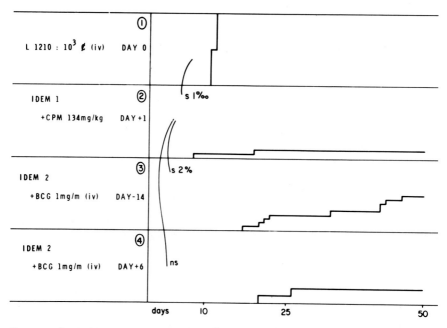

Figure 14. Survival times for mice injected with L1210 leukemia cells. BCG administered before cyclophosphamide deteriorates antileukemic effect of cyclophosphamide. (Reproduced from Mathé *et al.*, 1974a, with permission of Pergamon Press Ltd.)

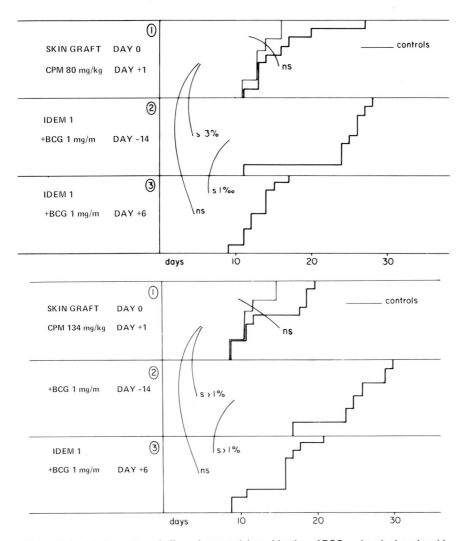

Figure 15. Cumulative curves of effect of sequential combination of BCG and cyclophosphamide (CPM) on survival of C3H skin graft on (DBA/2 × C57BL/6)F1 mice recipients. Top, cyclophosphamide dose, 80 mg/kg. Bottom, cyclophosphamide dose, 134 mg/kg. (Reproduced from Mathé *et al.,* 1974b, with permission of *Transplantation Proceedings,* Grune & Stratton, Inc.)

experiment using RFCNU, the only derivative of nitrosoureas that, among all those available in practice and a dozen of sugar derivatives synthesized by Imbach in Montpellier, France, and shown to be strongly oncostatic by our experiment screening, is not immunosuppressive at the minimal oncostatic dose (Imbach *et al.,* 1975). Figure 16 shows that the sequence BCG → RFCNU is more efficient than BCG or RFCNU alone (Mathé *et al.,* unpublished data).

Thus, we may conclude that the interspersion of immunotherapy and chemo-

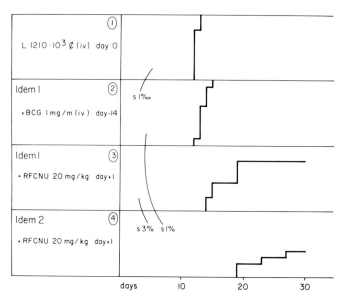

Figure 16. The sequence of BCG and RFCNU, a nonimmunosuppressive drug at the dose used (20 mg/kg), enhances effect of both agents, contrary to sequence of BCG and cyclophosphamide, an immunosuppressive agent.

therapy may be unfavorable or favorable, depending on at least one factor: the effect of the chemotherapy on immunity. Nonimmunosuppressive cytostatics must be chosen according to the available data. This effect on immunity does not eliminate the possible role of other factors, such as time, dose, phase dependency of the cytostatics, and the adjuvant used for immunotherapy (Mathé, 1976a).

IMMUNOTHERAPY APPLIED BEFORE OTHER CANCER TREATMENT(S)

If BCG applied before certain chemotherapy regimens may enhance the chemotherapy's immunosuppressive effect and hence enhance tumor growth (Mathé *et al.,* 1974a), the contrary may be obtained by applying immunotherapy before certain types of other cancer treatment. We showed that this is true for nonimmunosuppressive chemotherapeutic agents, such as RFCNU (Fig. 16) (Mathé *et al.,* unpublished data). Moreover, systemic immunity adjuvants may exert not only an immunostimulating effect on normal immune reactions, but also an immunorestoring effect (Simmler *et al.,* 1976). We showed in mice that a given chemotherapy is much less efficient in immunosuppressed animals than in animals with normal immune reactions (Mathé *et al.,* 1977c; Mathé, 1977).

The above data on the possible enhancing effect of BCG applied before certain treatments led us to study the effect of immunotherapy applied before surgery.

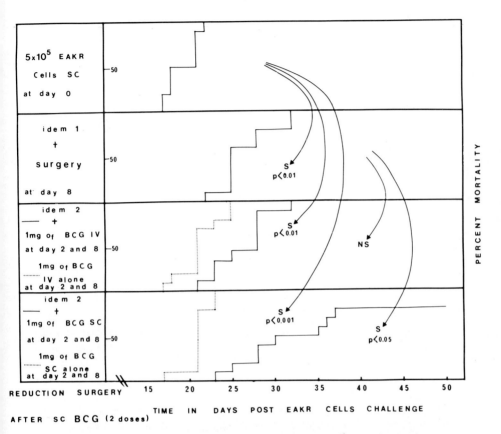

Figure 17. Effect of repeated BCG injections, combined with surgery, on survival of (C57BL/ 6 × DBA/2)F1 mice inoculated with 5 × 10³ EAKR lymphosarcoma cells. (Reproduced from Economides *et al.,* 1976, with permission of Masson.)

Figure 17 shows that BCG administered subcutaneously before tumor extirpation and between the tumor and draining lymph nodes in lymphosarcoma-bearing mice may significantly improve the effect of surgery (Economides *et al.,* 1976).

REGIONAL IMMUNOTHERAPY

The observation that preoperative BCG treatment may improve the effect of surgery (Economides *et al.,* 1976) draws our attention to a new form of immunotherapy, which we call regional immunotherapy. As a matter of fact, the results of this experiment should be compared with those of others in which BCG was applied after surgery for the same lymphosarcoma as mentioned above: After surgery, BCG works only if injected intravenously as in all our experiments on systemic immunotherapy (Mathé, 1976a), whereas BCG applied before surgery works only if injected subcutaneously near the tumor (Fig. 17) (Economides *et al.,* 1976).

The operational conditions of regional immunotherapy are not identical for all tumors. Applying BCG subcutaneously between a local inoculation of B16 melanoma and the draining lymph nodes invaded at time of treatment, we observed no effect, regardless of whether the lymph nodes were extirpated at the same time as the tumor. When combining this presurgical regional immunotherapy with postsurgical systemic BCG immunotherapy, however, we increased the proportion of cures obtained (40% versus 10%). Both systemic and systemic plus regional therapy worked only if adenectomy was performed at the same time as tumor exeresis (Economides *et al.,* in press). (It should be mentioned that draining lymph nodes were invaded at the time of surgery.) This observation should encourage the use of the same treatment for human melanoma and bronchus cancer with invaded lymph nodes.

Presurgical regional immunotherapy differs from local immunotherapy (Zbar and Tanaka, 1971), which consists of intratumoral injection of the agents, and may have many more clinical applications than local immunotherapy.

DEVELOPMENT OF THE CLINICAL TRIAL

In the preceding paragraphs are some of the experimental and clinical data that must be borne in mind before setting up any clinical trial. Experimentalists have submitted for study many questions regarding other aspects of immunotherapy, the answers to which also may be useful in developing clinical trials.

Can we improve the efficiency of specific immunotherapy with irradiated tumor cells by treating the cells with neuraminidase (Sedlacek *et al.,* 1977) or other enzymes, such as papain? We have not observed such a result with either grafted (Kiger, unpublished data) or spontaneous AKR leukemia (Mathé *et al.,* 1973a), and we have even noticed a growth enhancement of the EAKR leukemia (Doré *et al.,* 1974). Thus, this manipulation of the cells, if it works at all, does not work under all conditions and may facilitate tumor growth.

Can tumor cells produced by cultures in permanent lines replace cryopreserved cells and possibly be more efficient? We have several lines of cells produced from leukemic cell populations and which carry several markers of the original leukemic cells (Rosenfeld *et al.,* 1977). We are comparing in a randomized trial the uses of cultured and cryopreserved acute lymphoid leukemia cells in the active immunotherapy for this neoplasm (Mathé *et al.,* unpublished data).

The use of soluble tumor-associated antigens, which may be very effective under some experimental conditions, especially if administered early (Martyré, 1976), may be inefficient in others, for example, if antigen is injected later than in the preceding experimental condition. These antigens may induce tumor rejection or tumor growth enhancement, depending on the modality of preparation (Fig. 18) (Martyré *et al.,* 1974).

Can we improve the efficiency and the facility of use of the nonspecific manipulation made with adjuvants? Can we replace living BCG by mycobacterial extracts? We have observed that most extracts, including hydrosoluble ones, are efficient in an antibody production test and in macrophage activation, but only

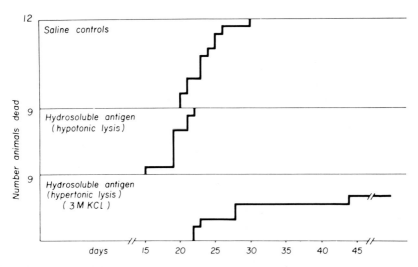

Figure 18. Effect of soluble tumor-associated antigen in immunoprophylaxis of RC-19 leukemia. (Reproduced from Martyré *et al.,* 1974, with permission of Springer-Verlag.)

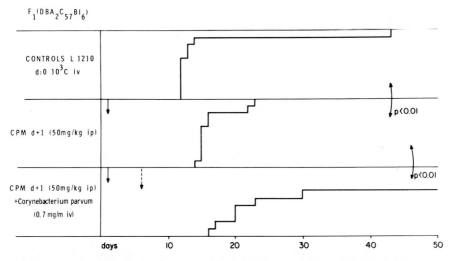

Figure 19. Immunotherapeutic effect of *C. parvum* after cyclophosphamide (CPM) treatment of (DBA/2 × C57BL/6)F1 mice inoculated with 10^3 L1210 cells. Cyclophosphamide (50 mg/kg) was administered on day 1, and *C. parvum* (0.7 mg per mouse), on day 6. (Reproduced from Mathé, 1976a, with permission of Springer-Verlag.)

the methanol extraction residue fraction of tubercle bacilli (MER) is active in tumor growth inhibition (Table 3) (Mathé *et al.,* 1976). However, its local tolerance is rather poorer than that of living BCG.

What about other dead organisms? I shall not comment on corynebacteria, which have been studied extensively by many other workers (Halpern *et al.,* 1973; Woodruff, 1974); they have given us only a moderate (Fig. 19) and irregular

Table 3. *Effects of BCG and Mycobacterium smegmatis Extracts on Tumor Growth and Survival**

| | Jerne Test | | | Immunoprophylaxis of | | | | | |
| | | | | L1210 | | | Lewis Lung Tumor | | |
Agent	Injection Route, Day†	Index of Effect†	p§	Injection Route, Day†	Index of Effect#	p§	Injection Route, Day†	Index of Effect#	p**
MER (BCG extract)	i.d., +1	2.4	.02↑	s.c., −3	1.5	.05↑	i.v., −3	1.2	.04↑
AE (BCG extract)	i.v., −3	0.5	.05↓	...	...	NS	...	...	NS
HIU II (BCG extract)	i.v., −3	1.6	.05↑	...	...	NS	...	...	NS
WSA F3684 (*M. smegmatis* extract)	i.v., −3	9.0	.01	...	...	NS	...	...	NS

Abbreviations and symbols: ↑, results consistent with immunostimulatory effect; ↓, results consistent with immunosuppressive effect; NS, not significant.

* Reproduced from Mathé *et al.*, 1976, with permissior of the *Israel Journal of Medical Sciences*. Only significant results are indicated.

† After or before antigen.

‡ Mean no. of plaque-forming cells in spleen of treatec mice/mean no. of plaque-forming cells in spleen of control mice.

§ Determined by Student-Fisher test.

Median survival time of treated mice (days)/median survival time of control mice (days).

** Determined by Wilcoxon's nonparametric test.

Table 4. *Effect of* Brucella abortus *on Tumor Growth and Survival*

B. abortus Strain, Dose (μg/mouse)	Route of Administration*	Jerne Test		L1210		Lewis Lung Tumor	
		Index of Effect†	p‡	Index of Effect§	p#	Index of Effect§	p#
B19S, 500	i.v.	0.95	NS	1.17	NS	1.11	NS
	s.c.	0.47	0.001ᵥ	0.92	0.02ᵥ	1.03	NS
B19R, 500	i.v.	1.28	NS	0.92	NS	1.09	NS
	s.c.	1.98	0.05↗	0.92	NS	1.11	NS
1,500	i.v.	2.82	0.02↗	1.00	NS	. . .	. . .
	s.c.	2.4	0.05↗	1.19	0.05↗	. . .	. . .

Abbreviations and symbols: ↗, results consistent with immunostimulatory effect; ᵥ, results consistent with immunosuppressive effect; NS, not significant.
* Injection 2.5 days before antigen.
† Mean no. of plaque-forming cells in spleen of treated mice/mean no. of plaque-forming cells in spleen of control mice.
‡ Determined by Student-Fisher test.
§ Median survival time of treated mice (days)/median survival time of control mice (days).
# Determined by Wilcoxon's nonparametric test.

effect on experimental tumors (Mathé *et al.*, 1975a). This may be explained by their known deteriorating effect on T cell immunity under certain conditions (Scott, 1972), which makes their use imprudent until we have a way of monitoring their effect. In a randomized clinical trial for acute lymphoid leukemia, the combination of *Corynebacterium granulosum*, BCG, and leukemic cells was not shown to be more efficient than the binary combination of BCG and leukemic

Table 5. *Immunopreventive Effect of* Pseudomonas aeruginosa *on L1210 Leukemia**

Injection		Dose (ml)					
		0.5		0.2		0.1	
Day†	Route	Index of Effect‡	p§	Index of Effect‡	p§	Index of Effect‡	p§
−10	i.v.	1.00	NS#	1.14	0.01	1.00	NS
	s.c.	1.00	NS	1.00	NS	1.00	NS
−7	i.v.	1.27	0.01	1.00	NS	1.00	NS
	s.c.	1.00	NS	1.27	0.01	1.25	0.01
−4	i.v.	1.14	0.01	1.14	0.01	1.00	NS
	s.c.	0.91	NS	1.14	NS	1.00	NS
−2.5	i.v.	1.27	0.01	1.00	NS	1.27	0.01
	s.c.	1.27	0.001	1.27	0.01	1.00	NS

* Reproduced from Mathé *et al.*, 1977a, with permission of Masson.
† Before L1210.
‡Median survival time of treated mice (days)/median survival of control mice (days).
§ Determined by Wilcoxon's nonparametric test. All statistically significant results were consistent with immunostimulatory effect.
# Not significant.

Table 6. *Effect of Heat-Killed* Pseudomonas aeruginosa *Preparation** *on Immune Status of (DBA/2 × C57BL/6)F1 Mice*

	Effect After Injection		
Day	3	7	10
Humoral immunity			
Response to thymus-dependent antigens			
SRBC	↘	→	↗
Trinitrophenylated KLH	→	→	↗
Response to thymus-independent antigens			
Trinitrophenylated POL	↗	↗	↘
Cell-mediated immunity			
Response to T cell mitogen (PHA, ConA)	→	→	→
Response to B cell mitogen (DS, LPS)	↗	↗	→
Induction of nonspecific suppressor cells	None	None	None
Macrophage activation	↗ (slight)	↗ (slight)	→

Abbreviations and symbols: ↗, results consistent with immunostimulatory effect; ↘, results consistent with immunosuppressive effect; →, results not significantly different from control values; ConA, concanavalin A; DS, dextran sulfate; KLH, keyhole limpet hemocyanin; LPS, lipopolysaccharide; PHA, phytohemagglutinin; POL, polymerized flagellin; SRBC, sheep red blood cells.

* Dose, 0.1 ml/mouse intravenously of preparation from Pasteur Insititute containing 10^9 heat-killed bacilli per milliliter.

cells (Mathé *et al.,* 1978). Conversely, we are enthusiastic about the action of *Brucella* (Toujas *et al.,* 1972), which, in our screening summarized in Table 4 (Mathé *et al.,* unpublished data), again illustrates the importance of a phenomenon we noted for BCG, namely that the adjuvant action depends on the strain of microorganism used. Only the strain B19R is efficient, and only at certain doses, whereas the strain B19S is immunosuppressive and enhances tumor growth. Finally, we have recently obtained promising results with *Pseudomonas*

Table 7. *Action of Lipopolysaccharide, 250 µg/mouse,** *in EORTC-ICIG Screening for Systemic Immunity Adjuvant*

	Index of Effect	
Assay	i.v.	s.c.
Jerne test	5.23† (*p* > 0.001‡)↗	6.55† (*p* > 0.001‡)↗
L1210 immunoprophylaxis	0.92§ (NS #)	0.92§ (NS #)
Lewis lung tumor immunoprophylaxis	0.84§ (*p* < 0.03 #)↘	0.88§ (*p* < 0.05 #)↘
Macrophage stimulation	71% (inhibition)	. . .

Abbreviations and symbols: ↗, results consistent with immunostimulatory effect; ↘, results consistent with immunosuppressive effect; NS, not significant.

* Injected 2.5 days before antigen.

† Mean no. of plaque-forming cells in spleen of treated mice/mean no. of plaque-forming cells in spleen of control mice.

‡ Determined by Student-Fisher test.

§ Median survival time of treated mice (days)/median survival time of control mice (days).

Determined by Wilcoxon's nonparametric test.

aeruginosa (Tables 5 and 6), both in our study with mice (Mathé *et al.,* 1977b; Florentin *et al.,* 1977) and in clinical study on the immunorestoration of immuno-suppressed patients (Mathé *et al.,* 1977a).

The possibility of tumor growth enhancement by certain modalities of immunointervention underlines the fact that immunotherapy is not homeopathy and must be based on experimental data. Table 7 shows that lipopolysaccharide increases antibody production and enhances tumor growth (Mathé *et al.,* unpublished data).

In conclusion, we have a strong, experimental background of knowledge for clinical immunotherapy, which should be considered carefully before establishing any protocol for clinical trials.

REFERENCES

Bernard, J. 1975. Panel discussion on classification and prognostic features in relation to clinical trials of therapy in acute leukemias. Third Meeting of International Society of Haematology, European-African Division, London.

Brinkley, D., and Haybittle, J. L. 1975. The curability of breast cancer. Lancet, 2:95–97.

Bruce, M. R., Meeker, B. E., and Valeriote, F. A. 1966. Comparison of the sensitivity of normal hematopoietic and transplanted lymphoma colony-forming cells to chemotherapeutic agents administered in vivo. J. Natl. Cancer Inst., 37:233–245.

Clarysse, A., Kenis, Y., and Mathé, G. 1976. Cancer Chemotherapy. Its Role in the Treatment Strategy of Hematologic Malignances and Solid Tumors. New York, Springer-Verlag.

Doré, J. F., Hadjiyannakis, M. J., Coudert, A., Guibout, A., Marholev, L., and Imai, K. 1974. Use of the enzyme-treated cells in immunotherapy of leukaemia. In Mathé, G., and Weiner, R. (eds.): Investigation and Stimulation of Immunity in Cancer Patients. New York, Springer-Verlag, vol. 47, pp. 387–393.

Economides, F., Bruley-Rosset, M., Florentin, I., and Mathé, G. 1977. Treatment of the B16 melanoma with tumorectomy combined or not with adenectomy, systemic and/or regional BCG immunotherapy. Med. Oncol., 3:5–34.

Economides, F., Bruley-Rosset, M., and Mathé, G. 1976. Effect of pre- and post-surgical active BCG immunotherapies on murine EAkR lymphosarcoma. Biomedicine, 25:372–375.

Florentin, I., Bruley-Rosset, M., Bourut, C., Davigny, M., and Mathé, G. 1977. Effects of systemic administration of heat-killed Pseudomonas aeruginosa on immune responses in mice. Applications to cancer immunotherapy. Read before the Third Medical Oncology Society Meeting, Nice.

Geffard, M., and Orbach-Arbouys, S. 1976. Enhancement of T-suppressor activity in mice by high doses of BCG. Cancer Immunol. Immunother., 1:41–44.

Gutterman, J. U., Mavligit, G. M., Reed, R. D., and Hersh, E. M. 1974. Immunochemotherapy of human cancer. Semin. Oncol., 1:409–423.

Halpern, B., Fray, A., Crepin, Y., Platica, O., Lorinet, A. M., Rabourdin, A., Sparrow, L., and Isac, R. 1973. Corynebacterium parvum, a potent immunostimulant in experimental infection and malignancies. In Wolstenholme, G. E. W., and Knight, J. (eds.): Immunopotentiation (Ciba Foundation Symposium 18). Amsterdam, Associated Scientific Publishers, pp. 217–236.

Imbach, J. L., Montero, J. L., Moruzzi, A., Serrou, B., Chenu, E., Hayat, M., and Mathé, G. 1975. The oncostatic and immunosuppressive action of new nitrosourea derivatives containing sugar radicals. Biomedicine, 23:410–413.

Khalil, A., Rappaport, H., Bourut, C., Halle-Pannenko, O., and Mathé, G. 1975. Histologic reactions of the thymus, spleen, liver, lymph-nodes to i.v. and s.c. BCG injections. Biomedicine, 22:112–121.

Martin, M., Bourut, C., Halle-Pannenko, O., and Mathé, G. 1975a. BCG immunotherapy of Lewis tumor residual disease left by local radiotherapy. Biomedicine, 23:337–338.

Martin, M., Bourut, C., Halle-Pannenko, O., and Mathé, G. 1975b. Routes other than i.v. injection to mice for BCG administration in active immunotherapy of L1210 leukemia. Biomedicine, 23:339–340.

Martyré, M. C. 1976. Attempt at specific immunotherapy of RC_{19} leukemia with soluble tumor antigen extracts. Biomedicine, 25:360–362.

Martyré, M. C., Weiner, R., and Halle-Pannenko, O. 1974. The in vivo activity of soluble extract obtained from RC_{19} leukemia: The effect of the method of extraction. In Mathé, G., and Weiner, R. (eds.): Investigation and Stimulation of Immunity in Cancer Patients. New York, Springer-Verlag, vol. 47, pp. 405–407.

Mathé, G. 1968. Immunothérapie active de la leucémie L1210 appliquée après la greffe tumorale. Rev. Fr. Etud. Clin. Biol., 13:881–883.

Mathé, G. 1974. Prevention of chemotherapy complications: Time, toxicity, pharmacokinetics, pharmacodynamic and logistic factors. In Mathé, G., and Oldham, R. K. (eds.): Complications of Cancer Chemotherapy. New York, Springer-Verlag, vol. 49, pp. 124–139.

Mathé, G. 1975. Active immunotherapy as a treatment for minimum residual disease left by chemoradiotherapy in acute lymphoid leukemia. In: Immunological Aspects of Neoplasia (The University of Texas System Cancer Center M. D. Anderson Hospital and Tumor Institute 26th Annual Symposium on Fundamental Cancer Research, 1973). Baltimore, Williams & Wilkins Co., pp. 640–641.

Mathé, G. 1976a. Cancer Active Immunotherapy, Immunoprophylaxis and Immunorestoration: An Introduction. New York, Springer-Verlag.

Mathé, G. 1976b. Side effects and possible harmful action of immunomanipulation. In Duncan, W. A. M., Leonard, B. J., and Brunaud, M. (eds.): The Prediction of Chronic Toxicity from Short Term Studies. Amsterdam, Excerpta Medica, pp. 67–82.

Mathé, G. 1977. Immune status and cancer chemotherapy efficacy. Cancer Immunol. Immunother., 2:81–83.

Mathé, G., De Vassal, F., Gouveia, J., Simmler, M. C., and Misset, J. L. 1977a. Comparison of the restoration effect of Pseudomonas aeruginosa, BCG, and poly I:poly C in cancer patients non responsive to recall antigen delayed hypersensitivity. Biomedicine, 27:328–330.

Mathé, G., Florentin, I., Bruley-Rosset, M., Hayat, M., and Bourut, C. 1977b. Heat-killed Pseudomonas aeruginosa as a systemic adjuvant in cancer immunotherapy. Biomedicine, 27:368–373.

Mathé, G., Halle-Pannenko, O., and Amiel, J. L. 1975a. Results obtained in our adjuvant screening model with *C. parvum* and *C. granulosum*. In Halpern, B. (ed.): *Corynebacterium parvum:* Application in Experimental and Clinical Oncology. New York, Plenum Press, vol. 1, pp. 48–58.

Mathé, G., Halle-Pannenko, O., and Bourut, C. 1973a. Active immunotherapy in spontaneous leukemia of AKR mice. Exp. Hematol., 1:110–114.

Mathé, G., Halle-Pannenko, O., and Bourut, C. 1973b. BCG in cancer immunotherapy. II. Results obtained with various BCG preparations in a screening study for systemic adjuvants applicable to cancer immunoprophylaxis or immunotherapy. Natl. Cancer Inst. Monogr., 39:107–112.

Mathé, G., Halle-Pannenko, O., and Bourut, C. 1974a. Immune manipulation by BCG administered before or after cyclophosphamide for chemo-immunotherapy of L1210 leukaemia. Eur. J. Cancer, 10:661–666.

Mathé, G., Halle-Pannenko, O., and Bourut, C. 1974b. Potentiation of a cyclophosphamide-induced immunodepression by the administration of BCG. Transplant. Proc., 6:431–433.

Mathé, G., Halle-Pannenko, O., and Bourut, C. 1977c. Effectiveness of murine leukemia chemotherapy according to the immune state. Reconsideration of correlations between chemotherapy, tumor cell-killing and survival time. Cancer Immunol. Immunother., 2:139–141.

Mathé, G., Halle-Pannenko, O., and Bourut, C. 1977d. Interspersion of cyclophosphamide and BCG in the treatment of L1210 leukaemia and Lewis tumor. Eur. J. Cancer, 13:1095–1098.

Mathé, G., Halle-Pannenko, O., Florentin, I., Bruley-Rosset, M., Kamel, M., Hiu, I. J., and Bourut, C. 1975b. The second generation of EORTC-ICIG experimental screening for systemic immunity adjuvants. Its significance for cancer immunotherapy. A comparison of BCG and its hydrosoluble extract. Eur. J. Cancer, 11:801–807.

Mathé, G., Hiu, I. J., Halle-Pannenko, O., and Bourut, C. 1976. Methanol extraction residue fraction of tubercle bacilli (MER) and other mycobacterial extracts as systemic immunity adjuvants in cancer immunotherapy. Isr. J. Med. Sci., 12:468–471.

Mathé, G., Kamel, M., Dezfulian, M., Halle-Pannenko, O., and Bourut, C. 1973c. An experimental screening for "systemic adjuvants of immunity" applicable in cancer immunotherapy. Cancer Res., 33:1987–1997.

Mathé, G., and Kenis, Y. 1976. La Chimiothérapie des Cancers (Leucémies, Hématosarcomes et Tumeurs Solides), third edition. Paris, Expansion Scientifique Française.

Mathé, G., Pouillart, P., and Lapeyraque, F. 1969. Active immunotherapy of L1210 leukaemia applied after the graft of tumour cells. Br. J. Cancer, 23:814–824.

Mathé, G., Pouillart, P., and Lapeyraque, F. 1971. Active immunotherapy of mouse RC 19 and EoK1 leukemias applied after the intravenous transplantation of the tumor cells. Experientia, 27:446–447.

Mathé, G., Schwarzenberg, L., De Vassal, F., Delgado, M., Pena-Angulo, J., Belpomme, D., Pouillart, P., Machover, D., Misset, J. L., Pico, J. L., Jasmin, C., Hayat, M., Schneider, M., Cattan, A., Amiel, J. L., Musset, M., and Rosenfeld, C. 1978. Chemotherapy followed by active immunotherapy in the treatment of acute lymphoid leukemias for patients of all ages: Results of ICIG acute lymphoid leukemia protocols 1, 9, and 10; prognosis factors and therapeutic implications. In Terry, W. D., and Windhorst, D. (eds.): Immunotherapy of Cancer: Present Status of Trials in Man. New York, Raven Press, pp. 451–469.

Olsson, L., Florentin, I., Kiger, N., and Mathé, G. 1977. Cellular and humoral immunity to leukemia cells in BCG-induced growth control of a murine leukemia. J. Natl. Cancer Inst., 59:1297–1306.

Olsson, L., and Mathé, G. 1977. A cytokinetic analysis of bacillus Calmette-Guérin-induced growth control of a murine leukemia. Cancer Res., 37:1743–1749.

Parr, I. 1972. Response of syngeneic murine lymphomata to immunotherapy in relation to the antigenicity of the tumor. Br. J. Cancer, 26:174–182.

Pouillart, P., Palangie, T., Schwarzenberg, L., Brugerie, H., Lheritier, J., and Mathé, G. 1975. Effect of BCG on haematopoietic stem cells. Biomedicine, 23:469–471.

Pouillart, P., Palangie, T., Schwarzenberg, L., Brugerie, H., Lheritier, J., and Mathé, G. 1976. Effect of BCG on hematopoietic stem cells: Experimental and clinical study. Cancer Immunol. Immunother., 1:163–169.

Rosenfeld, C., Goutner, A., Venuat, A. M., Choquet, C., Pico, J. L., Doré, J. F., Liabeuf, A., Durandy, A., Desgranges, C., and De Thé, G. 1977. An effective human leukaemic cell line: Reh. Eur. J. Cancer, 13:377–379.

Scott, M. T. 1972. Biological effects of the adjuvant "Corynebacterium parvum." I. Inhibition of PHA, mixed lymphocyte and GVH reactivity. Cell. Immunol., 5:459–468.

Sedlacek, H. H., Seiler, F. R., and Schwick, H. G. 1977. Neuraminidase and tumor immunotherapy. Klin. Wochenschr., 55:199–214.

Simmler, M. C., Schwarzenberg, L., and Mathé, G. 1976. Attempts at nonspecific cell-mediated immunorestoration of immunodepressed cancer patients with BCG. Cancer Immunol. Immunother., 1:157–162.

Skipper, H. E., Schabel, F. M., and Wilcox, W. S. 1964. Experimental evaluation of potential anticancer agents. XIII. On the criteria and kinetics associated with "curability" of experimental leukemia. Cancer Chemother. Rep., 35:1–111.

Skipper, H. E., Schabel, F. M., and Wilcox, W. S. 1965. Experimental evaluation of potential anticancer agents. XIV. Further study of certain basic concepts underlying chemotherapy of leukemia. Cancer Chemother. Rep., 45:5–28.

Skipper, H. E., Schabel, F. M., and Wilcox, W. S. 1967. Experimental evaluation of potential anticancer agents. XXI. Scheduling of arabinocytosine to take advantage of its S-phase specificity against leukaemic cells. Cancer Chemother. Rep., 51:125–165.

Toujas, L., Sabolovic, D., Dazord, L., Legarrec, Y., Toujas, J. P., Guelfi, J., and Pilet, C. 1972. The mechanism of immunostimulation induced by inactivated Brucella abortus. Eur. J. Clin. Biol. Res., 17:267–273.

van Putten, L. M. 1972. The kinetics of cell kill and cell proliferation in relation to curability of malignant disease. In Staquet, M. (ed.): The Design of Clinical Trials in Cancer Therapy. Brussels, Editions Scientifiques Européennes, pp. 115–131.

Woodruff, M. F. A. 1974. Nonspecific effects of Corynebacterium on systemic immunity responses. In Mathé, G., and Weiner, R. (eds.): Investigation and Stimulation of Immunity in Cancer Patients. New York, Springer-Verlag, vol. 47, pp. 272–274.

Zbar, B., and Tanaka, T. 1971. Immunotherapy of cancer: Regression of tumors after intralesional injection of living Mycobacterium bovis. Science, 172:271–273.

IMMUNOLOGIC AND CLINICAL BASIS
OF IMMUNOTIIERAPY

Immunotherapy of Human Cancer,
The University of Texas System Cancer Center
M. D. Anderson Hospital and Tumor Institute.
Raven Press, New York © 1978.

Principles of Immunology with Relevance to Immunotherapy

J. L. Fahey, M.D.

*Department of Microbiology and Immunology, UCLA School of Medicine,
Los Angeles, California*

In man, intense delayed hypersensitivity reactions in the vicinity of dermal neoplasms will induce rejection of superficially located tumors (Klein *et al.,* 1976). Reactions are induced by strong delayed hypersensitivity immunogens, not by tumor antigens. The mechanism by which this effect is achieved is not known exactly, although we do know that T cell immune reactions are involved. Intense amplification processes include macrophages and their release of enzymes and other tumoricidal substances. The regenerative capacity of normal cells allows the skin to regrow, and the skin tumors usually do not recur in the area where an induced delayed hypersensitivity reaction has caused initial rejection and successful eradication of tumor. Such local reactions have not been demonstrated in sites other than skin. Unfortunately, an intense reaction in superficial locations does not affect tumor that has already spread to lymph nodes or visceral organs.

IMMUNE RESPONSE TO TUMOR

A scheme conveying some key aspects of the immune system's response to tumors is shown in Figure 1. The essential points are that (1) both T and B lymphoid cells can respond to tumor antigens; (2) the response of T cells can involve both direct cytotoxicity and production of lymphokines, which involve macrophages and other lymphocytes in a reaction at the site of a tumor; (3) the T cell population contains suppressor cells, which influence the dimensions of immune reactions and can effectively inhibit immune response; and (4) antibody, through the mechanism of antibody-dependent, cellular cytotoxicity, can effectively involve macrophages and lymphocytes in the reaction against tumors. Not shown in the figure, but potentially important, is the fact that macrophages, in addition to assisting immune rejection reactions, can be suppressive and inhibitory of T cell responses to antigen.

The diagram shown in Figure 1 will serve as a reference for the discussion of immune malfunctions and potential immunotherapy.

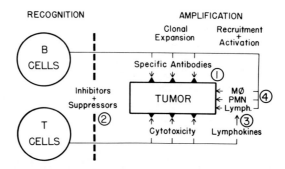

Figure 1. Diagrammatic representation of immune response to tumor antigens.

Immunosurveillance

Normal immune functions are associated with resistance against tumors. Data from studies in mice pointed to the importance of T cell functions in the resistance to cancer, but the resistance was largely to certain, virally induced neoplasms and did not seem to apply to all carcinogens. In man, immune deficiency diseases of B cells (e.g., immunoglobulin deficiencies) and of T cells are associated with increased frequency of tumors, primarily lymphosarcoma and related neoplasms (Kersey *et al.,* 1973; Penn, 1974; Melif and Schwartz, 1975). Also, patients with kidney transplants who are receiving immunosuppressive drugs have a 400-fold likelihood of tumor development, as compared to normal persons.

Several immune systems are likely to be involved in resistance to cancer. In addition to the T and B cell systems, a system involving natural cytotoxicity or spontaneous killer (SK) cell activity against tumor cell lines may be significant. Observations in nude (nu/nu) mice that have deficiencies of T cell function indicate no unusual frequency of neoplasms or susceptibility to oncogenic viruses or carcinogens (Stutman, 1977). In these mice, however, there is a normal amount of spontaneous, natural cytotoxicity. Thus, the SK cells may represent a form of natural cellular immunity and may play a significant role in the resistance to the earliest stages of neoplastic cell development and establishment.

Extension of these observations to testing for SK activities in man has led to appreciation of the fact that this immunity may be relatively specific and that several forms of cells may be involved (Takasugi *et al.,* 1977; Jondal *et al.,* unpublished data). Indeed, SK activity generally is coming to be viewed as a reflection of several immune cell systems.

FAILURE OF IMMUNE RESISTANCE

Human tumors develop from single cells that grow to clinically discernible masses (usually more than 10^9 cells) without exciting a sufficient or appropriate immune rejection reaction. This failure of immune responsiveness in man may be due to failure of immune resistance or to poor tumor immunogenicity. Several possible mechanisms for these defects and means of correcting the disorders are discussed in the following sections.

Excess Antigen—Immune Paralysis

Low doses of antigen (hapten and soluble proteins) given repeatedly over a long period induce immune unresponsiveness (low-dose tolerance) to subsequent challenge (Weigle, 1973). Large doses of antigen can overwhelm immune responsiveness and induce immune paralysis (or high-dose tolerance). These phenomena may apply to human tumor systems. The slow development of many human tumors allows for continuing presentation of gradually increasing amounts of antigen.

Immunotherapy is based on murine studies with soluble protein antigens, which have indicated that tolerance can be broken by drastic modification of the tolerogenic molecules with addition of new, highly immunogenic or other suitable carrier molecules. This, of course, is one rationale for chemically modifying tumor cells in immunotherapy efforts (Fig. 1, no. 1). If tolerance is firmly established, replacement of the immune system may be necessary. Bone marrow transplantation provides a means of eradicating the preexisting immune system and introducing stem cells for development of a new immune system.

Blocking Antibody

Tissue transplantation studies indicate that graft survival can be ensured by administration and maintenance of antibody directed against the histocompatibility antigens of the new graft. Furthermore, work of Mullen and associates (1977) indicates that the minor histocompatibility antigen differences are relatively easily protected from rejection reaction by specific antihistocompatibility antibodies of the immunoglobulin G class. The possibility that some tumor antigens are equivalent to minor histocompatibility antigens makes this a logical consideration. Evidence for blocking antibody as a significant factor in human tumor development, however, is lacking.

Antigen–Antibody Complexes

Antigen in the circulation of tumor-bearing animals is often complexed with antibodies (Hellström and Hellström, 1977). Antigen–antibody complexes can react with immune competent cells and cause decreased immune responsiveness to the specific antigen. Searches for circulating antigen-antibody complexes in patients with tumors indicate that such complexes are present in some tumor patient groups (Rossen *et al.,* 1977). Identification of specific antigen, however, has been difficult in human tumor systems, and the tests, themselves, for immune complexes are complex. Not all studies support the notion of circulating immune complexes in human cancer, and the matter is still in early stages of investigation.

Suppressor Cells

The T lymphoid cells regulate B cell function, e.g., antibody production, by means of helper and suppressor T cell subpopulations (Fig. 1, no. 2). Suppressor (and helper) T cells regulating immunoglobulin formation by human B cells have been demonstrated. Soluble factors are released from the suppressor T lymphoid cells as well as the helper T cells and help to mediate the T and B cell regulatory systems. Evidence to date indicates that the suppressor factors do not serve to neutralize helper cells but act on other stages of B cell maturation. Cells that suppress immune response to tumor antigens have been identified as T cells (Fujimoto *et al.,* 1976; Takei *et al.,* 1977) or adherent cells (macrophages) (Kirchner *et al.,* 1975).

Immunotherapy could be directed against the suppressor cell population by utilizing the specific cell-surface antigens of these cells. Production of specific heterologous antisera would allow destruction of this class of cells. Direct attack of the whole group of suppressor cells, however, might lead to general immune disorders. Thus, selective attack on a particular category of suppressor cells would be desirable. This might be achievable by directing antisera against idiotypic determinants on particular suppressor cell clones (reacting against tumor antigens). This type of suppressor cell idiotypic specificity has been identified in a hapten antigen system by Nisonoff and colleagues (Owen *et al.,* 1977), indicating that such an approach to tumor immunotherapy might be eventually feasible.

Impaired Amplification Mechanisms

Cellular immune manifestations are effectively initiated by a few T lymphoid cells. These, in turn, are able to enlist many other cells (Fig. 1, no. 3) in the intense reaction that can cause allograft and tumor rejection. Soluble mediators, the lymphokines (Yoshida and Cohen, 1977), from the immune lymphocytes act as chemotactic factors, and as migration inhibitory factors, and also as activation agents for lymphocytes and macrophages. These soluble factors are important in the intercellular cooperation that results in effective, normal, cellular immune responses.

Inflammatory response capability is often reduced in man by cancer, particularly advanced cancer (Hersh *et al.,* 1977). This impairment occurs in addition to the delayed hypersensitivity, T cell-mediated immune impairment. Because the inflammatory response is an important amplification mechanism for T cell-mediated cellular immune reactions, inflammatory constraints have serious consequences for effective immune reactions. The mechanisms responsible for the reduced function of key amplification mechanisms, particularly those involving macrophages, are not yet defined. Monocyte chemotaxis, however, is impaired in many patients with neoplastic diseases. As investigations of the monocyte and macrophage population are extended, more insight certainly will be gained.

Empiric approaches to the correction of these defects already have been taken. Agents such as bacillus Calmette-Guérin (BCG), *Corynebacterium parvum,* and levamisole are all capable of stimulating monocyte and macrophage activities (Fig. 1, no. 4). Stimulating these cells to increased activity may be critical for adequate rejection reactions. Potentially undesirable side effects, such as exhaustion and further impairment of a crucial system, also must be considered as potential effects of repeated or intensive stimulation. Careful clinical and laboratory evaluation of these modes of immunotherapy are indicated as they are explored in man.

Tumor Isolation from Immune Systems

The tumor may well be located in such a way that blood and lymph flow are greatly different from that in normal tissues. Furthermore, fluid-bathing tumors might be expected to contain a relatively large concentration of soluble antigen, either secreted or shed from the surface of tumor cells. The exact implications of this relatively high, local concentration of antigens for tumor immunology remain to be determined, but the tolerogenic effects of excess antigen in haptenic systems have been noted.

The geographic location of tumor in relation to the immune system may reduce the number of immune cells that can reach the tumor and engage the normal amplification processes necessary for effective rejection reactions. Investigations of this general aspect are warranted, but the technology for sampling fluids and cells immediately adjacent to tumors is not frequently practiced by immunologists.

Immunotherapeutic approaches to correct relative tumor isolation may involve efforts to induce acute inflammation in the vicinity of tumors in order to change the blood flow or lymphokine production or to present tumor antigens via more effective immunization routes and schedules (e.g., intralymphatic immunotherapy).

Quantitative Consideration

Investigations in animals clearly indicate that a large number of tumor cells can overcome an otherwise effective immune response. Thus, tumors that in small doses would excite an immune response sufficient to cope with the tumor (and cause rejection before the tumor becomes well established) are not rejected if a tenfold greater number of cells are given.

The therapeutic implications of this are well recognized. In most current immunotherapeutic regimens, surgery, radiotherapy, and/or chemotherapy for tumor reduction are incorporated prior to initiation of immunotherapy. One aspect, however, that probably has not been carefully considered or investigated relates to the effect of conventional therapy on immune responsiveness. For example, chemotherapy and immunotherapy often have been administered on the same days. This may be a convenience for outpatients who must make frequent hospital visits. Many chemotherapeutic agents, themselves, are immunosuppressive and will abrogate the desired immunologic effects and reduce immune potential. More attention to the scheduling of immune active agents in relation to other forms of therapy is warranted.

POOR IMMUNE STIMULATION

Antigen Lack or Low Immunogenicity

Human tumors that become clinically evident fail to evoke a readily discernible, cellular immune rejection reaction. This could be due to (1) lack of any tumor-specific antigens, (2) absence of tumor-specific transplantation (rejection) antigens, (3) expression of fetal antigens, or antigens that are normally present on other adult tissues and that fail to evoke a cellular rejection type of response, (4) antigens that are poor or weak immunogens because of their chemical composition, or (5) lack of critical "second signals" needed for effective immune response. Examination of the possibilities for low antigenicity or absence of antigens or for poor immunogenicity are complicated by a poor understanding of all the factors needed to excite a good immune response and difficulties in establishing methods for defining specific cellular immunity to tumor-associated antigens in man.

Second Signal Hypotheses

Effective immunogenicity of many antigens requires (in addition to specific antigen) the presence of an appropriate second signal, e.g., a signal to the responding cells that facilitates proliferation and maturation of immune competent cells (Lafferty and Woolnough, 1977; Davidson, 1977). At present, it is difficult to tell if tumor cells are nonimmunogenic because the antigen is lacking or there is a second-signal deficiency (or inhibitor). Some mitogens act as second signals. Soluble factors generated by induced cell-mediated lympholysis also may act as second signals. With further data and availability of large amounts of such materials, it may be possible in the future to add them to immunotherapeutic regimens at appropriate times and locations and thus achieve a stimulation of immune response that is not now feasible. In studies with human leukemic blast cells, Sondel *et al.* (1976) provided evidence that for some patients, a second signal is needed to render the leukemic cells immunogenic.

Cell Recognition Systems (Syngeneic Preference)

The development of murine cell-mediated lympholysis against virus-induced antigens, minor histocompatibility antigens, or haptens introduced onto the cell surface is facilitated by antigen presentation on syngeneic cells (Doherty *et al.,* 1976; Shearer *et al.,* 1976). Much has been made of the difference between presentation of antigen on syngeneic and allogeneic cells in the murine systems; often overlooked, however, is that some cytotoxicity response is induced in the allogeneic system but that greater responses are induced in the syngeneic system. Thus, an absolute requirement for syngeneic cell presentation may not exist (Ting and Law, 1977).

In man, cell-mediated cytotoxicity against allogeneic and syngeneic B lymphoblastoid human cell line cultures can be readily induced in vitro (Ling *et al.,* 1974; Spina *et al.,* unpublished data). Thus, the dimensions of the restrictions imposed by histocompatibility and other components of the cell surface on the response to tumor-associated antigens are important but will require further investigation to allow a clear insight into their significance and how they can be manipulated to therapeutic advantage. From an immunotherapeutic standpoint, modification of the cell surface to amplify cell interaction as well as to involve supplementary or accessory cells that may be helpful in promoting rejection types of immune response could be useful. Most approaches at present are empiric chemical modifications of tumor cells or extracts, but supplementation with lymphokines may be of value.

Intralymphatic Immunotherapy

Antigen is usually envisioned as leaving the tumor region as soluble molecules or larger components that flow primarily into the lymphatic channels and on to the regional lymph nodes. Direct entry into the serum is not ruled out. After antigens are released from viable, dying, or dead tumor cells, enzyme action can be expected to alter them. This action may reduce the antigen content or alter the presentation to the lymph node lymphocytes and other components of the immune system.

Intralymphatic antigen administration, as investigated by Juillard and Boyer (1977) and associates (in press), has been an effective form of immunotherapy for several canine tumors, especially lymphosarcoma. This mode of therapy alone apparently instigates effective containment of tumors. In some cases, animals are surviving two years or more with no other therapy. Extension of this approach to man has begun. Juillard and colleagues (1977) have shown that the administration of autologous or allogeneic tumor homogenates via the lymphatic channels in man are well tolerated, with minor, if any, toxicity. Several patients appear to have experienced tumor reduction with this form of therapy. With the completion of phase I trials, immunotherapeutic protocols are being initiated for selected human tumors.

SUMMARY

Starting from the evidence that immunologic reactions can kill cancers in man, several facets of immune function that may be relevant to the success or failure of immune rejection of tumors have been considered. Immunologic reactions, to be effective, need not be specifically directed at the tumor but can be in the immediate vicinity of the cancer. Clearly, tumor cells can be more susceptible than normal cells to damage of the type produced during an intense, T cell-mediated, delayed hypersensitivity reaction. Human tumors, however, develop without sufficient or appropriate immune rejection reactions. This failure may represent inadequate immune response or poor tumor immunogenicity. Possible causes of inadequate immune response are immune tolerance, blocking antibody, antigen-antibody complexes, suppressor cells, impaired amplification mechanisms, and tumor isolation. Poor immune stimulation may reflect antigen lack, low immunogenicity, deficient second signals, cell recognition systems, or modes of antigen presentation. Intralymphatic immunotherapy has potential value in treatment of human tumors.

ACKNOWLEDGMENTS

The author gratefully acknowledges many helpful discussions with colleagues in the UCLA Immunobiology Group. This work was made possible by grants CA-12800 and CA-16880 and contract CB-53939 from the National Institutes of Health, U.S. Public Health Service, Department of Health, Education, and Welfare.

REFERENCES

Davidson, W. F. 1977. Cellular requirements for the induction of cytotoxic T cells in vitro. Immunol. Rev., 35:263–304.

Doherty, P. C., Blanden, R. V., and Zinkernagel, R. M. 1976. Specificity of virus-immune effector T cells for H-2k or H-2D compatible interactions: Implications for H-antigen diversity. Transplant. Rev., 29:89–124.

Fujimoto, S., Greene, M. I., and Sehon, A. H. 1976. Regulation of the immune response to tumor antigens. II. The nature of immunosuppressor cells in tumor-bearing hosts. J. Immunol., 116(3):800–806.

Hellström, K. E., and Hellström, I. 1977. Immunologic enhancement of tumor growth. In Green, I., Cohen, S., and McCluskey, R. T. (eds.): Mechanisms of Tumor Immunity. New York, John Wiley and Sons, pp. 147–174.

Hersh, E. M., Mavligit, G. M., and Gutterman, J. U. 1976. Immunodeficiency in cancer and the importance of immune evaluation of the cancer patient. Med. Clin. North Am., 60:623–640.

Juillard, G. J. F., and Boyer, P. P. J. 1977. Intralymphatic immunization: Current status. Eur. J. Cancer, 13:439–440.

Juillard, G. J. F., Boyer, P. P. J., and Yamashiro, C. H. 1978. A phase I study of active specific intralymphatic immunotherapy (ASILI). Cancer Res. (in press).

Juillard, G. J. F., Boyer, P. P. J., Yamashiro, C. H., Snow, H. D., Weisenburger, T. H., McCarthy, T., and Miller, R. J. 1977. Regional intralymphatic infusion (ILI) of irradiated tumor cells with evidence of distant effects. Cancer, 39:126–130.

Kersey, J. H., Spector, B. D., and Good, R. A. 1973. Immunodeficiency and cancer. Adv. Cancer Res., 18:211.

Kirchner, H., Muchmore, A. V., Chused, T. M., Holden, H. T., and Herberman, R. B. 1975. Inhibition of proliferation of lymphoma cells and T lymphocytes by suppressor cells from spleens of tumor-bearing mice. J. Immunol., 114:206–210.

Klein, E., Holterman, O., Milgrom, H., Case, R. W., Klein, D., Rossner, D., Djerassi, I. 1976.

Immunotherapy for accessible tumor utilizing delayed type hypersensitivity reactions and separated components of the immune system. Med. Clin. North Am., 60(3):389–418.

Lafferty, K. J., and Woolnough, J. 1977. The origin and mechanism of the allograft and reaction. Immunol. Rev., 35:231–262.

Ling, N. R., Steel, C. M., Waliin, J., and Hardy, D. A. 1974. The interaction of normal lymphocytes and cells from lymphoid cell lines (LCL). V. Cytotoxic properties of activated lymphocytes. Immunology, 26:345.

Melif, C. J. M., and Schwartz, R. S. 1975. Immunocompetence and malignancy. In Becker, F. F. (ed.): Cancer: A Comprehensive Treatise. New York, Plenum Press, vol. 1, pp. 121–160.

Mullen, Y., Raison, R., and Hildemann, W. 1977. Cytotoxic versus immunoblocking effects of specific alloantibodies. Transplantation, 24:99–105.

Owen, F. F., Ju, S., and Nisonoff, A. 1977. Presence on idiotype-specific suppressor T cells of receptors that interact with molecules bearing the idiotype. J. Exp. Med., 145:1559–1566.

Penn, I. 1974. Occurrence of cancer in immune deficiencies. Cancer, 34:858.

Rossen, R. D., Reisberg, M. A., Hersh, E. M., and Gutterman, J. U. 1977. The C1Q binding test for soluble immune complexes: Clinical correlations with cancer. J. Natl. Cancer Inst., 58:1205–1215.

Shearer, G. M., Rehn, T. G., and Schmitt-Verhulst, A. 1976. Role of the murine major histocompatibility complex in the specificity of in vitro T-cell mediated lympholysis against chemically-modified autologous lymphocytes. Transplant. Rev., 29:222–248.

Sondel, P. M., O'Brien, C., Porter, L., Schlossman, S. F., and Chess, L. 1976. Cell-mediated destruction of human leukemic cells by MHC identical lymphocytes: Requirement for a proliferative trigger in vitro. J. Immunol., 117:2197–2203.

Stutman, O. 1977. Immunodeficiency and cancer. In Green, I., Cohen, S., and McCluskey, R. T. (eds.): Mechanisms of Tumor Immunity. New York, John Wiley and Sons, pp. 27–53.

Takasugi, M., Koide, Y., Akira, D., and Ramseyer, A. 1977. The specificities in natural cell-mediated cytotoxicity by the cross-competition assay. Cancer, 19:291–297.

Takei, F., Levy, J. G., and Kilburn, G. G. 1977. Characterization of suppressor cells in mice bearing syngeneic mastocytoma. J. Immunol., 118:412–417.

Ting, C., and Law, L. W. 1977. Studies of H-2 restriction in cell-mediated cytotoxicity and transplantation immunity to leukemia associated antigens. J. Immunol., 118:1259.

Weigle, W. O. 1973. Immunological unresponsiveness. Adv. Immunol., 16:61.

Yoshida, T., and Cohen, S. 1977. Lymphocytes in tumor immunity. In Green, I., Cohen, S., and McCluskey, R. T. (eds.): Mechanisms of Tumor Immunity. New York, John Wiley and Sons, pp. 87–108.

Immunotherapy of Human Cancer,
The University of Texas System Cancer Center
M. D. Anderson Hospital and Tumor Institute.
Raven Press, New York © 1978.

Host Mechanisms for Control of Tumor Growth That Can Be Modulated by Nonspecific Immunotherapy

David W. Weiss, Ph.D., D.Phil.Med.

Lautenberg Center for General and Tumor Immunology, Hebrew University-Hadassah Medical School, Jerusalem

Cognizant of the adage that fools rush in where angels fear to tread, I must begin any discussion of tumor immunology with several disclaimers, and with a clarion emphasis on the major restrictions placed on us by the large uncertainties that today characterize this aspect of tumor biology. I shall attempt this admonitory introduction by focusing on several of the cardinal questions that face investigators who seek ways of modulating host immunologic reactions against tumor cells for therapeutic ends, questions to which answers have proved most elusive.

Are there, in fact, host mechanisms of immunologic kind operative in surveillance against neoplasia in nature? The laboratory tumor models on which an affirmative reply was based some years ago may be, in large part, devoid of relevance. We have chosen to work with those tumors that *are* immunogenic, but we have come to recognize that their immunogenicity may be artifactual. The causative oncogenic stimuli that elicit most of the growths that have become the stock in trade of the experimental oncologist must be suspected of inducing neoplasms whose pronounced antigenic and immunogenic characteristics are exaggerated and possibly even incidental to their neoplastic properties, and which for other reasons do not serve as veracious models of spontaneously occurring neoplasms. Chemical carcinogens applied in large quantities, strong doses of ionizing radiation, powerfully oncogenic viruses originating in inbred strains and propagated in the laboratory, and passaged tumor cell lines of ancient origin all constitute circumstances that can readily make for the expression of cell surface deviations representing mutational and adaptive events that are not necessarily a condition or unexpendable attribute of neoplastic growth as such. The low or absent immunogenicity of spontaneously arising animal tumors (Weiss, 1977) and, apparently, of many human malignant growths (Weiss, 1977, unpublished data) stands in sharp contrast to these supposed animal models, and argues against the likelihood of a prevalent immune surveillance *in nature* against progressive neoplasia.

The counter-argument that immune surveillance, in fact, does exist and contributes appreciably to the infrequency of neoplastic disease in normal young animals and human beings—the classic example, perhaps, is the extreme rarity of polyoma tumors in nonimmunosuppressed rodents—may be of much theoretical interest but of little pertinence to the immunotherapist. We are concerned with those tumors that do appear, not with those prevented from arising by immunologic or other mechanisms, and the operative question thus remains: Are those neoplasms that do occur, and that threaten host survival, in any way the manifestations of a breakdown in normally effective immunologic control, or of active means of tumor escape from the control mechanisms? Or, are most spontaneously developing tumors essentially beyond the scope of immunologic concern because they lack immunogenicity in the autochthonous organism?

In reply, we perhaps might be justified in formulating a minimal hypothesis of tumor antigenicity on theoretical and indirect grounds (Weiss, 1977), and thereby provide ourselves with a viable justification for pursuing attempts at cancer immunotherapy. This minimal hypothesis holds that in the course of even spontaneous neoplastic transformations, a sufficient degree of alteration in cell surface structures occurs to create the potential for immunologic response by the host; that if these changes are too limited to afford active immunogenicity on the transformed cells in an unstimulated host, they nonetheless represent an antigenic quality that can be translated into frank immunogenicity by artificial manipulations of the tumor cell surface and the immunologic apparatus of the organism.

A number of considerations can be advanced in support of this expectation. Neoplasms occurring in nature do not manifest morphologic and physiologic aspects that would lead one to differentiate them categorically from the laboratory neoplasms of known immunogenicity; although the etiologic circumstances of the former may be greatly different, quantitatively if not qualitatively, the assumption of some similarities of antigenicity between spontaneous and intentionally induced tumors may not be unwarranted, even if the range of antigenic potency is skewed in the direction of paucity for the spontaneous growths. Moreover, morphologic and physiologic properties are often similar for tumors developing as a random event in the natural history of an organism and for analogous neoplasms arising only after decisive immunosuppression. Then, the "nonimmunogenicity" of many spontaneous tumors may not be the total immunologic neutrality maintained by Hewitt *et al.* (1976), but rather, as indicated by Baldwin (in press), a poor capacity to elicit protective immunologic responses even though detectable changes in antigenicity have taken place. The behavior of certain neoplasms in the host of origin is also suggestive of at least a fluctuating, moderate capability of the host to mount defenses, of seeming immunologic type; and, as pointed out elsewhere (Weiss, 1977, unpublished data), the altered structure and functionality of neoplastic variants is highly suggestive of macromolecular changes of concomitant immunologic import.

However, even assuming that immunologic interactions are part of the host-tumor confrontation in nature, or that they can be brought into being by intervention directed at tumor cell structure or host reactivity, we still face two basic questions: What are the immunologic mechanisms of tumor cytostasis and cytotoxicity in those experimental systems in which tumor immunogenicity and host reactivity are established, and how are these mechanisms to be modulated and focused?

Little in return can be offered with certainty. Various investigators today advance the candidacy of different key mediators and effectors of tumor immunity, cellular and humoral, but the claims are distinguished more by modishness than by fact derived from comparative analyses. It would appear most likely, indeed, that a variety of immunologic defense mechanisms are at play, to different extents and in different combinations and sequences with regard to different tumors, and perhaps variously at different moments in the progression of a neoplastic process. It seems most dangerous to advocate favorite candidates as inclusive, central pillars of tumor immunity, such as it be.

Even more formidable a task than the definition of the effectors of antitumor reactivity in a given situation is the attempt to intervene selectively toward a strengthening of resistance. Immunologic responsiveness must be viewed today as an intricate network of positive and rescinding signals, and even in the most defined systems of hapten-antibody interactions, we have only begun to learn the pathways through this maze. To this must be added the consideration that those immunomodulator (or adjuvant) substances available today that have a demonstrated capacity to heighten antitumor resistance in different models are, for the most part, crude microbial entities of complex and undefined composition. Immunotherapeutic intervention in malignant diseases is thus rather like the attempt to alter an exceedingly delicate equilibrium between multicomponental living interactants—host immunocytes on the one hand, neoplastic variants on the other—by means of a crowbar.

This holds true for both specific and nonspecific immunologic intervention. Because the nonspecific approach to cancer immunotherapy nonetheless holds certain advantages over the specific, at this stage of our efforts to potentiate host resistance (Weiss, in press, unpublished data), it will be to this aspect that the present discussion is directed.

Under some circumstances, every known arm of the immunologic response to tumor-associated antigens has been shown capable of inhibitory action against transformed cells, in vitro and, in some instances, also in vivo. Included in this spectrum of effector mechanisms are several classes of free antibody; K cells; natural killer (NK) cells; mature T cells; macrophages in their "native state," armed with specific antibody or T cell recognition factors, activated nonspecifically by lymphokines, or "excited" after prior contact with target antigens against which the cells were specifically armed; and B-lymphocytes following blast transformation or other activation. Each of these categories of immunocytes may be composed of multiple subpopulations with distinct predilections for effector, mediator, and suppressor activity. The chain of events that leads to stimulated or depressed activity of any of these arms of reactivity following nonspecific immunomodulation remains largely unknown. All that can be said at this point is that a given immunomodulator, under defined conditions, can bring about effects on particular tumors that are due to, or paralleled by, altered reactivity of certain effector arms in specified tests.

Depressingly unsatisfactory as such a conditioned, guarded statement of our insights into nonspecific immunomodulation may be, it does indicate that broad and profound effects may be elicited by such means. To control these effects and to intervene in neoplastic diseases with precision and foreknowledge is a hope for the future. A step in that direction is to classify accurately the effects attained, to enlarge the test systems in which they are looked for, and to build a catalogue of information that, albeit still largely descriptive, eventually may reveal certain inclusive principles and thereby permit ultimately the dissection of modalities of action and the inductive design of a strategy of immunotherapy.

Resorting to MER (methanol extraction residue fraction of tubercle bacilli) (Weiss, 1972, 1976a) as a model, I will exemplify some of the broadly expressed proclivities of microbial immunomodulators in influencing immunologic function, to illustrate the range of possibilities before us. Although beyond our means of precision control at this time, the breadth and extent of the effects that can be evoked show the tools of immunomodulation to be, for all their present bluntness, potentially powerful indeed (Weiss *et al.,* 1976).

IMMUNOMODULATION WITH MER

Polyclonal Mitogenicity

As reported by Ben-Efraim and Diamantstein (1975), MER acts as a polyclonal lymphocyte mitogen (Table 1). Its mitogenicity for spleen and peripheral blood leukocytes of BALB/c mice is greater than that of the known B cell mitogens dextran sulfate, gram-negative bacterial lipopolysaccharide (here employed in optimum stimulatory quantities), and purified protein derivative, but far less than that of phytohemagglutinin and concanavalin A. On the other hand, neither of these latter substances is mitogenic for splenocytes of T cell-deficient nude (nu/nu) mice, whereas MER is reactive. Moreover, depletion of glass-adherent cells from splenocyte cultures or addition of syngeneic peritoneal exudate cells, largely macrophages, to the depleted cultures exerts no effect on the mitogenic responsiveness to the agent (Table 2). It thus appears that MER serves as a polyclonal B cell mitogen in mice, and apparently without the intermediacy of macrophagic cells. In further studies by Ben-Efraim *et al.* (1976), MER also emerged as a B cell mitogen in guinea pigs.

It is not yet certain if MER exerts a direct, polyclonal, mitogenic effect on T-lymphocytes. Some findings in this direction have been reported (Mitchell *et al.,* 1975), but the possibility remains that the effect is an indirect one, mediated by macrophages or other cells (Ben-Efraim, 1977).

Table 1. *Polyclonal Mitogenicity of MER and Other Substances on Mouse Lymphoid Cells In Vitro**

| Mitogen‡ | Amount (µg/culture) | Stimulation Index in Cell Cultures† | | | | nu/nu Spleen |
| | | BALB/c | | | | |
		Spleen	Lymph Node	Bone Marrow	Blood	
None (control)	...	1	1	1	1	1
PHA	10	55	42	3	ND§	2
ConA	10	67	80	3	ND	3
MER	10	4	1	1	ND	4
	30	6	2	2		8
	100	9	2	2	3	15
	300	13	2	1	9	17
PPD	10	2	ND	1	11	2
	30	3	1	1	ND	3
	100	3	1	2	2	4
	300	5	1	2	2	5
DS	50	9	3	2	1	13
LPS	50	5	4	1	3	8

* Adapted from Ben-Efraim and Diamantstein, 1975.
† Each culture consisted of 3 × 10^5 cells. Values shown are means of three determinations; standard error < 10%.
‡ ConA, concanavalin A; DS, dextran sulfate; LPS, lipopolysaccharide; PHA, phytohemagglutinin; PPD, purified protein derivative.
§ Not done.

Table 2. *Polyclonal Mitogenicity of MER and Other Substances on BALB/c Spleen Cells In Vitro. Role of Glass-Adherent Cells**

		Stimulation Index in Spleen Cultures[†]		
Mitogen[‡]	Amount (μg/culture)	Original	Nonadherent	Nonadherent +3% PE Cells[§]
None (control)	...	1	1	1
MER	100	9	12	12
PPD	300	8	5	7
LPS	50	9	9	9

* Adapted from Ben-Efraim and Diamantstein, 1975.
† Values shown are means of three determinations; standard error < 10%.
‡ LPS, lipopolysaccharide; PPD, purified protein derivative.
§ 6×10^4 peritoneal exudate cells (mostly macrophages)/2×10^6 nonadherent splenocytes.

Stimulation of Antibody Production to Defined Antigens

As has been reviewed in several recent communications (Weiss, 1972, 1976a), MER can heighten markedly the antibody response of experimental animals and cancer patients to a variety of defined antigens, especially when the specific immunizing stimulus is weak. Under defined experimental conditions, it has been possible by means of MER to direct the response to such antigens preferentially toward cellular or humoral antibody reactivity (Ben-Efraim, 1973). In further experiments, the modulatory propensities of MER on antibody formation were studied in vitro, employing Marbrook tissue cultures (Ben-Efraim and Diamantstein, 1975; Ben-Efraim, 1977), to obtain more discriminating information on the kinetics and loci of the effects. Table 3 presents data from initial experiments that reveal that MER can strongly potentiate the plaque-forming

Table 3. *Effect of MER on Primary Antibody Response In Vitro of Mouse Splenocytes to Sheep Red Blood Cells (SRBC). Kinetics of Response**

		No. of Plaque-Forming Cells (19S) per Culture[†]			
		nu/nu	BALB/c		
Mitogen Added to Cultures	SRBC Added	Day 4	4	5	6
None	No	430	160	160	75
	Yes	700	1,700	1,650	1,200
MER, 10 μg	No	200	330	220	90
	Yes	1,780	16,500	17,900	10,100
PPD,[‡] 100 μg	No	200	170	110	80
	Yes	1,350	5,060	13,000	7,040

* Adapted from Ben-Efraim and Diamantstein, 1975.
† Determined on indicated day after onset of incubation. Values shown are means of three determinations, performed on three distinct splenocyte cultures; standard error < 6%.
‡ Purified protein derivative.

cell response to sheep red blood cells. This was evident as well with regard to the levels of free antibody and responsiveness to the hapten, trinitrophenol (Ben-Efraim and Diamantstein, 1975; Ben-Efraim, 1977). The amounts of MER effective in increasing antibody-forming capacity of both BALB/c and nu/nu splenocytes were far below those required for a polyclonal mitogenic effect; indeed, elevation of the amount to 70 μg per culture abolished the stimulation of specific antibody synthesis. The excipient actions on antibody formation and polyclonal mitogenicity thus appear to be at least partially independent.

In subsequent work (Ben-Efraim *et al.,* unpublished data), it was found that macrophage depletion abrogates the ability of mouse spleen cultures to synthesize antibody against sheep red blood cells in Marbrook cultures, but that addition of MER to the depleted cultures restores reactivity. It thus appears that MER may be able to substitute for macrophage or adherent T cell helper function by somehow providing the "second signal" to B cells required for antibody synthesis.

Among further studies under way on the potentiation of antibody formation in vitro by MER, experiments are being conducted to ascertain if the agent can preferentially direct antibody responsiveness to the production of different categories of immunoglobulins with different biologic activities.

Stimulation of T Cell Functions

MER has been shown to stimulate a variety of immunologic reactions in vivo—delayed hypersensitivity to defined antigens, allograft immunity, and resistance to syngeneic tumors—in which T-lymphocytes appear to play a major role (Kuperman *et al.,* 1972; Weiss, 1976a; Ben-Efraim, 1977). It is not certain, however, whether the agent affects T cells directly or exerts its influence on cell-mediated immunity via other pathways, with T cells involved only secondarily or their function preempted entirely by other effector mechanisms. To cast further light on this question, we have conducted a number of studies in which the influence of MER on cell-mediated immunity is assessed in vitro.

In one series of experiments, we measured splenocyte effector function against allogeneic tumor cells by a ^{51}Cr release assay (Kuperman *et al.,* 1973). C57BL mice were immunized with allografts of a BALB/c plasmacytoma, and in addition were treated with MER or saline, and with normal rabbit serum or absorbed rabbit antilymphocytic serum. The splenocytes of immunized mice were cytotoxic to the tumor; this effect was vitiated wholly or in part by treatment of the spleen donors with antilymphocytic serum. When these animals were given MER, the cytotoxic potency of their spleen cells increased, and their capacity to attack the plasmacytoma was resistant to antilymphocytic serum action. This and other aspects of the splenic cytotoxic reactivity suggested that it was executed by T-lymphocytes (Kuperman *et al.,* 1973).

In more recent experiments, we have analyzed the ability of MER to influence the in vitro generation of effector cells cytotoxic to syngeneic and allogeneic

Table 4. *Cytotoxic Activity of In Vitro Sensitized Allogeneic and Syngeneic Lymphocytes for Normal and Leukemic Target Cells**

Sensitization Cell Mixture	Percent Specific Lysis of			
	EL4 Leukemia	YAC Leukemia	C57BL/6 Blasts[†]	BALB/c Blasts[†]
BALB/c ⟶ EL4 (H − 2[d]) (H − 2[b])	98	7	90	3
C57 ⟶ EL4 (H − 2[b]) (H − 2[b])	43	5	2	2
BALB/c ⟶ YAC (H − 2[d]) (H − 2[a])	6	96	3	ND[‡]

* Adapted from Kedar *et al.*, 1977.
† Normal splenocytes transformed by concanavalin A or lipopolysaccharide.
‡ Not done.

mouse neoplasms. The methodology of the in vitro sensitization procedures has been described elsewhere (Kedar *et al.*, 1976, 1977; Kedar and Lupu, unpublished data), as have the first results obtained in vitro and in vivo with the sensitized effector cells. A major aim of these experiments is to explore the possibilities of adoptive-passive specific immunotherapy with effector cells educated to antitumor cytotoxicity in mixed lymphoid-tumor cell (MLTC) cultures, employing mitomycin-inactivated neoplastic stimulator cells, and MER as an excipient in the education process. At the same time, however, this work also promises to clarify the loci of action of MER effects on cell-mediated immunity.

Table 4 depicts the results obtained in a representative protocol, in which the activity of specifically sensitized effector cells is measured in vitro by the ^{51}Cr method. The pronounced cytotoxic capacity of the cells was highly specific (although it must be said that such specificity was not evident in all effector-tumor cell combinations tested).

The ability of in vitro sensitized effector cells to neutralize in vivo the tumor cells to which they were exposed in culture is illustrated by an experiment in which allogeneic spleen cells educated to react against the YAC lymphoma of strain A mice prevented growth of that tumor in a large majority (35/42) of the syngeneic recipient animals following subcutaneous introduction of the tumor challenge inoculum (2×10^4 leukemia cells) admixed with 2 to 4×10^6 effector cells (Winn test); in contrast, 28/29 control animals developed rapidly growing tumors, to which they succumbed within 35 days. Effector cells sensitized to the unrelated C57BL EL4 leukemia afforded no protection; neither did normal splenocytes. In parallel experiments, the protective ability of syngeneic as well as allogeneic spleen cells was demonstrated with five different mouse lymphomas and leukemias, as ascertained by Winn assays; joint introduction of the tumor-effector cell mixture by routes other than subcutaneous was also seen to reveal tumor-neutralizing capacity of the in vitro activated cells. [It may be questioned whether the Winn test truly affords an in vivo assay, or whether the test animal serves as little more than a convenient, passive test tube for assessing tumor neutralization. A degree of host involvement in such tests is suggested, however, by the observation that the antitumor potency of transferred effector cells is diminished in immunosuppressed test animals (Kedar *et al.*, unpublished data).]

When these cells were tested for immunotherapeutic efficacy against an already implanted tumor, prolongation of the life of the challenged animals was found commonly, but cures only occasionally (Kedar *et al.*, unpublished data). We then turned to chemoimmunotherapy procedures, treating animals challenged with leukemic and lymphomatous isografts with both sensitized cells and various chemotherapeutic substances. From results of treatment by protocols in which cyclophosphamide is used (Kedar *et al.*, 1978a in press), it is evident that the combination of cyclophosphamide and sensitized cells is more effective than cyclophosphamide alone in effecting "permanent" cures (tumor-free survival for more than 90 days). In these and in a large number of similar, repeated experiments in which all control animals rapidly died of extensive neoplastic disease, 90% to 100% of the animals could be cured by such combined therapy, even when other routes of challenge and treatment were employed and when treatment was introduced as late as four to seven days after tumor implantation. In many instances, the specificity of the in vivo therapeutic action of the sensitized effector cells was also clearly demonstrable (Kedar *et al.*, 1978a in press, unpublished data).

Subsequently, we learned that removal of most of the glass-adherent cells from the splenocyte population at the outset of in vitro sensitization does not abrogate the education process; however, small numbers of such cells, i.e., those remaining after one glass-bead absorption procedure, may be necessary. Similarly, removal of most of the adherent cells at the end of in vitro sensitization does not reduce effector capacity. In contrast, this ability is abrogated when the spleen cells are exposed to purified, absorbed anti-theta serum and complement. It thus appears that the effector cells in this system are predominantly of the T-lymphocyte series, although the possibility that macrophages participate in the sensitization process has not yet been excluded.

Addition of small quantities of MER to the in vitro sensitization cultures potentiates markedly the generation of cytotoxic reactivity (Kedar *et al.*, 1978b in press). This is exemplified by the experiment outlined in Table 5: As little as 0.8 μg MER per culture increased the cytotoxic capacity of the splenocytes, as assessed by chromium liberation at effector:target cell ratios of 100:1 and 30:1. This incremental effect disappeared when the amount of MER was raised to 66 μg per culture, and a negative action became evident at the 200-μg concentration.

An identical excipient influence of small quantities of MER on the in vitro education of effector cells was observed in all the tumor-effector cell combinations tested, with both spleen and lymph node effectors and both allogeneic and syngeneic MLTC. The suppressive action of larger amounts of the agent also was observed consistently. Moreover, incubation of lymphoid tissue cells with MER

Table 5. *Effect of MER on In Vitro Generation of Antitumor Cytotoxic Effector Cells. C57BL Splenocytes* Against EL4 Leukemia†*

MER (μg) Added to Culture§	Specific Lysis (%) of EL4 Target Cells‡ at Effector/Target Cell Ratios of	
	100:1	30:1
0 (control)	20	15
200	12	6
66	19	14
22	40	38
7	60	39
2.5	62	47
0.8	60	49

* Pooled from four to five normal donors.

† Adapted from Kedar *et al.*, 1978b in press.

‡ Determined by chromium release test. Values represent mean of three determinations performed with effector cells six days after incubation of culture.

§ 5 ml mixed lymphocyte-tumor cell culture.

alone, in the absence of any neoplastic stimulator cells, also elicited a degree of cytotoxic reactivity, wholly nonspecific in direction. This was evident in both mouse lymphoid cell and human peripheral blood leukocyte cultures. It appears that the stimulating influence of MER in the presence of specifically sensitizing tumor cells is twofold: the magnification of specific reactivity and the induction of a component of nonspecific reactivity (Kedar *et al.,* 1978b in press).

Figure 1 illustrates the kinetics of effector cell generation in both allogeneic and syngeneic cell mixtures under the influence of graded amounts of MER. With a responder-to-stimulator cell ratio of 10:1, maximum reactivity in the chromium liberation assay was found after six days of incubation, more strongly in these and all other such experiments for allogeneic than for syngeneic effector cells. MER at high concentration was inhibitory in every instance, but stimulated reactivity at limited doses.

It was also noted that MER in concentrations that furthered the generation of cytotoxic effector cells in MLTC cultures prevented the development of suppressor cell activity in lymphoid tissue cultures incubated alone (Kedar *et al.,* 1978b in press). This preventive action of the agent could be one mechanism of its excipient influence in these systems. Further information on the modality of the MER effect is still lacking, and it is not known as yet whether the greater in vitro cytotoxicity of effector cells produced in the presence of the substance accrues from an increased number of reactive cells or from an increased reactivity of each active cell. Neither is it certain that the effectors are, in fact, exclusively mature T-lymphocytes. Some participation of NK cells has not been ruled out entirely, and note must be taken of recent work (Henney

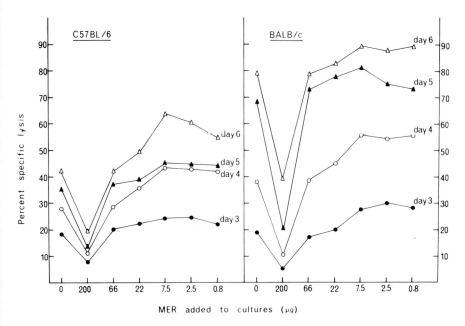

Figure 1. Kinetics of development of cytotoxic effector cells (C57BL/6 and BALB/c splenocytes) influenced by addition of MER on day 0, as measured by chromium liberation assay. EL4 stimulator and target cells. Responder-to-stimulator cell ratio, 10:1. (Adapted from Kedar *et al.,* 1978b in press.)

et al., in press) that indicates that mycobacterial immunomodulators can potentiate NK cytotoxic reactivity.

Experiments are now under way to ascertain if the in vivo antitumor potency of effector cells generated with the help of MER differs appreciably from that of effector cells sensitized without the help of the fraction. Having observed consistently a close correlation between in vitro and in vivo cytotoxic strengths of effector cell populations sensitized under different conditions, we are now screening the comparative in vitro and in vivo reactivities of lymphoid cells sensitized specifically with and without the aid of MER.

A recent observation of considerable interest is that the spleens of mice that survive Winn test assays with in vitro sensitized effector cells, and that display a much increased resistance to massive rechallenge with the corresponding neoplasms, have categorically greater cytotoxic capacity after in vitro sensitization than do corresponding lymphoid cells from normal donors (Kedar *et al.,* unpublished data). In some instances, indeed, splenocytes derived from Winn test survivors and sensitized in vitro showed curative powers in immunotherapy tests, even without joint chemotherapy. This elevation in the ability to undergo more effective sensitization in vitro was evident even in spleen cells obtained from survivors several months after challenge, and even when the protective effector cells in the Winn test were of allogeneic origin. These findings suggest that the implanted effector cells may be able to bring about a recruitment or other form of initiation of host lymphoid cells to potential cytotoxic reactivity against the tumor initially used to sensitize the passively employed effectors.

Stimulation of Macrophage Activities

Our first studies on the impact of MER on macrophage function dealt with the lysosomal enzyme activities of the peritoneal washing macrophages of mice treated with MER (Yagel *et al.,* 1975). It was found that both intraperitoneal and intravenous administration of MER heightened appreciably the activities of four lysosomal enzymes of peritoneal washing macrophages harvested several days to weeks after treatment. In subsequent experiments, the methodology of which is detailed elsewhere (Gallily *et al.,* 1977), we observed a marked potentiation of the phagocytic, bacteriostatic, and bactericidal capabilities of such cells from MER-treated donors. Representative protocols illustrating the potentiated activities of peritoneal washing macrophages vis-à-vis *Staphylococcus albus* are shown in Tables 6, 7, and 8.

As seen in Table 6, the peritoneal washing macrophages of strain A and C57BL mice given 0.4 or 1.0 mg MER three to 14 days before cell harvesting displayed an increment of 33% to 77% in uptake capacity for labeled *S. albus* under standard test conditions. When the amount of MER administered to the animals was reduced to 0.25 mg, no activation was evident. With incorporation of labeled thymidine by the phagocytized microorganisms as a criterion of bacterial mitotic capability 30 and 60 minutes after ingestion, a marked depressive effect was evident in macrophages obtained from donors treated with 0.4

Table 6. *In Vitro Uptake of ³H-TdR-Labeled* Staphylococcus albus *by Mouse Peritoneal Macrophages**

Macrophage Donor Strain	IP MER Treatment of Donors (mg)	Bacteria Phagocytized (%)†	Increase in Macrophages (%) from Treated Donors
A	0	5.5	
	0.25	5.8	6
	0	3.6	
	0.4	6.3	75
	0	6.6	
	1.0	10.4	58
C57BL	0	13.1	
	0.4	17.4	33
	0	6.5	
	1.0	11.5	77

* Adapted from Gallily *et al.,* 1977.
† Values represent averages of two to three identical experiments, calculated from the means of three determinations in each.

Table 7. *³H-TdR Incorporation by* Staphylococcus albus *Engulfed In Vitro by Peritoneal Macrophages from Strain A Mice (Bacteriostasis)* *

IP MER Treatment of Donors (mg)	Incorporation of ^{3}H-TdR per 10^6 Intracellular Bacteria†			
	30 min		60 min	
	cpm	Decrease (%) in MER Group	cpm	Decrease (%) in MER Group
0	750		ND	
0.25	730	3	ND	...
0	2,598		4,602	
0.4	765	70	1,460	68
0	644		1,519	
0.4	140	78	434	71
0	2,085		ND	
0.4	339	84	ND	...
0	704		1,006	
1.0	226	68	393	61
0	3,283		ND	
1.0	607	81	ND	...

* Adapted from Gallily *et al.*, 1977.
† Values represent mean of three determinations for each macrophage pool, in each experiment.

or 1.0 mg, but not with only 0.25 mg, MER; this is illustrated in Table 7 for strain A mice, and was evident as well for animals of other inbred strains. When bacterial viability was ascertained by colony counts performed on macrophage lysates 30 and 180 minutes after phagocytosis, a pronounced reduction in the numbers of ingested viable staphylococci was seen in the macrophages

Table 8. *Viability of* Staphylococcus albus *Within Peritoneal Macrophages of Strain A Mice Following Phagocytosis In Vitro (Bactericidal Effect)* *

IP MER Treatment of Donors (mg)	No. of Viable Bacteria per Macrophage†		Difference (%) During 150-min Interval
	30 min	180 min	
0	2.1	4.9	+ 133
0.25	2.3	5.1	+ 122
0	5.0	14.4	+ 188
0.25	6.1	3.7	− 39
0	4.0	9.6	+ 140
0.4	9.0	6.0	− 33
0	1.0	1.0	0
0.4	9.1	4.5	− 50
0	8.1	22.2	+ 177
1.0	15.5	19.2	+ 24

* Adapted from Gallily *et al.*, 1977.
† Values represent mean of three determinations for each macrophage pool, in each experiment.

taken from donors exposed to MER, sometimes even when the smaller amount was used (Table 8). Such an effect was equally evident in macrophages from animals of other strains, and could be demonstrated even at 24 hours after bacterial uptake by the cells. Similar findings were made in repeated experiments, and with other microorganisms as well (Gallily *et al.,* 1977).

We next attempted to test for such effects of MER on macrophage function by exposing purified populations of peritoneal washing macrophages from normal donors to the agent in vitro. Unexpectedly, little or no effect on lysosomal enzyme functions or on any of the antibacterial activities could be found. However, when T-lymphocytes were added to the macrophage-MER mixture, or when supernatants of T-lymphocytes incubated with MER were introduced to macrophages cultured alone, magnified macrophage functionality again appeared. It thus seems that in these test systems, the stimulating influence of MER on macrophage capacity is mediated by T-lymphocyte product(s).

Studies are now under way to test the antitumor reactivity of macrophages of peritoneal and other origin under the influence of MER administered to the donor animals and to cell cultures. We encountered considerable difficulty in this work because of the high background cytotoxic capacity of macrophages from supposedly normal animals; this "normalcy" must be questioned, however, as our animals, despite their specific pathogen-free status, are indigenously under the influence of a variety of microbial substances and many other antigens that may trigger the release of nonspecific activating factors (Fidler, in press) from sensitized T cells. More recently, we have begun to overcome this technical difficulty by resorting to bone marrow macrophages, which have a much lesser background reactivity for tumor cells; preliminary data suggest that MER injection of the donors does indeed elevate macrophage cytotoxicity to tumor cell lines in vitro.

Summation

The investigations briefly described above underline the broad influence of MER, a model of microbial immunomodulators, on the immunologic apparatus of experimental animals, and indicate that potentiation of various facets of the immunologic response can be considerable under appropriate circumstances.

Little solid information is available so far on the primary loci of action of MER and similarly acting agents, and neither is it clear which effect(s) on immunologic function play the central role in the heightened resistance against a given tumor, in a given host, at a given moment in the evolution of neoplastic disease. The findings obtained do provide encouragement, however, that continued work designed to supply answers to these questions is both worthwhile and feasible, at least in light of the magnitude of the effects that can be attained. Newer approaches in this direction are now indicated, for instance, the study of immunomodulator action on purified, identified immunocyte populations in vitro and the utilization of cells so exposed in reconstitution experiments with irradiated or otherwise immunosuppressed hosts challenged with neoplastic cells.

IMMUNOTHERAPEUTIC ACTIVITIES OF MER IN RECENTLY STUDIED ANIMAL TUMOR MODELS

An experimental tumor model that has attracted much attention is the transplantable, chemical carcinogen-induced hepatoma of strain 2 guinea pigs (Rapp, 1973). It appears that effective nonspecific immunotherapy for this neoplasm is conditioned on intralesional or proximal application of the agent, and that both living BCG and several nonliving mycobacterial preparations are effective (Rapp, in press). The therapeutic efficacy of MER in this model is exemplified by the experiments (depicted in Table 9) with guinea pigs of this line bred at the Weizmann Institute and National Jewish Hospital; strain 2 guinea pigs raised at the National Institutes of Health evince MER curative effects seemingly to a much lesser extent (Wainberg *et al.*, 1977). As seen in Table 9, MER treatment effected cures in approximately 40% of the animals when injected into an established tumor focus, but not when injected distally (although the survival times of animals so treated were prolonged; not shown in table). Prophylactic administration of MER by the intradermal route, even as early as six months before challenge and even when administered at a site contralateral to the eventual tumor implant, was effective in approximately 50% of the subjects (see also Minden *et al.*, 1974; Wainberg *et al.*, 1976a,b). Prophylactic and therapeutic intervention with the same material thus may comprise different modes of action, an "innocent bystander" effect perhaps contributing importantly to the therapeutic use. The development of cell-mediated immunity to the tumor cells in surviving animals and the interesting observation of a passive

Table 9. *Effect of MER on Development of Line 10 Hepatoma Isografts in Strain 2 Guinea Pigs**

Route†	MER Treatment Day‡	Dose (mg)	No. Cured/ No. Treated
IL	+7	0, saline only	0/10
		1.0, in saline	2/8
		in IFA§	4/8
		0.5, in saline	2/4
		in IFA	2/4
Distal, ID	−180#	1.0, in saline	3/6
	+7	in saline	0/4
	+7	in IFA	0/4
	+7 & +14	0.5, in saline	0/4
IL + distal, ID	+7	0.5, in saline, × 2	1/4
		in IFA, × 2	2/4

* Adapted from Wainberg *et al.*, 1976a,b; 1977.
† IL, intralesional; ID, intradermal.
‡ Relative to tumor challenge.
§ Incomplete Freund's adjuvant.
# Prophylactic.

Table 10. *Rous Sarcoma Regression in Chickens Pretreated with MER and Challenged with Rous Sarcoma Virus (10^6 Focus-Forming Units)**

MER Pretreatment			Complete Tumor Regression (%)
Dose (mg)	Day†	Injection Site‡	
0.5	14 & 3	same	38
		other	0
	14	same	13
		other	0
	3	same	58
0.25	14 & 3	same	7
		other	0
	14	same	6
		other	0
1.0	14	same	18
0 (saline controls)		same or other	0

* Adapted from Markson *et al.,* in press. Each treatment group consisted of 20 to 50 birds.
† Before RSV challenge.
‡ Same or other wing as used for RSV challenge.

transfer of immunity to the offspring of successfully treated females are described in other publications (Wainberg *et al.,* 1976a,b,c; 1977).

The requirement of local application of MER for therapeutic purposes has been seen also in another model recently developed in our laboratories (Markson *et al.,* in press): Rous sarcoma virus (RSV) injected into the wing web of White Leghorn chickens results invariably in the development of local sarcomas, which grow progressively, spread, and kill their hosts. Pretreatment of the birds with MER under given conditions results in regression of the tumors and permanent cures in a significant proportion. This is shown by the series of experiments summarized in Table 10. Introduction of 0.5 mg MER into the same wing (and the same area) used for subsequent RSV challenge was effective in 58% of the birds (20 to 50 animals per group) when administration of the agent preceded viral infection by only three days; considerably fewer animals were saved when treatment with this amount, or with 1.0 mg, was two weeks earlier. Two injections of 0.5 mg on days 14 and 3 before challenge were also effective; two prophylactic treatments with only 0.25 mg were ineffective in bringing about cures, but did prolong survival (not shown in table). Contralateral application of the agent failed in every instance, regardless of dosage and timing.

In further experiments, MER was given only after palpable tumors had developed following RSV injection. Contralateral treatment sometimes prolonged survival but was not curative; neither was injection directly into the tumor, or adjacent to it, when the MER inoculum was suspended in a small volume (0.05 ml) of fluid. However, when large volumes containing the same amount of MER (0.5 mg in 1.0 cc) were injected into the tumors, permanent regressions were obtained in the majority of the subjects; similar volumes of the suspending

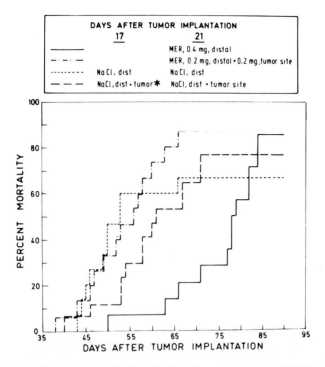

Figure 2. Effect of different routes of MER administration on survival of BALB/c mice bearing syngeneic implants of mammary carcinoma D7T4S (* tumor site). NaCl, physiologic saline. (Reproduced from Cohen *et al.,* 1975, with permission of H. K. Lewis & Co. Ltd.)

fluid alone exerted no effect. We tend to ascribe this therapeutic efficacy of intralesional MER injected with a large amount of fluid to a saturation of the tumor site with the agent, but other explanations can be entertained. In any event, intimate association of tumor cells, and perhaps of host immune elements in the vicinity, with the immunomodulator appears to be requisite in both the guinea pig hepatoma and chicken Rous sarcoma therapy test models.

That this condition does not apply as a general rule is evident from the many studies reported by various investigators on the systemic efficacy of immunomodulator treatment in leukemic and some solid neoplasms; similar findings have been made in clinical trials (Cuttner *et al.,* in press; Mathé, in press). A case in point with regard to solid tumors of experimental animals are mammary adenocarcinomas of mice. These cancers, in most instances, cannot be cured with immunomodulator treatment, but a highly significant retardation of tumor growth and prolongation of life of the hosts can be achieved. This is illustrated by experimental results presented in Figure 2. In that study, groups of 20 BALB/c mice each were given implants of the syngeneic transplantable mam-

Table 11. *Effect of Treatment with MER and Chemotherapy on Tumor Growth and Survival of BALB/c Mice with Simulated, Locally Recurrent Implants of Mammary Carcinomas**

Treatment‡	Proportion of Test Groups Experiencing Benefits†	
	MTV^+ Tumor	D7T4S Tumor
MER alone	7/15	1/12
Cyclophosphamide alone	2/2	0/2
5-FU alone	3/4	1/2
Methotrexate alone	1/2	0/2
Cyclophosphamide + MER	4/4	0/4
5-FU + MER	5/7	4/4
Methotrexate + MER	1/4	1/4

* Adapted from Yron *et al.,* 1973; Cohen *et al.,* 1975.

† Treatment groups had 20 to 50 animals each. Benefits include significant retardation of tumor growth and prolongation of host survival. In each distinct experiment, comparison is made between the several treatment groups and the placebo controls. Differences considered significant if $p \leq 0.05$, as ascertained by parametric or nonparametric analysis.

‡ After removal of initial syngeneic tumor implant and immediate reimplantation in situ.

mary tumor designated D7T4S (Weiss *et al.,* 1971), free of the mammary tumor virus (MTV). On days 17 and 21 after implantation, the animals received injections of isotonic saline or MER at the tumor site or subcutaneously at a contralateral location, or both. Figure 2 shows that distal administration only was more effective than injection of the same amount divided into distal and tumor-adjacent inocula; adjacent or intralesional injection without distal administration also was found inferior to distal injection only (Cohen *et al.,* 1975).

The therapeutic efficacy, albeit of limited extent, of subcutaneous, distal injection of MER for mammary carcinomas in mice has been demonstrated also in another series of experiments, in which simulated, locally recurrent tumors were treated (Table 11). BALB/c mice were given subcutaneous, syngeneic implants of the D7T4S tumor or of a spontaneous mammary adenocarcinoma that had recently arisen in a BALB/cfC3H mouse. When the growths reached palpable size, they were removed surgically, and a small fragment of each tumor was immediately reimplanted in situ (Yron *et al.,* 1973, 1975). The animals then were randomized to groups of 20 to 50 mice each, and treated with MER or a chemotherapeutic agent, or both. Differences in tumor growth rate and host survival were considered significant if $p \leq 0.05$, as ascertained by parametric or nonparametric analysis. Treatment with MER or chemotherapy alone effected a significant retardation of growth of the MTV-positive tumor in many instances, but not of the MTV-negative D7T4S neoplasm. Combined treatment with MER and 5-fluorouracil, in contrast, was effective for both tumors. A proportion of the mice subjected to chemoimmunotherapy was cured permanently; few such cures were seen when treatment was by either modality alone. In all these experiments, chemotherapy was administered intraperitoneally, and MER, subcutaneously contralateral to the site of tumor removal and reimplantation (Cohen *et al.,* 1976).

CONCLUSION

The results of studies here described leave no doubt as to the potent immuno-modulatory and resistance-heightening abilities of MER. Other microbial immu-nomodulators also have shown powerful capacity in both respects, and although MER is an agent holding some advantages over most of the other adjuvants in use today (Weiss, 1976a), it is probable that substances of still greater potential, and perhaps of far less complex composition, will be developed in the future (Chedid, in press).

On the other hand, every modality of cancer therapy available today is accom-panied by considerable uncertainty and risk. This is assuredly true for immuno-logic manipulation, specific as well as nonspecific. Neoplastic cells, for all their deviations and excesses, remain close relatives of the analogous normal tissues of an organism. Every attempt to alter the exceedingly delicate equilibria that mark immunologic function, and which are the basis of normal relationships between the multiple cell systems that make up the individual, is accompanied by serious dangers of precipitating pathogenetic departures from immunologic homeostasis. Such distortions, moreover, are not unlikely to afford avenues for still further escape of the neoplastic variants from host defenses, immunologic and other (Weiss, 1976b); whereas the chances of creating a changed immuno-logic environment in host tissues decisively hostile to the tumor are limited as long as our knowledge of the immunologic maze is confined largely to a gross phenomenology. These cautionary verses must be invoked whether immune surveillance has evolved indeed as an important line of defense against some forms of neoplasia in nature, or whether it must be structured artificially by intervention at the hands of the therapist, based on minimal changes in the surface antigenicity of transformed clones. The task before us, then, is to over-come the salient difficulties of matching, in the reality of the clinic, the successes reached with (nonspecific) immunotherapy in the rarefied circumstances of the laboratory model (Weiss, 1978a).

The various forms of nonspecific immunologic intervention that suggest them-selves and the mechanisms that may be involved are discussed elsewhere (Weiss, in press, unpublished data). The purpose of this review of the scope of activities of MER is illustrative, to point to the dimensions of the potential inherent in the nonspecific approach to immunotherapeutic intervention.

ACKNOWLEDGMENT

The hospitality of Drs. George Bekesi and James Holland, in whose laborato-ries this paper was prepared while the author served as visiting professor, is acknowledged with the greatest appreciation.

REFERENCES

Baldwin, R. 1978. Immunological adjuvants in tumor immunotherapy. In Sela, M. (ed.): The Role of Nonspecific Immunity in the Prevention and Treatment of Cancer. Amsterdam, North-Holland Publishing Co. (in press).

Ben-Efraim, S. 1977. Methanol extraction residue: Effects and mechanisms of action. Pharmacol. Ther. [A], 1:383–410.

Ben-Efraim, S., Constantini-Sourojon, M., and Weiss, D. W. 1973. Potentiation and modulation of the immune response of guinea pigs to poorly immunogenic protein-hapten conjugates by pretreatment with the MER fraction of attenuated tubercle bacilli. Cell. Immunol., 7:370–379.

Ben-Efraim, S., and Diamantstein, T. 1975. Mitogenic and adjuvant activity of a methanol extraction residue (MER) of tubercle bacilli on mouse lymphoid cells in vitro. Immunol. Commun., 4:565–577.

Ben-Efraim, S., Ulmer, A., Schmidt, M., and Diamantstein, T. 1976. Differences between lymphoid cell populations of guinea pigs and mice as determined by the response to mitogens in vitro. Int. Arch. Allergy Appl. Immunol., 51:117–130.

Chedid, L. 1978. Therapeutic potential of immunoregulating synthetic glycopeptides. In Sela, M. (ed.): The Role of Nonspecific Immunity in the Prevention and Treatment of Cancer. Amsterdam, North-Holland Publishing Co. (in press).

Cohen, D., Yron, I., Haber, M., Grover, N., and Weiss, D. W. 1976. Chemoimmunotherapy of syngeneic mouse mammary carcinomas employing MER. Ann. NY Acad. Sci., 277:195–208.

Cohen, D., Yron, I., Haber, M., Robinson, E., and Weiss, D. W. 1975. Effect of treatment with the MER tubercle bacilli fraction on the survival of mice carrying mammary tumor isografts: Injection of MER at the tumor site or at a distal location. Br. J. Cancer, 32:483–489.

Cuttner, J., Glidewell, O. J., and Holland, J. F. 1978. A controlled trial of chemoimmunotherapy in acute myelocytic leukemia (AML). Proc. Am. Soc. Clin. Oncol. (in press).

Fidler, I. J. 1978. Recognition and destruction of target cells by tumoricidal macrophages. In Weiss, D. W. (ed.): Immunological Parameters of Host-Tumor Relationships, vol. 5. New York, Academic Press (in press).

Gallily, R., Duchan, Z., and Weiss, D. W. 1977. Potentiation of mouse peritoneal macrophage antibacterial functions by treatment of the donor with the methanol extraction residue (MER) fraction of tubercle bacilli. Infect. Immun., 18:405–411.

Henney, C. S., Tracey, D. E., and Wolfe, S. E. 1978. BCG induced natural killer cells: Immunotherapeutic implications. In Weiss, D. W. (ed.): Immunological Parameters of Host-Tumor Relationships, vol. 5. New York, Academic Press (in press).

Hewitt, H. B., Blake, E. R., and Walder, A. S. 1976. A critique of the evidence for active host defense against cancer, based on personal studies of 27 murine tumors of spontaneous origin. Br. J. Cancer, 33:241–259.

Kedar, E., Nahas, F., Schwartzbach, M., Unger, E., Raanan, Z., and Weiss, D. W. 1978a. Generation in vitro of cytotoxic effector cells against syngeneic and allogeneic mouse leukemias and lymphomas. In: Proceedings of the Milano Conference on Tumor-Associated Antigens and Their Specific Immune Response. New York, Academic Press (in press).

Kedar, E., Nahas, F., Unger, E., and Weiss, D. W. 1978b. In vitro induction of cell-mediated immunity to murine leukemia cells. III. Effect of the methanol extraction residue (MER) fraction of tubercle bacilli on the generation of anti-leukemia cytotoxic lymphocytes. J. Natl. Cancer Inst. (in press).

Kedar, E., Schwartzbach, M., Raanan, Z., and Hefetz, S. 1977. In vitro induction of cell-mediated immunity to murine leukemia cells. II. Cytotoxic activity in vitro and tumor-neutralizing capacity in vivo of anti-leukemia cytotoxic lymphocytes generated in macrocultures. J. Immunol. Methods, 16:39–58.

Kedar, E., Unger, E., and Schwartzbach, M. 1976. In vitro induction of cell-mediated immunity to murine leukemia cells. I. Optimization of tissue culture conditions for the generation of cytotoxic lymphocytes. J. Immunol. Methods, 13:1–19.

Kuperman, O., Feigis, M., and Weiss, D. W. 1973. Reversal by the MER tubercle bacillus fraction of the suppressive effects of heterologous antilymphocytic serum (ALS) on the allograft reactivity of mice. Cell. Immunol., 8:484–489.

Kuperman, O., Yashphe, D. J., Ben-Efraim, S., Sharf, S., and Weiss, D. W. 1972. Nonspecific stimulation of cellular immunological responsiveness by a mycobacterial fraction. Cell. Immunol., 3:277–282.

Markson, Y., Doljanski, F., and Weiss, D. W. 1978. Effects of prophylactic treatment with the MER tubercle bacillus fraction on the development of Rous sarcomas of chickens following challenge with the Rous sarcoma virus. Isr. J. Med. Sci. (in press).

Mathé, G. 1978. From experimental to clinical cancer active immunotherapy. In Sela, M. (ed.): The Role of Nonspecific Immunity in the Prevention and Treatment of Cancer. Amsterdam, North-Holland Publishing Co. (in press).

Minden, P., Wainberg, M., and Weiss, D. W. 1974. Protection against guinea pig hepatomas by pretreatment with subcellular fractions of Mycobacterium bovis (BCG). J. Natl. Cancer Inst., 52:1643–1645.

Mitchell, M. S., Birnbaum-Mokyr, M., and Kahane, I. 1975. Stimulation of lymphoid cells by components of BCG. J. Natl. Cancer Inst., 55:1337–1343.

Rapp, H. J. 1973. A guinea pig model for tumor immunology. A summary. In Weiss, D. W. (ed.): Immunological Parameters of Host-Tumor Relationships. New York, Academic Press, vol. 2, pp. 162–170.

Rapp, H. J. 1978. Animals, test-tubes, and cancer immunotherapy: *In vivo* veritas, *in vitro* mendacium. In Sela, M. (ed.): The Role of Nonspecific Immunity in the Prevention and Treatment of Cancer. Amsterdam, North-Holland Publishing Co. (in press).

Wainberg, M. A., Deutsch, V., and Weiss, D. W. 1976a. Stimulation of anti-tumor immunity in guinea pigs following immunoprophylactic treatment with the methanol extraction residue of BCG. Br. J. Cancer, 34:500–508.

Wainberg, M. A., Margolese, R. G., and Weiss, D. W. 1976b. Tumor immunoprophylaxis and immunotherapy in guinea pigs treated with the methanol extraction residue (MER) of BCG. In Lamoureux, G., Turcotte, R., and Portelance, V. (eds.): BCG in Cancer Immunotherapy. New York, Grune and Stratton, pp. 38–50.

Wainberg, M. A., Margolese, R. G., and Weiss, D. W. 1977. Differential responsiveness of various substrains of inbred strain 2 guinea pigs to immunotherapy with the methanol extraction residue (MER) of BCG. Cancer Immunol. Immunother., 2:101–108.

Wainberg, M. A., Minden, P., and Weiss, D. W. 1976c. Vertical transmission of tumor resistance in guinea pigs. Nature, 259:213–215.

Weiss, D. W. 1972. Nonspecific stimulation and modulation of the immune response and of states of resistance by the MER fraction of tubercle bacilli. Natl. Cancer Inst. Monogr., 35:157–171.

Weiss, D. W. 1976a. MER and other mycobacterial fractions in the immunotherapy of cancer. Med. Clin. North Am., 60:473–497.

Weiss, D. W. 1976b. Neoplastic disease and tumor immunology from the perspective of host-parasite relationships. Natl. Cancer Inst. Monogr., 44:115–122.

Weiss, D. W. 1977. The questionable immunogenicity of certain neoplasms: What then the prospects for immunological intervention in malignant disease? Cancer Immunol. Immunother., 2:11–19.

Weiss, D. W. 1978a. Discussions. In Terry, W. D., and Windhorst, D. (eds.): Immunotherapy of Cancer: Present Status of Trials in Man. New York, Raven Press.

Weiss, D. W. 1978b. Role of nonspecifically heightened resistance in the prevention and treatment of cancer. In Sela, M. (ed.): The Role of Nonspecific Immunity in the Prevention and Treatment of Cancer. Amsterdam, North-Holland Publishing Co. (in press).

Weiss, D. W., Kuperman, O., Fathallah, N., and Kedar, E. 1976. Mode of action of mycobacterial fractions in anti-tumor immunity: Preliminary evidence for a direct nonspecific stimulatory effect of MER on immunologically reactive cells. Ann. NY Acad. Sci., 276:536–549.

Weiss, D. W., Sulitzeanu, A., Young, L., Adelberg, M., and Segev, Y. 1971. Studies on the immunogenicity of preneoplastic and neoplastic mammary tissues of BALB/c mice free of the mammary tumor virus (MTV). Isr. J. Med. Sci., 7:187–201.

Yagel, S., Gallily, R., and Weiss, D. W. 1975. Effect of treatment with the MER fraction of tubercle bacilli on hydrolytic lysosomal enzyme activity of mouse peritoneal macrophages. Cell. Immunol., 19:381–386.

Yron, I., Cohen, D., Robinson, E., Haber, M., and Weiss, D. W. 1975. Effects of methanol extraction residue and therapeutic irradiation against established isografts and simulated local recurrence of mammary carcinomas. Cancer Res., 35:1779–1790.

Yron, I., Weiss, D. W., Robinson, E., Cohen, D., Adelberg, M. G., Mekori, T., and Haber, M. 1973. Immunotherapeutic studies in mice with the methanol extraction residue (MER) fraction of BCG: Solid tumors. Natl. Cancer Inst. Monogr., 39:33–54.

Immunotherapy of Human Cancer,
The University of Texas System Cancer Center
M. D. Anderson Hospital and Tumor Institute.
Raven Press, New York © 1978.

Experimental Basis of Immunotherapy for Metastatic Disease

Isaiah J. Fidler, D.V.M., Ph.D.

Biology of Metastasis Section, Cancer Biology Program, Frederick Cancer Research Center, Frederick, Maryland

Successful approaches to immunotherapy for micrometastases may be more forthcoming once the underlying pathobiology of cancer metastasis is more clearly understood. The eventual outcome of the metastatic process depends on both host and tumor properties, and the balance of these relative contributions may vary among tumor systems. This suggests that useful animal tumor models, designed to answer a clearly defined question, can be selected by considering this interplay of tumor and host properties. However, whether induced or transplantable animal tumor systems, of which there are many, are valid models for therapeutic modalities for human cancer has been the subject of considerable debate (Bartlett *et al.,* 1976; Alexander, 1977). In studies of experimental immunotherapy, as in other aspects of cancer biology, specific questions can be answered only with a suitable model. Too often, investigations are conducted in experimental tumor systems in which inherent limitations almost seem designed to hamper results and interpretations.

Are animal tumors relevant or realistic as models for human disease? Can therapeutic modalities developed for one animal tumor system necessarily predict the success of comparable treatment applied to another system? Do results of immunotherapy for experimental animals injected with highly antigenic tumors parallel those for animals injected with weak or nonimmunogenic tumor cells (Weiss, D. W., 1977)? Obviously, the answer to such questions is no. Not even in human clinical oncology do therapeutic modalities exhibit a spectrum of efficacy against a range of different neoplasms. Thus, neither in experimental animals nor in human patients can the therapy for one type of tumor be predictive for another type. The failure of animal tumor models to serve as predictive models for human cancer does not necessarily diminish their usefulness, but might reflect the choice of an unsuitable model to answer a specific question.

Animal models have proved invaluable in the elucidation of host and tumor

---

Abbreviations used in this chapter: ^{125}IUdR—^{125}I-5-iodo-2'-deoxyuridine; ^{3}H-TdR—tritiated thymidine.

properties involved in tumor metastasis, and the utilization of such models may considerably enhance our knowledge of the immunotherapy for metastatic disease. The prime intent of the following discussion is to answer a specific question: Does successful tumor dissemination in a weakly immunogenic tumor system occur because of host deficiency, or does it depend on a constant interplay of properties of the host and the metastatic cells?

GENERAL CONSIDERATIONS

The development of tumor metastasis involves several sequential steps: (1) invasion of cells from the primary tumor into the surrounding tissue, with penetration of blood and/or lymph vessels; (2) detachment or release of single or multiple tumor cell emboli into the circulation; (3) arrest of the circulating emboli in small, vascular beds of organs; (4) tumor cell invasion of the wall of the arresting vessel, infiltration into adjacent tissue, and multiplication; and (5) growth of vascularized host stroma. The subsequent growth of the arrested tumor emboli leads to the formation of multiple tumor colonies. Here, too, the processes of invasion, embolization, arrest, and cell multiplication can take place once again to yield other metastases (Fidler, 1975a; Weiss, L., 1977; Sugarbaker and Ketcham, 1977).

Whether or not neoplasms arise from one cell, at the time of diagnosis they contain subpopulations with differing biological behavior. Nowell (1976) proposed that during the process of tumor progression, variants (mutants) may arise within a developing neoplasm and be subjected to host or environmental selection pressure, and new sublines with increased survival, i.e., malignant potential, thus emerge. The rate of the stepwise progression could differ from tumor to tumor, but the biologic behavior of neoplasms appears to parallel their stages of genetic evolution. Malignant tumors are characterized by fast-growing pleomorphic cells with a variety of abnormal chromosomes and various degrees of anaplasia. Indeed, tumor cell populations have been shown to be heterogeneous in regard to their cell kinetics (Schabel, 1975), metabolic characteristics (Kircutta *et al.,* 1965), ploidy (Rabotti, 1959), sensitivity to chemotherapeutic agents (Hakansson and Trope, 1974a,b), antigenic characteristics (Prehn, 1970; Pimm and Baldwin, 1977), and metastatic potential (Fidler and Kripke, 1977). The morphologic and cellular structure of a tumor can serve as a rough guide to its potential clinical course, but in the final analysis, the only two major characteristics unique to malignant cells are their invasive and metastatic properties.

As outlined above, the process of metastasis is highly selective, and the final growth of tumors in various distant organs represents the end point of several destructive events, which few tumor cells survive. Only a few tumor cells within a primary neoplasm may actually invade blood vessels, and of those, even fewer may survive in the hostile circulation. Similarly, not all malignant cells that survive transport can be arrested in the microcirculation, undergo extravasation into the parenchyma, escape host defense mechanisms, and grow into secondary tumor colonies (metastases) (Fidler, 1975a; Sugarbaker and Ketcham, 1977).

What role does the host defense (homeostatic) mechanism play in the development of cancer metastasis? Two explanations have been postulated. The first proposes that cancer in general, and metastasis in particular, occurs only if the host is deficient in its defense mechanism. Thus, if such a deficiency (peculiar to the tumor-bearing host) can be identified and overcome, cancer metastasis can be prevented or even cured. The second explanation takes into account the heterogeneous nature of malignant neoplasms and suggests that at every step of the metastatic cascade, the rules of "survival of the fittest" apply with regard to the dynamic interplay of tumor cell and host properties. Thus, metastasis occurs when a few selected tumor cells evade host defense mechanisms or even use normal host homeostatic mechanisms to their own gain. The possible heterogeneous nature of tumor cell populations, i.e., their antigenicity and invasive and metastatic potential, therefore becomes of paramount importance. If, indeed, tumors are heterogeneous and a selection process in metastasis formation is a real phenomenon, comparative studies of primary versus secondary tumors should allow for characterization of metastatic subpopulations. This would further our understanding of and suggest new approaches to the therapy for metastasis.

TUMOR CELL PROPERTIES THAT ALLOW FOR METASTASIS

To study the various steps and directly compare properties that may be important in the metastatic process, one should have sets of highly metastatic, weakly metastatic, and nonmetastatic tumor cells. Fortunately, such systems exist where tumor cell line variants have been selected in vivo in syngeneic hosts for their enhanced ability to implant and survive to form gross organ tumors after intravenous injection of suspended, individual tumor cells. Using C57BL/6 mice, I selected for tumor cell variants of the syngeneic B16 melanoma, which yield pulmonary metastases (Fidler, 1973c, 1975b). The ability of the highly metastatic variants (designated B16-F10), but not the weakly metastatic variants (designated B16-F1), to form exclusively lung colonies after injection suggested that selection for organ preference of B16 melanoma variants was possible (Fidler and Nicolson, 1976) (Table 1).

The B16 melanoma has been a useful tool in experimental studies on tumor and host properties in metastasis. Some of the advantages of the B16 variant system are: The tumor arose spontaneously in skin of inbred C57BL/6 mice and has been maintained in syngeneic hosts; the tumors can be readily identified because of the presence of melanin; comparisons with dubious, "normal" counterpart cells are unnecessary because B16 variants of low and high metastatic potential are available; the B16F cells can be grown easily in vivo at various sites or in vitro in tissue cultures; and the B16 melanoma is weakly immunogenic.

The importance of tumor-cell adhesive properties in metastatic tumor spread

Table 1. *Arrest, Distribution, and Fate of 100,000 Viable ^{125}IUdR-Labeled B16 Melanoma Cell Lines Injected Intravenously into Normal C57BL/6 Mice*

Time of Death	Viable Injected Tumor Cells in Lungs (%)*			
	Line F1†	F1^{Lr-6}	F10‡	F10^{Lr-6}
2 min	64.0 ± 6.00	55.8 ± 4.00	99.0 ± 6.2	82.00 ± 5.20
1 hr	57.0 ± 4.20	50.5 ± 3.20	97.1 ± 7.1	80.40 ± 6.10
3 hr	32.0 ± 2.70	28.1 ± 1.90	88.2 ± 4.9	75.60 ± 4.80
1 day	1.2 ± 0.20	0.5 ± 0.06	12.5 ± 0.8	5.10 ± 0.30
3 days	0.6 ± 0.04	0.3 ± 0.06	3.4 ± 0.6	0.87 ± 0.20
7 days	0.6 ± 0.02	0.2 ± 0.04	3.3 ± 0.4	0.46 ± 0.10
14 days§	0.4 ± 0.03	0.2 ± 0.04	1.6 ± 0.2	0.37 ± 0.04

* Mean percent of labeled tumor cells ± standard deviation. Five animals per time interval.
† Differences between animals given injections of cells from line F1 and line F1^{Lr-6} were significant ($p < 0.01$).
‡ Differences between animals given injections of cells from line F10 and line F10^{Lr-6} were significant ($p < 0.01$).
§ On day 14, gross pulmonary metastases in mice given injections of cells from line F1 averaged 66 ± 11; line F1^{Lr-6}, 29 ± 9 ($p < 0.05$); line F10, 269 ± 37; and line F10^{Lr-6}, 54 ± 6 ($p < 0.001$).

has been stressed by Coman (1954) and Weiss (1976). When we examined the homotypic (tumor:tumor) rates of adhesion of the B16 variant lines in qualitative or quantitative assays, the highly metastatic B16 lines always adhered to each other at faster rates than did the less metastatic lines. Similarly, examinations of the heterotypic (tumor:host cell) rates of adhesion of B16 variant cells to platelets, lymphocytes, and an endothelial cell line indicated that the highly metastatic B16 lines also adhered at greater rates to circulating and noncirculating host cells (Fidler and Nicolson, 1978). These results suggest that target organ recognition by tumor cells may occur through cell-surface adhesive interactions. Evidence for organ-specific determinants on vascular endothelial cells has been obtained by Pressman and Yagi (1964) using anti-organ antibodies.

IN VITRO SELECTION FOR TUMOR VARIANTS. MALIGNANT PROPERTIES OF TUMOR CELLS AND THEIR RELATIVE ANTIGENICITY (IMMUNOGENICITY)

The selection of tumor cells with increased capacity for metastasis by successive cycling in animals was achieved as a result of either the adhesive properties of the tumor cells (Nicolson and Winkelhake, 1975), their biochemical and biophysical growth-related differences (Bosmann *et al.,* 1973), or their interaction with the host immune mechanism (Fidler, 1974). In vivo selection of metastatic tumor cells could have been also a result of tumor cell-lymphocyte interaction, which has been reported to be important in the pathogenesis of experimental metastasis. Was the in vivo selection of metastatic tumor cells a direct result of such interaction? Specifically, could the in vivo selection process for metastatic cells be duplicated by in vitro procedures, in which the interaction can be limited to tumor cells and lymphocytes alone, thereby eliminating factors such as tumor-cell adhesiveness to other host cells?

In studying particular interactions, it is often desirable to select resistant cell variants in culture. Selection of cells that are resistant to killing by chemical and viral agents after they have been exposed continuously and/or repeatedly to those agents in culture is common practice. It follows, then, that cells resistant to killing by whole cells, i.e., syngeneic lymphocytes, can be selected by a similar approach. Two B16 melanoma lines, F1 (low metastasis) and F10 (high metastasis), were cultured with lymphocytes from C57BL/6 mice immunized against B16. The selection procedure involved repeated exposure of the tumor cells to lymphocytes in vitro. After each interaction, the viable tumor cells were trypsinized, replated, and designated lines $F1^{Lr-1}$ and $F10^{Lr-1}$. The procedure was repeated five times, yielding lines $F1^{Lr-6}$ and $F10^{Lr-6}$, which resisted in vitro cytolysis by syngeneic lymphocytes even at the ratio of 10,000:1.

Mice were injected subcutaneously or intravenously with cells from line F1, $F1^{Lr-6}$, F10, or $F10^{Lr-6}$. Tumor growth patterns were the same for all four lines when the cells were injected subcutaneously; however, the incidence of pulmonary metastases differed significantly after intravenous injection. Line F10 cells yielded more pulmonary metastases than did an equal number of line F1 cells ($p < 0.01$). $F1^{Lr-6}$ cells yielded significantly fewer metastases than did an equal number of line F1 cells ($p < 0.01$). A similar difference between $F10^{Lr-6}$ and F10 cells was observed. The incidence of artificial metastases after intravenous injection of $F10^{Lr-6}$ cells was similar to that with F1 cells. The quantitative organ distribution, arrest, and survival of intravenously injected tumor cells were studied by using $^{125}IUdR$-labeled cells. There were significantly more cells from line F10 than from line F1, which were arrested and survived in the lungs for 14 days. In contrast, cells from both lines $F1^{Lr-6}$ and $F10^{Lr-6}$ had a lower incidence of arrest and survival than that of their lymphocyte-sensitive counterparts (Fidler *et al.*, 1976b) (Table 1).

The resistance of $B16-F1^{Lr-6}$ and $B16-F10^{Lr-6}$ to lysis by syngeneic lymphocytes was not associated with loss of H-2 antigens, for the variants were lysed in vitro by sensitized allogeneic lymphocytes and did not grow in allogeneic recipients. In addition, $B16-F^{Lr-6}$ cells were destroyed in vitro by syngeneic and allogeneic macrophages, indicating that their resistance to syngeneic lymphocytes does not correlate with resistance to syngeneic macrophages.

Cocultivation experiments were carried out to determine if the state of tumor cell resistance to syngeneic lymphocytes was due to shedding of cell surface antigens into the culture media, which could be absorbed by specific lymphocyte receptors and thus interfere with or "block" lymphocyte reactivity (Alexander, 1974; Vaage, 1974; Bonavida, 1976). If the resistance to lymphocyte-mediated cytolysis was due to blocking of lymphocytes, then $B16-F10^{Lr-6}$ cells should be able to protect cocultivated lymphocyte-susceptible B16-F10 cells from destruction. The data demonstrated that this was not the case. Lymphocytes from B16-immune mice were highly cytotoxic to the B16-F10 cells (62%, $p < 0.005$). Neither B16-F10^{Lr} nor unrelated but syngeneic fibrosarcoma UV-112 cells were affected by the B16-immune lymphocytes. An excess of unlabeled B16-F10 cells, when added to ^{3}H-TdR-labeled B16-F10 cells and immune lymphocytes, successfully blocked the cytotoxicity against the labeled cells. The degree of cytotoxicity (62%) against ^{3}H-TdR-labeled B16-F10 cells was reduced to 0% by the addition of 10^6 unlabeled B16-F10 cells. In contrast, the addition of either B16-F10^{Lr} or UV-112 cells at the same dose had no significant effect on the level of cytotoxicity mediated by immune lymphocytes against the labeled B16-F10 cells. We thus concluded that even a 100-fold excess of B16-F10^{Lr} cells did not protect B16-F10 cells from destruction by syngeneic immune lymphocytes (Fidler and Bucana, 1977).

To determine if lymphocyte-resistant B16 variants were immunogenic, we conducted cross-immunization and challenge experiments. C57BL/6 mice were immunized with either B16-F10 or B16-F10^{Lr} cells and challenged subcutaneously with a lethal dose of B16-F10 cells. Immunization with B16-F10 cells successfully protected mice against challenge with B16-F10 cells. However, mice immunized with B16-F10^{Lr} were not protected against B16-F10 challenge. B16-F10^{Lr} cells grew poorly following subcutaneous injection and also were not immunogenic when tested under these conditions. Clearly, whereas B16-F10 cells were immunogenic in vivo, B16-F10^{Lr} cells were not.

The possibility that B16-F^{Lr} cells may be deficient in lymphocyte-binding sites was examined by light scanning and electron microscopy (Fidler and Bucana, 1977). We investigated the in vitro heterotypic clumping of the B16-F10 line and its lymphocyte-resistant counterpart, B16-F10^{Lr}, with syngeneic lymphocytes. Our earlier study (Fidler, 1975b) demonstrated that the degree of in vitro lymphocyte:tumor clumping (clump size) was related to properties of both cells. Our present studies agree in that the tumor:lymphocyte clump size was 14 ± 4 for line B16-F10, in contrast to 2 ± 1 for line B16-F10^{Lr}. Also, an occasional homotypic clump was observed. Microscopic examination demonstrated lymphocyte clustering around B16-F10, but not around B16-F10^{Lr}. These data suggest that resistance to lysis of the B16-F^{Lr} cells by syngeneic lymphocytes is associated with decreased lymphocyte binding. Whether lymphocyte-binding sites are synonymous with tumor-specific transplantation antigens remains unclear.

Collectively, the above data demonstrate the importance of tumor cell properties in their interaction with host cells, which determine the extent and location of experimental metastasis. In our B16 melanoma system, which is weakly immunogenic, host circulating cells, such as lymphocytes, platelets (Gasic et al., 1973), and host endothelial cells (Nicolson and Winkelhake, 1975; Fidler and Nicolson, 1978), appear to enhance rather than inhibit the formation of metastases. This enhancement might be due to the aggregation effects of host cells on melanoma cells while the latter are invading a blood vessel or are blood-borne.

The formation of a large tumor embolus may lead to increased cell arrest and survival in a capillary bed.

HOST IMMUNITY AND OUTCOME OF METASTASIS

One factor that is not well understood in the metastatic process is host immunity. Host response to tumor-associated antigenic determinants in many experimental systems may result in tumor cell destruction, but in other animal models, it may enhance tumor growth. Experiments designed to test if the host's immune system can effectively stop the spread of tumors by monitoring the survival of tumor cells introduced into the circulation have been inconclusive. For example, treatment of animals with agents reported to depress immune responses, such as L-asparaginase (Deodhar, 1971) and antilymphocyte serum (Fisher *et al.,* 1969), often resulted in greater numbers of metastatic foci, but this same outcome also occurred when host immune responses were stimulated or augmented by immunization (Duff *et al.,* 1973) or when there was a transfer of a low number of immune cells (Fidler, 1974).

For many years, investigators have suspected that some circulating tumor cells may be destroyed by specific host immune mechanisms, but the evidence for such a hypothesis is inconclusive. Some studies actually have contradicted the view that a patient's resistance to tumor is related to the activity of the reticuloendothelial system (Fisher and Fisher, 1965). Borberg *et al.* (1972) reported that intravenous injection of lymphocytes from immunized syngeneic or allogeneic mice or even sheep brought about inhibition of tumor grafts (activation of reticuloendothelial system?) in mice. On the other hand, Fisher *et al.* (1972) did not find that tumor transplant growth (in mice) was inhibited following injection of sensitized lymphocytes. It would appear that the outcome of such experiments may be related directly to the number of lymphocytes transferred (i.e., a high number of lymphocytes is necessary to achieve tumor growth inhibition in vivo) and the antigenicity of the tumor cell itself.

Many immunologic and nonimmunologic functions have been attributed to cells of the lymphoreticular system. Data on the "trephocytic" function of lymphocytes as a possible source of essential growth substances for various organs were reported by Carrell in 1922. Several investigators have suggested that the lymphoreticular system regulates the growth of other normal tissue (for review, see Prehn and Lappé, 1971; Prehn, 1976). Stimulation of tumor and normal cell growth in vitro was clearly demonstrated in our studies with mouse tumors and transplantation systems (Fidler, 1973a) and with spontaneous dog tumors of various histologic types (Fidler, 1975a). Results of these studies agreed closely with those of earlier reports by Medina and Heppner (1973) and Heppner *et al.* (1973).

Observations similar to these led Prehn (1971, 1972, 1976) and Prehn and Lappé (1971) to propose that the host immune response to neoplasia can have a dual role: stimulation of tumor growth during the early development of cancer or when tumors are weakly antigenic; and tumor growth inhibition at the later stages of development, when the immune response is more active or when the tumors are strongly antigenic. The dual response of host immune mechanisms has been shown in an experimental metastasis system in which B16 melanoma cells with varying ratios of lymphocytes are injected intravenously into syngeneic C57BL/6 mice (Fidler, 1974). Injections of tumor cells mixed in low ratios with syngeneic lymphocytes yield significantly fewer lung tumor colonies.

Thus, our experiments demonstrated again that circulating host cells (lymphocytes, in particular) are involved in the formation of heterotypic, multicell aggregates. It appeared reasonable to further investigate the effect of host lymphocytes in the formation of metastasis when specific immunosuppressed mice were used as recipients for the metastatic B16-F1 or -F10 cells (Gersten and Fidler, unpublished data). Adult thymectomized X-irradiated (ATX), sham-thymectomized X-irradiated (STX), normal X-irradiated, and/or normal C57BL/6 mice were injected intravenously with syngeneic lymphocytes 24 hours prior to or 24 or 48 hours after intravenous tumor cell injection. All mice were killed 18 days later, and the number and location of tumor colonies were determined. The data indicated that ATX mice had a lower incidence of lung metastasis than STX mice or normal X-irradiated control animals, and all lymphocyte-reconstituted mice had a higher incidence of lung metastasis than their controls. Thus, even ATX mice injected with syngeneic lymphocytes 48 hours following intravenous injection of tumor cells had increased incidence of tumor colonies and thus were indistinguishable from normal mice (Table 2).

Obviously, the role of lymphocytes in promoting tumor growth is not restricted

Table 2. *Number of Lung Tumor Colonies in C57BL/6 Mice Untreated or Treated Once with Intravenous Injection of 10^7 Syngeneic Lymphocytes*

| | Average No. of Pulmonary Metastases* | | | |
| | | Lymphocyte-Treated | | |
Mice	Untreated	−24 hr	+24 hr	+48 hr
Normal controls[†]	42 ± 5	246 ± 10	44 ± 4	55 ± 6
Thymectomized, X-irradiated[†‡]	16 ± 2§	166 ± 23	60 ± 11	39 ± 3
Sham-thymectomized, X-irradiated[†]	60 ± 11	239 ± 18	47 ± 8	90 ± 14
Normal mice injected with lymphocytes alone	0	0	0	0

* Mean ± standard deviation. Ten mice per group. Pulmonary metastases were counted with the aid of a dissecting microscope 21 days after tumor cell injection.
† Injected intravenously with 50,000 viable B16-F1 melanoma cells.
‡ Thymectomized at four to five weeks of age prior to tumor cell injection; 450 R total body irradiation four weeks prior to tumor cell injection.
§ Number of lung tumor colonies differed from controls ($p < 0.001$).

to the phase of tumor cell arrest and implantation only, but also to later stages of the process, such as establishment of microenvironment and perhaps stimulation of vascularity.

SURVIVAL AND GROWTH OF TUMOR CELLS INJECTED INTRAVENOUSLY INTO CONGENITALLY ATHYMIC MICE

An interesting animal model, which we assumed could be used to study the contribution of host immune status to the outcome of experimental metastasis, is the congenitally athymic (nude) mouse. Nude (nu/nu) mice accept subcutaneous implants of normal and neoplastic grafts from allogeneic and xenogeneic donors. Although such tumor implants grow, they rarely invade host tissue and metastasize (Skov et al., 1976). We first tested the response of nu/nu mice and heterozygous littermates (nu/+) on an N.NIH(S) background to C57BL/6 skin and B16 melanoma tumor allografts. Skin allografts from C57BL/6 mice were rejected by nu/+ mice in ten to 12 days, but were intact on the nu/nu mice at the end of the observation period of seven weeks. In all nu/nu mice, subcutaneous tumor allografts grew progressively.

The nu/nu mice and their heterozygous littermates were injected intravenously with ^{125}IUdR-labeled B16 cells. Tumor cell arrest, distribution, and fate were then determined. In addition, nu/nu or control nu/+ mice were reconstituted with 10^7 lymphocytes from normal nu/+ syngeneic mice 24 hours prior to tumor cell injection. The data, shown in Table 3, permitted the following conclusions: (1) Although nu/nu mice were unable to reject skin grafts or subcutaneous tumor allografts, they did not support the growth of the same tumor cells injected intravenously. (2) On the other hand, nu/+ littermates resisted both skin and subcutaneous tumor allografts, yet permitted the growth of allogeneic tumor cells in the lung. (3) Nu/nu mice injected intravenously with 10^7 nu/+ lymphocytes 24 hours prior to tumor challenge rejected a subcutaneous injection of B16 melanoma cells. (4) The same lymphocyte-reconstituted nu/nu mice did not support the growth of lung tumor colonies, although initial arrest of tumor

Table 3. *Number of Lung Tumor Colonies in Nude Mice and Heterozygous Littermates Untreated or Treated with Intravenous Injection of 10^7 Syngeneic Lymphocytes from Heterozygous Mice*

Mice†	Average No. of Lung Tumor Colonies*	
	Untreated	Lymphocyte-Reconstituted‡
Nude	2 ± 1§	0
Heterozygous	12 ± 3	30 ± 8

* Mean ± standard deviation. Ten mice per group. Pulmonary metastases were counted with the aid of a dissecting microscope 14 days after tumor cell injection.
† Injected intravenously with B16 melanoma cells.
‡ 24 hours prior to tumor cell injection.
§ $p < 0.001$.

emboli in the lungs was indeed increased in these mice as compared with nu/nu mice that were not lymphocyte-treated. (5) Lastly, this study suggests that nonimmunologic factors are responsible for the poor growth of hematogenously disseminated, allogeneic tumor cells in nu/nu mice (Fidler *et al.,* 1976a).

RELATIONSHIP OF HOST IMMUNE STATUS TO TUMOR CELL ARREST, DISTRIBUTION, SURVIVAL, AND GROWTH

The naive, normal animal has been used in the past as an experimental model for all-inclusive studies of tumor spread. The possibility that such animals may not be a suitable model for studies of the metastatic process analogous to that in cancer patients has been recognized by Weiss *et al.* (1974), Glaves and Weiss (1975), and Wexler *et al.* (1975). We therefore have analyzed the patterns of tumor cell arrest, survival, and growth in normal, tumor-bearing, immunized, and immunosuppressed syngeneic recipients as well as normal allogeneic mice. Groups of mice were injected intravenously with ^{125}IUdR-labeled B16-F1 cells. At intervals after injection, mice were killed and their organs monitored for radioactivity. The number of originally injected cells was thus determined (Fidler, 1970) (Fig. 1–3).

The following conclusions can be made from the data: Initial tumor cell arrest in organs is influenced by the host immune status, but it is not an indication

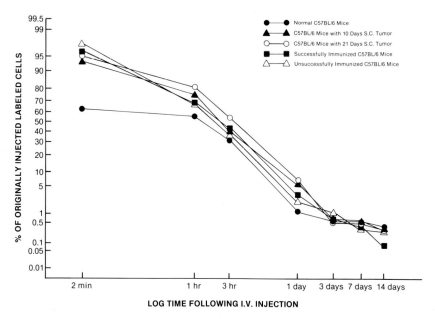

Figure 1. Percent of originally ^{125}IUdR-labeled, intravenously injected tumor cells that are viable in the lungs at various times after injection into C57BL/6 mice.

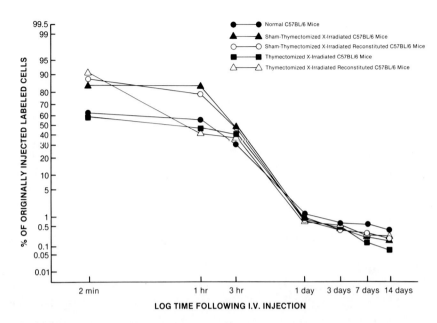

Figure 2. Percent of originally [125]IUdR-labeled, intravenously injected tumor cells that are viable in the lungs at various times after injection into X-irradiated, thymectomized or sham-thymectomized, and/or lymphocyte-reconstituted C57BL/6 mice.

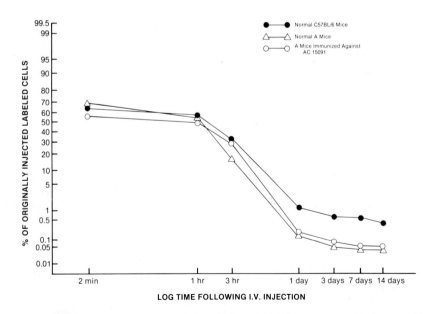

Figure 3. Percent of originally [125]IUdR-labeled, intravenously injected tumor cells that are viable in the lungs at various times after injection into normal C57BL/6 mice, normal strain A mice, and strain A mice immunized against AC15091 (syngeneic to strain A mice).

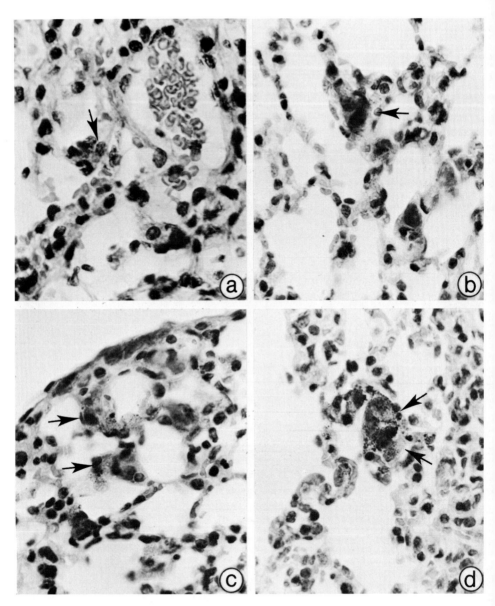

Figure 4. Formation of micrometastasis in lungs of C57BL/6 mice injected intravenously with viable B16 melanoma cells. Note melanin-containing tumor cells in lung parenchyma and steady growth of tumor colony (arrows). Time after tumor injection: *a-d,* one to four days, respectively (× 400); *e,* seven days (note cells invading blood vessel) (× 400); *f,* 14 days (note large tumor colony surrounding blood vessel) (× 100).

of nor does it correlate with the cells' survival kinetics or development into tumor colonies. The same tumor cells, which were rejected in mice after a subcutaneous tumor challenge, grew in the lungs after intravenous injection. Therefore, rejection of a subcutaneous challenge as the sole criterion of host immunity to neoplasms should be questioned. Allogeneic animals are not appropriate for use as a model system for the study of experimental metastasis. Animals sensitized to a tumor exhibit kinetic patterns of tumor cell arrest and survival that differ from those of normal (naive) syngeneic hosts. Therefore, based on the data, we must question the validity of using normal animals in inclusive studies of the pathogenesis of metastasis. Alternative animal models for studies of experimental metastasis which take into account the interaction of host immune mechanisms must be considered (Fidler *et al.,* 1977).

The above studies also indicate that manipulation of the host immune response can affect tumor cell kinetics beyond the stage of initial arrest. For example, tumor cells were destroyed in immunized animals at a faster rate than in all syngeneic test groups. (Successfully immunized mice have been defined as animals capable of rejecting an ordinarily lethal challenge of tumor cells injected subcutaneously or intramuscularly.) Nevertheless, in our studies, successfully immunized animals did not reject an intravenous tumor challenge of 100,000 viable cells. This observation confirmed the previous reports by Wexler *et al.* (1972, 1975) regarding lung tumor colonies of so-called immune mice. This paradox also applied to the allogeneic mice, used in some of our studies, that ordinarily are capable of rejecting a subcutaneous tumor allograft of the B16-F melanoma; they all permitted the growth of the same tumor following an intravenous chal-

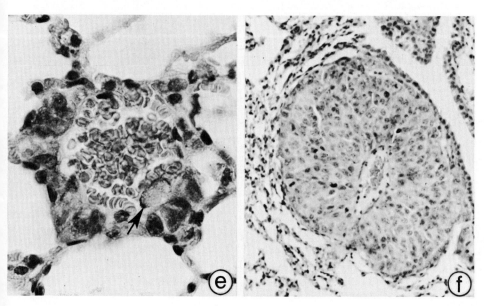

lenge. In contrast to intravenous administration, intramuscular and subcutaneous tumor injections have in common the existence of discrete tumor foci. Tumor cells injected intravenously disseminate and are trapped or arrested in the capillary bed of an organ (the lung in the case of B16-F) in the form of multiple foci. By day 1 after intravenous tumor cell injection, tumor cells that may later develop into micrometastasis have extravasated into the parenchyma of the lung. Two days after intravenous dissemination and arrest, small microcolonies of tumor cells can be observed in histopathologic sections of the lung, and these colonies continue to grow (Fig. 4). One possible explanation for the difference in survival between tumor cells injected intravenously and those injected subcutaneously or intramuscularly is that although the host immune response is capable of rejecting tumors in a discrete focus, it is ineffective in dealing with tumors that are widely disseminated. Alternatively, the lung might be a more suitable "soil" than subcutaneous sites for growth of melanoma (Fidler, 1975a).

HOST-TUMOR INTERACTION

The mechanism of immune enhancement in metastasis is not well understood, possibly because of differing immune properties in each tumor system investigated. Tumor cell antigenicity and level of host response may also differ from one experimental system to another. In the B16-F melanoma variant system, immune enhancement can be attributed, at least in part, to increased tumor cell-lymphocyte interactions during circulation, leading to formation of large tumor cell:lymphocyte clumps, which should aid in tumor cell arrest and perhaps also subsequent survival.

Several observations suggest the importance of the interaction of tumor cells and circulating host cells in determining the efficiency of experimental metastases: (1) Variants of the B16-F melanoma with differing capacities to form experimental metastases have different propensities to form tumor cell:lymphocyte heterotypic aggregates in vitro (Fidler, 1974, 1975b). (2) Greater homotypic aggregation has been observed with the highly metastatic tumor cells (B16-F10 > B16-F5 > B16-F1) (Nicolson and Winkelhake, 1975; Nicolson *et al.,* 1976). (3) Homotypic tumor cell clumps of different sizes yield different numbers of tumor colonies when equal cell numbers are injected intravenously (Fidler, 1973b). (4) In vitro mixtures of tumor cells and lymphocytes injected intravenously compared with an equal number of tumor cells injected alone give rise to more tumors when the lymphocyte:tumor cell ratio is low, or fewer tumors when the ratio is high (Fidler, 1974). (5) Thrombocytopenia also has been observed to alter the outcome of experimental B16-F metastasis (Gasic *et al.,* 1973).

Thrombocytopenia occurs immediately after intravenous tumor cell injection and appears to be directly correlated to the successful outcome of experimental metastasis. Interestingly, the highly metastatic B16-F10 cells readily aggregated platelets and produced no extrapulmonary metastases, whereas the weakly metastatic B16-F1 tumor cells failed to aggregate platelets and produced extrapulmonary metastases in a large percentage of animals. It is reasonable to assume that if circulating tumor cell emboli bring about aggregation of platelets in vivo, then the release of vasopressive mediators from platelets may lead to a local pulmonary vasospasm. In the lung, such a vasospasm would begin primarily as a mechanical obstruction of vessels and then cause secondary local vasoconstriction, spreading to other lobes of the lung. The vasoconstriction would bring about a rise in pulmonary vascular pressure, which, in turn, would open preexisting arteriovenous communications (Avaido, 1965). The arrest of B16-F1 and B16-F10 tumor cells in the lungs by two minutes after injection is associated with leukopenia, which is accompanied by an accumulation of leukocytes in the lungs. Injections of both live and dead tumor cells, but not normal cells, result in leukopenia (Fidler et al., 1977).

Collectively, these observations suggest that the formation of an embolus (either homotypic or heterotypic) of some critical size could ensure the arrest of tumor cells in the lung capillary bed. A constriction of the vessel lumen also could enhance metastatic formation. Inflammatory agents, such as adrenergic hormones (Van den Brenk et al., 1976) and X-irradiation (Fidler and Zeidman, 1972), which serve to decrease the diameter of the capillary lumen, have been associated with an increase in the number of pulmonary tumor colonies following intravenous injection of tumor cells. Thus, any factors that will either increase tumor embolic size or constrict the vessel lumen, or both, could profoundly influence the outcome of experimental metastasis.

HETEROGENEITY OF METASTATIC POTENTIAL FOR CELLS IN A MALIGNANT NEOPLASM

An alternative to the theory that critical embolus size determines the success of experimental metastasis is the theory that each heterogeneous population of tumor cells may include a small, variant fraction that is destined to home to a specific site (i.e., lung), implant, and successfully yield gross tumors after intravenous injection. The actual size of such a variant tumor cell fraction might be determined by the relationship of tumor cell properties to the status of the host.

Studies with the B16 melanoma have demonstrated the heterogeneity of subpopulations within the tumor with regard to their survival in vivo (Fidler, 1973c), formation of organ-specific metastases (Brunson et al., in press), and resistance to destruction by syngeneic lymphocytes (Fidler et al., 1976b), as well as their immunogenicity (Fidler and Bucana, 1977). By performing an experiment similar to the fluctuation test devised by Luria and Delbrück (1943) to distinguish between selection and adaptation in the origin of bacterial mutants, we recently demonstrated that cells with different metastatic potential preexist in the population.

A cell suspension of the B16 melanoma parent line was divided into two parts. One aliquot was injected intravenously into syngeneic C57BL/6 mice. The other aliquot was used to produce clones, which were then also injected intravenously into groups of C57BL/6 mice. Eighteen days after the tumor cells were injected, the numbers of pulmonary tumor colonies and all extrapulmonary growths were determined. The B16 clones varied greatly in their ability to survive in the circulation and to form pulmonary tumor colonies. There was also considerable variation among the clones in the number and sites of extrapulmonary metastases. We therefore concluded that the cells with a high metastatic potential are present within the parent B16 line prior to injection into animals. From control subcloning experiments, we also concluded that the variability among the clones resulted not from the process of cloning, but from heterogeneity of the unselected parent tumor (Fidler and Kripke, 1977).

CONCLUSIONS

The pathogenesis of metastasis is a complex biologic phenomenon with many sequential steps. Many malignant neoplasms may consist of heterogeneous subpopulations of cells with differing capabilities of invasion, survival, and growth into secondary tumor foci. From the B16 melanoma tumor, syngeneic to the C57BL/6 mouse, tumor cell variants with increased capacity for survival and growth in the lungs were selected in vivo by successive culturing of cells from artificial metastases. In addition, variants of B16 melanoma, which are resistant to lysis mediated by syngeneic immune lymphocytes, were selected in vitro. The lymphocyte-resistant variants, which form few tumor colonies after intravenous injection, were found to be nonimmunogenic in vivo, and the mechanism of their resistance was attributed to lack of binding sites for syngeneic lymphocytes on their surfaces. The highly metastatic tumor variants were shown to preexist within the unselected parental B16 tumor. The main factors responsible for success of tumor spread could be the unique, inherent characteristics of tumor cells, including modifications in adhesive properties, cell motility, secretion of enzymes, and surface characteristics that allow for interaction with circulating and noncirculating host cells and survival during blood-borne transport. Our data suggest that host factors involving a possible immune stimulation-to-tumor spread are extremely important for the establishment of experimental metastases. B16-F cells, and thus the few selected tumor cells with metastatic capabilities, may, in fact, use host homeostatic mechanisms to their own gain.

ACKNOWLEDGMENTS

The author would like to thank Ian Hart and Elynor Sass for their help in preparation of this manuscript. This research was sponsored by the National Cancer Institute under contract NO1-CO-25423 with Litton Bionetics, Inc.

REFERENCES

Alexander, P. 1974. Escape from immune destruction by the host through shedding of surface antigens: Is this a characteristic shared by malignant and embryonic cells? Cancer Res., 34:2077–2082.

Alexander, P. 1977. Back to the drawing board, the need for more realistic model systems for immunotherapy. Cancer, 40:467–470.

Avaido, D. M. 1965. The Lung Circulation. London, Pergamon Press, vol. 2, p. 1405.

Bartlett, G. L., Kreider, J. W., and Purnell, D. M. 1976. Immunotherapy of cancer in animals: Models or muddles. J. Natl. Cancer Inst., 56:207–210.

Bonavida, B. 1976. Immune lymphocytes interaction with cancer cells. In Weiss, L. (ed.): Fundamental Aspects of Metastasis. Amsterdam, North-Holland Publishing Co., pp. 205–225.

Borberg, H., Oettgen, H. F., Choudry, K., and Beattie, E. J., Jr. 1972. Inhibition of established transplants of chemically induced sarcomas in syngeneic mice by lymphocytes from immunized donors. Int. J. Cancer, 10:539–547.

Bosmann, H. B., Bieber, G. F., Brown, A. E., Case, K. R., Gersten, D. M., Kimmerer, T. W., and Lione, A. 1973. Biochemical parameters correlated with tumour cell implantation. Nature, 246:487–489.

Brunson, K. W., Beattie, G., and Nicolson, G. L. 1978. *In vivo* selection of malignant melanoma for organ preference of experimental metastasis. J. Am. Soc. Cell Biol. (in press).

Carrell, A. 1922. Growth promoting function of leucocytes. J. Exp. Med., 36:385–391.

Coman, D. R. 1954. Cellular adhesiveness in relation to the invasiveness of cancer: Electron microscopy of liver perfused with a chelating agent. Cancer Res., 14:519–531.

Deodhar, S. D. 1971. Enhancement of metastasis by L-asparaginase in a mouse tumor system. Nature, 231:319–321.

Duff, R., Doller, E., and Rapp, F. 1973. Immunologic manipulation of metastases due to herpesvirus-transformed cells. Science, 180:79–81.

Fidler, I. J. 1970. Metastasis: Quantitative analysis of distribution and fate of tumor emboli labeled with ^{125}I-5-iodo-2'-deoxyuridine. J. Natl. Cancer Inst., 45:775–782.

Fidler, I. J. 1973a. *In vitro* studies of cellular-mediated immunostimulation of tumor growth. J. Natl. Cancer Inst., 50:1307–1312.

Fidler, I. J. 1973b. The relationship of embolic homogeneity, number, size and viability to the incidence of experimental metastasis. Eur. J. Cancer, 9:223–227.

Fidler, I. J. 1973c. Selection of successive tumor lines for metastasis. Nature (New Biol.), 242:148–149.

Fidler, I. J. 1974. Immune stimulation-inhibition of experimental cancer metastasis. Cancer Res., 34:491–498.

Fidler, I. J. 1975a. Patterns of tumor cell arrest and development. In Becker, F. F. (ed.): Cancer: A Comprehensive Treatise. New York, Plenum Press, pp. 101–131.

Fidler, I. J. 1975b. Biological behavior of malignant melanoma cells correlated to their survival *in vivo*. Cancer Res., 35:218–224.

Fidler, I. J., and Bucana, C. 1977. Resistance of tumor cells to lysis by syngeneic lymphocytes: A possible mechanism. Cancer Res., 37:3945–3956.

Fidler, I. J., Caines, S., and Dolan, Z. 1976a. Survival of hematogenously disseminated allogeneic tumor cells in athymic nude mice. Transplantation, 22:208–215.

Fidler, I. J., Gersten, D. M., and Budmen, M. B. 1976b. Characterization *in vivo* and *in vitro* of tumor cells selected for resistance to syngeneic lymphocyte-mediated cytotoxicity. Cancer Res., 36:3160–3168.

Fidler, I. J., Gersten, D. M., and Riggs, C. 1977. Relationship of host immune status to tumor cell arrest, distribution and survival in experimental metastasis. Cancer, 40:46–55.

Fidler, I. J., and Kripke, M. L. 1977. Metastasis results from preexisting variant cells within a malignant tumor. Science, 197:893–895.

Fidler, I. J., and Nicolson, G. L. 1976. Organ selectivity for survival and growth of B16 melanoma variant tumor lines. J. Natl. Cancer Inst., 57:1199–1202.

Fidler, I. J., and Nicolson, G. L. 1978. Tumor cell and host properties affecting the implantation and survival of blood-borne metastatic variants of B16 melanoma. Isr. J. Med. Sci., 14:38–51.

Fidler, I. J., and Zeidman, I. 1972. Enhancement of experimental metastasis by X-ray: A possible mechanism. J. Med., 3:172–177.

Fisher, B., Saffer, E. A., and Fisher, E. R. 1972. Experience with lymphocyte immunotherapy in experimental tumor systems. Cancer, 27:771–781.

Fisher, E. R., and Fisher, B. 1965. Experimental study of factors influencing development of hepatic metastases from circulating tumor cells. Acta Cytol. (Baltimore), 9:146–158.

Fisher, E. R., Soliman, O., and Fisher, B. 1969. Effect of antilymphocyte serum on parameters of growth of MCA-induced tumors. Nature, 221:287–288.

Gasic, G. J., Gasic, T. B., Galanti, N., Johnson, T., and Murphy, S. 1973. Platelet-tumor cell interaction in mice. The role of platelets in the spread of malignant disease. Int. J. Cancer, 11:704–718.

Glaves, D., and Weiss, L. 1975. Effect of host sensitization on patterns of metastasis. Transplant. Proc., 7:253–257.

Hakansson, L., and Trope, C. 1974a. On the presence within tumours of clones that differ in sensitivity to cytostatic drugs. Acta Pathol. Microbiol. Scand. [A], 82:35–40.

Hakansson, L., and Trope, C. 1974b. Cell clones with different sensitivity to cytostatic drugs in methylcholanthrene-induced mouse sarcomas. Acta Pathol. Microbiol. Scand. [A], 82:41–47.

Heppner, G. H., Stolbach, L., Byrne, M., Cummings, F. J., McDonough, E., and Calabresi, P. 1973. Cell mediated and serum blocking activity to tumor antigens in patients with malignant melanoma. Int. J. Cancer, 11:245–260.

Kircutta, I., Mustea, I., Rogozaw, I., and Simu, G. 1965. Relations between tumor and metastases. I. Aspects of the crabtree effect. Cancer, 18:978–984.

Luria, E. S., and Delbrück, M. 1943. Mutations of bacteria from virus resistance. Genetics, 28:491–511.

Medina, D., and Heppner, G. 1973. Cell mediated "immunostimulation" induced by mammary tumor virus-free BALB/c mammary tumors. Nature, 242:329–330.

Nicolson, G. L., and Winkelhake, J. L. 1975. Organ specificity of blood-borne tumour metastasis determined by cell adhesion? Nature, 255:230–232.

Nicolson, G. L., Winkelhake, J. L., and Nussey, A. C. 1976. An approach to studying the cellular properties associated with metastasis; Some *in vitro* properties of tumor variants selected *in vivo* for enhanced metastasis. In Weiss, L. (ed.): Fundamental Aspects of Metastasis. Amsterdam, North-Holland Publishing Co., pp. 291–303.

Nowell, P. C. 1976. The clonal evolution of tumor cell populations. Science, 194:23–28.

Pimm, M. V., and Baldwin, R. W. 1977. Antigenic differences between primary methylcholanthrene-induced rat sarcomas and post surgical recurrences. Int. J. Cancer, 20:37–43.

Prehn, R. T. 1970. Analysis of antigenic heterogeneity within individual 3-methylcholanthrene-induced mouse sarcomas. J. Natl. Cancer Inst., 45:1039–1045.

Prehn, R. T. 1971. Perspectives in oncogenesis: Does immunity stimulate or inhibit neoplasia? J. Reticuloendothel. Soc., 10:1–12.

Prehn, R. T. 1972. The immune reaction as a stimulator of tumor growth. Science, 176:170–171.

Prehn, R. T. 1976. Tumor progression and homeostasis. Adv. Cancer Res., 23:203–236.

Prehn, R. T., and Lappé, M. A. 1971. An immunostimulation theory of tumor development. Transplant. Rev., 7:26–54.

Pressman, D., and Yagi, Y. 1964. Chemical differences in vascular beds. In Spierstein, M. D., Colwell, A. R., and Meyer, K. (eds.): Small Blood Vessel Involvement in Diabetis Mellitus. Washington, D.C., American Institute of Biological Sciences, pp. 177–183.

Rabotti, E. 1959. Ploidy of primary and metastatic human tumors. Nature, 183:1276–1277.

Schabel, F. M., Jr. 1975. Concepts for systemic treatment of micrometastases. Cancer, 35:15–24.

Skov, C. B., Holland, J. M., and Perkins, E. H. 1976. Development of fewer tumor colonies in lungs of athymic nude mice after intravenous injection of tumor cells. J. Natl. Cancer Inst., 56:193–195.

Sugarbaker, E. V., and Ketcham, A. S. 1977. Mechanisms and prevention of cancer dissemination: An overview. Semin. Oncol., 4:19–32.

Vaage, J. 1974. Circulating tumor antigens versus immune serum factors in depressed concomitant immunity. Cancer Res., 34:2979–2983.

Van den Brenk, H. A. S., Stone, M. G., Kelly, H., and Sharpington, C. 1976. Lowering of innate resistance of the lungs to the growth of blood-borne cancer cells in states of topical and systemic stress. Br. J. Cancer, 33:60–78.

Weiss, D. W. 1977. The questionable immunogenicity of certain neoplasms. Cancer Immunol. Immunother., 2:11–19.

Weiss, L. 1976. Biophysical aspects of the metastatic cascade. In Weiss, L. (ed.): Fundamental Aspects of Metastasis. Amsterdam, North-Holland Publishing Co., pp. 51–70.

Weiss, L. 1977. A pathobiologic overview of metastasis. Semin. Oncol., 4:5–17.

Weiss, L., Glaves, D., and Waite, D. A. 1974. The influence of host immunity on the arrest of circulating cancer cells and its modification by neuraminidase. Int. J. Cancer, 13:850–862.

Wexler, H., Chretien, P. B., and Ketcham, A. S. 1972. Effect of tumor immunity on production of lung tumors after intravenous inoculation of antigenically identical tumor cells. J. Natl. Cancer Inst., 48:657–663.

Wexler, H., Chretien, P. B., Ketcham, A. S., and Sindelar, W. F. 1975. Induction of pulmonary metastases in both immune and nonimmune mice. Effect of the removal of a transplanted primary tumor. Cancer, 36:2042–2047.

Immunotherapy of Human Cancer,
The University of Texas System Cancer Center
M. D. Anderson Hospital and Tumor Institute.
Raven Press, New York © 1978.

Clinical Rationale for Immunotherapy and Its Role in Cancer Treatment

Evan M. Hersh, M.D., Jordan U. Gutterman, M.D., Giora M. Mavligit, M.D., Christine H. Granatek, Ph.D., Roger D. Rossen, M.D.,* Adan Rios, M.D., Allan L. Goldstein, Ph.D.,† Yehuda Z. Patt, M.D., Ernesto Rivera, M.D., Stephen P. Richman, M.D., Joseph C. Bottino, M.D., David Farquhar, Ph.D., Dexter Morris, B.A., and Khoji Ezaki, M.D.

*Department of Developmental Therapeutics, The University of Texas System Cancer Center M. D. Anderson Hospital and Tumor Institute, Houston, Texas; *Department of Microbiology and Immunology, Baylor College of Medicine, Houston, Texas; and †Department of Biochemistry, The George Washington University Medical Center, Washington, D.C.*

Immunotherapy is developing as the fourth major modality of human cancer treatment. Although it is in its earliest developmental phases and the immunotherapeutic agents available are, for the most part, crude and poorly defined, immunotherapy already has demonstrated activity in terms of increasing the remission rate or increasing the remission and survival durations in a variety of human malignancies: acute leukemia, chronic leukemia, soft tissue sarcoma, malignant melanoma, and the more common neoplasms, including carcinomas of the breast, colon, and lung (Hersh *et al.,* 1976a). The development of immunotherapy, in part, has been based on empirical experiments demonstrating activity of microbial adjuvants in a variety of animal systems (Mathé *et al.,* 1973) but increasingly is being based on an improved understanding of the immunologic characteristics of human malignant disease. Indeed, immunologic studies of human cancer are establishing a rational, scientific basis for the development of immunotherapy and its application to man. Furthermore, as the other conventional modalities of cancer treatment (surgery, radiotherapy, and chemotherapy) are improved and better defined, and the immunologic effects of these modalities of treatment are documented, a rational, scientific basis for the integration of immunotherapy into the overall strategy of cancer treatment can be developed.

The scientific basis of the clinical rationale for immunotherapy for human cancer is as follows: Most importantly, there is now abundant evidence that human malignant tumors contain cell surface antigens that are qualitatively and/or quantitatively different from those found on the analagous normal tissue.

Abbreviation used in this chapter: DTIC—dimethyl triazeno imidazole carboxamide.

These can be recognized as foreign by the tumor-bearing host, and can induce an immune response in that host (Baldwin and Price, 1975). Also important is the recognition that a progressive immunodeficiency is associated with progressively growing human tumors (Twomey *et al.,* 1974). This immunodeficiency is complex in its origin, and its characteristics have not been fully defined. However, a number of factors appear to be important. First is the presence of circulating blocking serum factors, including those that nonspecifically impair in vitro lymphocyte blastogenesis (Sample *et al.,* 1971), those that are tumor-specific and interfere with lymphocyte-tumor cell interaction (Hellström *et al.,* 1973), and circulating antigen-antibody complexes (Rossen *et al.,* 1977). There is also clearly a deficiency of effector cells in patients with malignant disease, particularly as the disease progresses (Aisenberg, 1966). Finally, recent observations in both experimental animals and man suggest that at least part of the immunodeficiency of cancer is associated with suppressor cells, either circulating or in the lymph nodes and spleen (Berlinger *et al.,* 1977). Whereas the immunodeficiency of cancer is most clearly associated with metastatic disease, it is seen also in certain circumstances in patients with primary tumors, especially lung cancer.

Another important contribution to the rationale for immunotherapy is the observation that the various modalities of cancer treatment are immunosuppressive. A period of profound immunodeficiency follows surgery and can be associated with skin test anergy lasting one month (Jubert *et al.,* 1973). The immunosuppressive effects of radiotherapy are well characterized (Hersh, 1974). Chemotherapy also is immunosuppressive (Patt *et al.,* 1978), particularly if chemotherapeutic agents are administered continuously. However, if chemotherapy is intermittent, rather than continuous, there is often a rebound, and overshoot, in immunologic reactivity (Cheema and Hersh, 1971) after the course of therapy is terminated. These immunosuppressive effects of therapy must be taken into account both in terms of being a legitimate target for immunotherapeutic manipulation and in terms of selection of the optimal timing of immunotherapy.

Finally, a critically important factor is the recognition that there is a relationship between immunocompetence and prognosis in cancer (Hersh *et al.,* 1975). At every stage of the disease and for almost every diagnosis, patients who are relatively immunocompetent have a better prognosis than patients who are relatively immunoincompetent. It has been hypothesized that if one could reverse the immunoincompetence associated with a poor prognosis, the prognosis would improve.

MATERIALS AND METHODS

Delayed-type hypersensitivity was evaluated by skin testing with the recall antigens dermatophytin (Hollister-Stier Laboratories); streptokinase, streptodornase, or Varidase (Lederle Laboratories); *Candida* (Hollister-Stier Laboratories); and purified protein derivative (PPD) (Merck Sharp & Dohme), as we have described in detail previously (Hersh *et al.,* 1974). Induration was measured at 24 or 48 hours, and the mean of the sum of two right-angled diameters was recorded as the degree of response. A negative response was defined as less than 2 mm of induration.

Lymphocyte blastogenic responses to the mitogens phytohemagglutinin (PHA), pokeweed mitogen (PWM), and concanavalin A (ConA), and to the antigen streptolysin O as well as the various tumor antigens were measured by the microlymphocyte culture system in Falcon microculture plates, with 1.5×10^5 lymphocytes per well in a volume of 0.2 ml complete medium, as described previously (Hersh *et al.,* 1976b). Lymphocyte blastogenesis was measured by thymidine incorporation (1 μCi per well) for eight hours (specific activity, 1.9 Ci/mmole) and recorded as counts per minute per well or as a stimulation index. All cultures were done in triplicate, and the mean of the triplicates was recorded. For studies of blocking of blastogenesis, cells were washed three times in ten volumes of medium with 5% fetal calf serum and resuspended at the appropriate volume in the appropriate serum.

T-lymphocytes were measured on peripheral blood leukocyte suspensions, purified by Ficoll-Hypaque density solution centrifugation by a fixed slide modification of the sheep erythrocyte rosette assay, which we have described previously (Schafer *et al.,* 1975). Cells with three or more attached erythrocytes were considered positive. B-lymphocytes or lymphocytes with surface immunoglobulin were measured on lymphocyte suspensions purified by differential centrifugation and removal of adherent (phagocytic) cells by passage through a column of gum arabic-coated glass beads (Gutterman *et al.,* 1973). These preparations, consisting of more than 99% small lymphocytes, were then incubated with fluorescein-conjugated anti-human IgG, IgM, or IgA (Melloy Laboratories), and the percentage of viable cells positive for surface or membrane immunofluorescence in a 100-cell count was determined by fluorescent microscopy.

The leukocyte migration inhibition assay was carried out with leukocytes separated by a modified Ficoll-Hypaque density solution gradient centrifugation method. These leukocytes were packed into capillary tubes, which were cultured in the presence or absence of appropriate antigen (100 to 1,000 μg/ml) in complete medium in Sykes-Moore chambers. The areas of leukocyte migration from the ends of the capillary tubes were recorded after 48 hours of culture, and the specific migration inhibition in control and antigen-treated cultures was calculated (Rivera *et al.,* unpublished data).

The fetal colony-forming unit assay was carried out by mixing normal or specifically sensitized BALB/c lymph node cells with 15-day-old BALB/c mouse fetal liver cells, incubating the cells at 37°C for 60 minutes in the presence or absence of the appropriate test serum (for blocking), injecting these mixtures into lethally irradiated mice (750 rads), counting the number of fetal liver cell colonies eight days later (Granatek *et al.,* in press), and comparing these to the same manipulations on bone marrow colonies in the spleen.

Circulating immune complexes were evaluated by measurement of the binding of ^{125}I-labeled C1q to serum samples (Rossen *et al.,* 1977). ^{125}I-labeled C1q was incubated with heat-inactivated serum for one hour at 22°C, after which immunoglobulin was precipitated with polyethylene glycol. After washing, the precipitated radioactivity was counted in a gamma counter. The percent C1q bound was calculated from the amount precipitated with polyethylene glycol, the total C1q precipitable by trichloracetic acid, and the appropriate background subtractions.

Tumor antigen was purified by the methods of Hollinshead *et al.* (1976). Briefly, fresh leukemic cells or the various cultured cell lines outlined below were exposed to progressive, stepwise, hypotonic lysis, and the membranes were collected by ultracentrifugation. These were subjected to low-frequency sonication, and the resultant solubilized antigens were used either directly or after fractionation by polyacrylamide gel electrophoresis and elution from the gels. Protein determinations were by the Lowry method.

Antipyrine half-time was measured as follows: At 8:30 A.M. on the test days, patients received a single intravenous dose of 250 mg/m^2 of antipyrine. Blood samples were drawn at 2, 4, 6, 8, and 24 hours. Plasma samples were assayed in triplicate for antipyrine by the methods of Brodie and Axelrod (1950).

The lymphokine generation assay was carried out as follows: For each experimental point, 12×10^6 Ficoll-Hypaque-separated peripheral blood lymphocytes were cultured in T35 Falcon plastic flasks with or without sepharose-bound ConA (Pharmacia Laboratories Inc.). After 48 hours of incubation, the supernatants were collected, concentrated ten times, and added to microwells containing 1.5×10^5 normal human monocytes in a final concentration of 10%. After an additional 24 hours of incubation, 0.037×10^6 HeLa cells (freshly collected from culture flasks) were added to each well, and after 24 hours, the thymidine incorporation was measured by a terminal eight-hour incubation with 1 μCi per well. The degree of cytotoxicity was calculated from the thymidine incorporation of HeLa cells alone, HeLa cells plus normal monocytes, and HeLa cells plus normal monocytes preincubated with control or ConA-induced lymphocyte culture supernatants. Cytotoxicity induced by patient and control lymphocyte supernatant was then compared.

RESULTS

The results presented are examples of the various immunologic determinations made in cancer patients by which a rational, scientific basis for immunotherapy can be developed. More extensive studies of these phenomena have been carried out in our group and are reported in detail elsewhere or are in preparation for report.

Tumor Immunity

Table 1 shows an example of specific tumor immunity in cancer (Rivera *et al.,* unpublished data). Tumor immunity in cervical cancer was measured by leukocyte migration inhibition. A control antigen was prepared from cells of a normal human lymphoblastoid cell line, and cervical cancer antigen was prepared from the Sykes cervical cancer cell line (kindly provided by Joseph Sinkovics, M.D.). In no cells from any of the groups, including cervical cancer, in situ carcinoma, normal controls, and other cancers, was there specific migration inhibition induced by the control antigen. In contrast, there was a highly significant migration inhibition induced by the cervical cancer cell line antigen among the lymphocytes of patients with cervical cancer. Thus, patients with frank cervical cancer appear to have tumor immunity. Of interest, patients with the premalignant lesion of in situ carcinoma apparently do not have sufficient exposure to the antigen, if indeed it is present, to develop tumor immunity. This suggests that in the circumstance of a small primary tumor, not only in cervical cancer but perhaps also in various other histologic types of malignancy, active-specific immunization with histologic type-specific tumor antigen might prolong remission and survival after conventional therapy.

Immunodeficiency in Cancer

Delayed hypersensitivity responses to the recall antigens dermatophytin, Varidase, and *Candida* in 152 malignant melanoma patients and 336 age- and environment-matched normal control subjects are compared in Table 2. The control subjects consisted of spouses, siblings, parents, children, and close contacts of the patients with malignant melanoma. For the dermatophytin antigen, significant immunodeficiency was observed in three of the four age groups. For the Varidase and *Candida* antigens, significant immunodeficiency was seen only in the older age groups. However, because the median age of these patients is approximately 50, this is a highly relevant observation. Because there is a relation-

Table 1. *Tumor Immunity in Cervical Cancer Measured by Leukocyte Migration Inhibition*

	Mean Migration Index*	
Cancer	Control Antigen	Cervical Cancer Antigen
Cervical cancer (n = 30)	0.89	0.68†
In situ carcinoma (n = 16)	0.99	1.2
Normal control (n = 19)	0.90	0.91
Other cancers (n = 40)	0.93	0.90

* Index < .75 is significant inhibition.
† $p = .001$.

Table 2. *Delayed Hypersensitivity to Recall Antigen in Age- and Environment-Matched Malignant Melanoma Patients (P) and Normal Controls (C)*

		Median Induration Diameter (mm)/Age (yr)			
Antigen	Group	25–34	35–44	45–54	55–64
Dermatophytin	P	0.4	0.2	0.4	0.3
	C	0.4	5.9	9.1	5.5
Varidase	P	14.6	14.0	9.7	1.5
	C	17.3	14.1	9.0	4.3
Candida	P	10.5	17.5	20.0	4.5
	C	12.5	17.7	18.7	12.0

ship between immunocompetence and prognosis, as will be shown later, and because immunotherapy with microbial adjuvants can boost delayed hypersensitivity, these immunodeficient patients are suitable candidates for this type of immunotherapy.

Immunosuppressive Serum Factors

Some circulating factors in the serum are either directly or indirectly associated with the immunodeficiency of cancer. Table 3 shows data on the lymphocyte blastogenic responses of 43 patients and paired normal subjects whose lymphocytes were cultured in either autologous or allogeneic serum. With PWM and ConA, which are predominantly B- and T-lymphocyte mitogens, respectively, patient serum had an immunosuppressive effect on cells of both normal control subjects and patients. The immunorestorative activity of normal serum is also evident. Even in normal serum, the blastogenic responses of patients' lymphocytes were weaker than those of the matched, normal control lymphocytes.

In Table 4 is data that exemplifies blocking in a system involving tumor-associated antigen (Granatek *et al.,* in press). Inhibition of mouse fetal liver

Table 3. *Blocking Serum Factors in Cancer Patients Measured by In Vitro Lymphocyte Blastogenic Responses*

		Blastogenic Response (cpm $\times$ 10³)* to	
Cells	Serum	PWM†	ConA‡
Patient	Patient	7.6	11.0
	Normal	9.2	19.3
Normal	Patient	14.0	24.1
	Normal	35.4	32.2

* Mean of data from 44 subjects.
† Pokeweed mitogen.
‡ Concanavalin A.

Table 4. *Blocking of Mouse Antifetal Immunity by CEA-Containing Human Cancer Sera*

CEA Concentration in Serum (ng/ml)	Inhibition of Fetal Colony Formation by Immune Spleen Cells (%)	Blocking by Serum (%)
15.8	52	0
21.0	51	0
28.5	22	44
39.5	11	77
52.5	9	81
158.0	9	82
210.0	3	94

colony formation in the spleens of lethally irradiated mice was induced by specifically sensitized mouse lymphocytes. The addition of human serum of increasing carcinoembryonic antigen (CEA) content (derived from patients with colon cancer) to the mixture of fetal colony-forming cells and immune lymphocytes blocked colony inhibition in direct proportion to the CEA content. This is not to be interpreted as blocking of antifetal antigen immunity by CEA, but only by a serum factor, the concentration of which parallels the CEA concentration. If these observations are correct, then it is logical to assume that the removal of blocking serum factors by either plasmapheresis or activation of the reticuloendothelial system (RES) should have beneficial immunotherapeutic effects.

We studied circulating immune complexes in 134 cancer patients and 85 normal control subjects by the C1q binding assay (Rossen *et al.,* 1977). Patients with malignant melanoma, breast cancer, lung cancer, colon cancer, acute leukemia, lymphoma, and other cancer diagnoses were studied. The vast majority had immune complex levels higher than normal. More recently, we have evaluated data on these patients according to C1q binding activity greater or less than 10% (Table 5). There was a highly significant correlation between binding activity greater than 10% and evident disease, disease present for less than five months, and poor prognosis in terms of tumor progression. Indeed, in a small group of melanoma patients, those with low levels of circulating immune complexes (less than 2% C1q binding activity) had a one-year survival rate of 75% compared with 25% for those with elevated levels. Again, if these complexes could be removed by plasmapheresis or RES activation, improvement in prognosis might ensue.

Effector Cell Deficiency

Deficient numbers or function of effector cells is associated with a poor prognosis in cancer. Table 6 demonstrates that patients with solid tumors or leukemia who have low numbers of B-lymphocytes or lymphocytes with surface immuno-

CLINICAL RATIONALE

Table 5. *Characteristics Associated with C1q Binding Activity GreaterThan 10%*

Characteristic	Patients No. (%)	p Value*
Untreated patients		
Evident disease	32/70 (45)	
No evident disease	8/33 (24)	<.05
Duration of disease (mo)		
<5	33/79 (41)	
>5	10/54 (18)	<.01
Prognosis		
Progression	20/40 (50)	
No progression	25/87 (29)	<.02

* Determined by chi-square test.

globulin have a poor prognosis in terms of remission duration, whereas patients with relatively high percentages of these cells have a significantly better prognosis. Lymphokine generation from ConA-stimulated cultures of lymphocytes of cancer patients is deficient, as determined by an assay in which monocytes from normal subjects cultured in microwells are stimulated to reduce the thymidine incorporation of HeLa cells after addition of macrophage activating factor derived from ConA-stimulated cultured lymphocytes of patients and controls. Twenty patients with solid tumors were studied, and the lymphocytes of only three were capable of generating macrophage activating factor, resulting in a mean cytotoxicity to the HeLa cells of 3.9%. In contrast, 14 of 24 normal subjects' lymphocytes were capable of generating macrophage activating factor, resulting in a 17.4% cytotoxicity to the HeLa cells. This difference is significant ($p = .01$).

Immunologic Boosting

Tables 7 to 11 show examples of the immunostimulatory effects of immunotherapy. Table 7 indicates that when bacillus Calmette-Guérin (BCG) is adminis-

Table 6. *Relationship of Circulating Lymphocytes with Surface Immunoglobulin to Prognosis in Patients with Solid Tumors and Leukemia*

Diagnosis	Surface Immunoglobulin	Percent of Cells	Remission Duration (mo)*	
			< Percent Cells	> Percent Cells
Solid tumor	IgM	5.0	8.5	>25
	IgA	1.0	8.3	18
Acute leukemia	Ig	6.5	9.7	>25
	IgM	2.0	7.6	>25

* All differences significant ($p < .05$).

Table 7. *Effect of BCG on Delayed Hypersensitivity to Dermatophytin in Patients with Melanoma*

Stage	Therapy*	n	Percent Conversion		
			1 mo	3 mo	6 mo
III, NED†	None	16	0	0	19
	BCG (Tice)	20	44‡	47‡	50
	BCG (Pasteur)	35	64	55‡	57‡
	BCG (frooh)	22	35	41†	41
	BCG + DTIC	39	43	58‡	62‡
IVA	BCG + DTIC	25	32	33	33
IVB	BCG + DTIC	83	13	15	15

* BCG administered weekly for three months, then every other week.
† Tumor removed by surgical extirpation.
‡ Significant ($p < .05$).

tered weekly for three months and then every other week to patients with stage III melanoma after surgical extirpation, there is significant boosting of delayed hypersensitivity to recall antigens. Patients and control subjects were repeatedly skin tested at intervals of approximately three months, and a cumulative conversion rate was calculated from the number of patients whose skin tests converted from negative to positive or who showed greater than 100% increase in diameter of induration. The boost in delayed hypersensitivity in stage III patients persists even when DTIC chemotherapy is added to the immunotherapy. In contrast, significant boosting is not seen in patients with stage IVA (distant metastasis removed surgically) or stage IVB disease (distant metastasis that cannot be removed surgically). This latter observation suggests that immunorestorative therapy with agents such as thymic hormones and levamisole may be necessary before immunostimulating therapy with BCG can be effective in these more advanced cases.

Table 8 illustrates related observations for immunotherapy with *Corynebacterium parvum*. In this study, patients with advanced, metastatic solid tumors received various doses of *C. parvum* administered either subcutaneously or intravenously on a weekly basis. Only patients receiving high doses of *C. parvum*

Table 8. *Effect of* C. parvum *on Delayed Hypersensitivity to Recall Antigens. Conversion of Patients from Anergic to Reactive State*

Dose (mg/m²)	No. Converting/No. Treated		p Value
	Injected s.c.	Injected i.v.	
<5	2/17	3/19	NS*
≥5	0/7	8/19	.03
Total	2/24 (8.3%)	11/38 (28.9%)	.03

* Not significant.

Table 9. *Active-Specific Immunization of AML Patients with Pooled Allogeneic Leukemia-Associated Antigen. Effect on Blastogenic Response to Autologous Leukemic Cells*

Lymphocyte Stimulant†	Blastogenic Response (cpm)*				
	Day 1	8	15	22	29
Autologous leukemic cells	1,295	3,077	2,016‡	3,687‡	2,367
PHA	60,900	52,400	61,900	53,700	58,000
ConA	17,100	20,500	21,100	22,100	21,600
PPD	500	400	300	300	300

* Mean response.
† PHA, phytohemagglutinin; ConA, concanavalin A; PPD, purified protein derivative.
‡ Significantly higher than preimmunization (day 1) value.

intravenously experienced conversion from anergy to reactivity to a battery of recall antigens (dermatophytin, *Candida,* Varidase, and mumps). Thus, both dose and route of administration are important to the immune boosting effects of *C. parvum.*

In a study of active-specific immunization, patients with acute myelogenous leukemia (AML) in complete remission were immunized with pooled, allogeneic, AML-derived leukemia-associated antigen in a dose of 100 to 400 μg mixed with 50 μg of BCG cell wall skeleton, administered on days 1, 8, and 15 of the study. Significant boosting of lymphocyte blastogenic responses to autologous leukemic cells resulted (Table 9). Specificity of this response was confirmed by the fact that there was no change in lymphocyte reactivity to PHA, ConA, or PPD (Ezaki *et al.,* in press). Of interest, the boosting of delayed hypersensitivity to leukemia-associated antigen was nonspecific in these patients, and patients also showed increases in responses to recall delayed-hypersensitivity antigens. This suggests that active-specific immunization with allogeneic tumor cells or tumor antigen may be useful in boosting specific tumor immunity and therefore may have a potential immunotherapeutic effect.

Thymosin and levamisole are examples of immunorestorative agents. In a phase I study, thymosin (fraction 5) was administered at various doses to patients with advanced, chemotherapy-refractory metastatic cancer. Twenty patients who

Table 10. *Effect of Single Oral Dose of Levamisole on Delayed Hypersensitivity to Serial Post-Therapy Skin Tests with Dermatophytin**

Skin Test Reaction	No. (%) of Skin Tests	
	Levamisole	Control
Positive change	31 (31)	13 (14)
Negative change	11 (11)	23 (25)
No change	57 (58)	55 (60)
Total	99	91

* Levamisole vs. control, $p = .0018$.

Table 11. *Effect of Intravenous BCG on Hepatic Microsomal Enzyme Functions in Rats**

Days After BCG Treatment	Pentobarbital-Induced Sleep (min)	DTIC Demethylase Activity (per mg protein)
3	152	75
6	136	72
10	169	65
14	148	80

* All values significantly different from control and/or pretherapy values.

had low numbers of T cells (mean, 34 ± 4) prior to therapy showed significant boosting of the number of T cells (mean, 46 ± 3) after therapy ($p < .001$). In contrast, thymosin immunotherapy had no significant effect on T cell levels in 11 patients who had normal numbers of T cells (mean, 63 ± 3 prior to therapy; 57 ± 4 after therapy) (Schafer *et al.,* 1976). Table 10 indicates that a single, oral dose of levamisole can significantly boost delayed hypersensitivity to dermatophytin and significantly suppress a negative change in reactivity to this antigen (Lewinski *et al.,* 1977). These two studies offer substantial hope that immunorestoration may indeed be effective in patients with advanced cancer and may be useful in correcting the immunologic deficiencies associated with that state.

Detrimental Effects of Immunotherapy

There is a need for precaution in the use of immunotherapy, particularly when combined with chemotherapy or other modalities of treatment. Table 11 indicates that the intravenous administration of BCG to rats can suppress the function of hepatic microsomal enzymes, as measured by prolongation of pentobarbital-induced sleeping time and depression of the activity of DTIC demethylase (Farquhar *et al.,* 1976). A similar phenomenon appears to occur in man, as indicated in Table 12. In patients receiving a ten-day course of

Table 12. *Effect of Daily Intravenous C. parvum on Antipyrine Half-Time in 18 Melanoma Patients*

Parameter	Day After Start of Therapy		
	0	5–6	10
Mean half-time (hr)	11.71	14.31	10.67
Standard deviation	4.65	7.64	4.50
Change from day 0 (no. of patients)			
Increase	. . .	13	3
Decrease	. . .	4	11
None	. . .	1	4

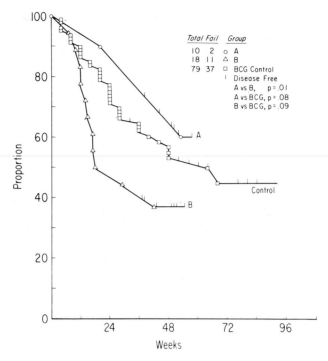

Figure 1. Relationship of immunocompetence to disease-free interval for stage IIIB and IIIAB melanoma patients treated with BCG and thymosin with or without DTIC. Group A: PHA stimulation index (SI) $\geq$ 50, thymosin 4 mg/m²; SI < 50, thymosin 40 mg/m². Group B: PHA SI $\geq$ 50, thymosin 40 mg/m²; SI < 50, thymosin 4 mg/m².

intravenous *C. parvum,* antipyrine half-time (which is metabolized by hepatic microsomal enzymes) was measured before, during the middle of, and at the end of the course. There was an increase in the half-time, representing decreased metabolic activity, at the five- to six-day point and a return to normal or below normal, indicating activation of hepatic microsomal enzymes, at the ten-day point. Because many chemotherapeutic agents are either activated or degraded by hepatic microsomal enzymes, these observations must be taken into account during the design of chemoimmunotherapy trials.

The combination of two immunotherapeutic agents also must be approached with caution. Figure 1 shows the results of a study of immunotherapy with BCG and thymosin, with or without chemotherapy with DTIC, for patients with no evident disease after surgical removal of stage III malignant melanoma. We observe a complex but important relationship between immunocompetence and thymosin dose. Immunocompetent patients receiving high doses of thymosin and immunoincompetent patients receiving low doses of thymosin had poor prognoses relative to immunocompetent and immunoincompetent patients receiving low doses and high doses, respectively. (Immunocompetence was measured by PHA response.) Thus, immunotherapy may have deleterious as well as beneficial effects. An improved understanding of important dose-response relationships and determination of the immunoreactive state of the patient will be important in the design of combination immunotherapy trials.

DISCUSSION

From the immunologic phenomena described, the objectives of immunotherapy can be defined. If a patient is immunodeficient, one should attempt to restore his immunocompetence. If the patient is receiving immunosuppressive therapy, that is, surgery, radiotherapy, or chemotherapy, one can attempt to prevent or reverse that immunosuppression. Many patients with progressive malignancy do not have severe immunodeficiency, and it may be necessary to hyperactivate the intact, but relatively ineffective, nonspecific host defense mechanisms. Because active immunization is effective in some cancer patients, it should be possible to induce or heighten specific tumor immunity by active-specific immunization. Circulating blocking factors seem to be of increasing importance; it may be possible to remove these by plasmapheresis or RES activation. Also, it may be possible to reduce the numbers or interfere with the function of suppressor cells, which have been shown to be increased in tumor-bearing animals and humans.

The currently available approaches to immunotherapy can, at least in part, achieve these objectives. Thus, active-nonspecific immunotherapy with BCG, *C. parvum,* methanol extraction residue of BCG (MER), BCG cell wall skeleton plus P_3, or endotoxin can boost delayed hypersensitivity; expand the population of peripheral blood, lymph node, or spleen lymphocytes; and activate the RES. Active-specific immunotherapy is possible by immunization with tumor cells, or tumor antigen alone or mixed with adjuvant. Adoptive immunotherapy can transfer the immunocompetence or specific immunity of an immune or immunocompetent donor to the appropriate nonimmune or immunodeficient recipient. Immunorestoration of the immunodeficient patient with levamisole or thymic hormones is possible, and plasmapheresis can be utilized for immunomodulation to remove circulating blocking factors.

Finally, these observations must be included in the development of principles of immunotherapy. Because immunodeficiency is directly related to the tumor burden, reduction of the tumor burden is essential for the development of effective immunotherapy. Furthermore, the immunologic status of the subject is critical. If he is immunodeficient, he should receive immunorestoration; if he is immunocompetent, then immunostimulation, either active-nonspecific or active-specific, may be effective. The location and extent of the tumor are also critical in the design of immunotherapy trials and in the dose, route, and schedule of administration of immunotherapeutic agents. Immunotherapy-chemotherapy interactions may be exceedingly important because of the potential effects of immunotherapy on hepatic microsomal enzyme function. Therefore, intravenous immunotherapeutic agents must be investigated in this regard. We have demonstrated that immunorestorative therapy may be detrimental to the immunocompetent patient; thus, monitoring of immunologic effects of the therapy is essential in guiding its course and evaluating new approaches. Development of these principles and evaluation of approaches will be greatly augmented by the development of appropriate and relevant animal models of immunotherapy in tumor systems as closely as possible related to those of man.

SUMMARY

The immunologic characteristics of cancer, including the presence of tumor antigens and tumor immunity, the presence of immunodeficiency, the immunosuppressive effects of circulating serum factors and of cancer treatment, and the relationship between immunocompetence and prognosis, have led to the development of a rational clinical basis for immunotherapy. These observations have led to certain principles and objectives for immunotherapy development, which we hope will guide the clinical utilization of this fourth major modality of cancer treatment in the future.

ACKNOWLEDGMENT

This work was supported by contract NO1-CB-33888 and grants CA-05831 and CA-14984 from the National Cancer Institute.

REFERENCES

Aisenberg, A. C. 1966. Immunological status of Hodgkin's disease. Cancer, 19:385–394.

Baldwin, R. W., and Price, M. R. 1975. Neoantigen expression in chemical carcinogenesis. In Becker, F. F. (ed.): Cancer: A Comprehensive Treatise. New York, Plenum Press, pp. 353–383.

Berlinger, N. T., Lopez, C., Lipkin, M., Vogel, J. E., and Good, R. A. 1977. Defective recognitive immunity in family aggregates of colon carcinoma. J. Clin. Invest., 59:761–769.

Brodie, B. B., and Axelrod, J. 1950. The fate of antipyrine in man. J. Pharmacol. Exp. Ther., 98:97.

Cheema, A. R., and Hersh, E. M. 1971. Patient survival after chemotherapy and its relationship to in vitro lymphocyte blastogenesis. Cancer, 28:851–855.

Ezaki, K., Hersh, E. M., Keating, M., Dyre, S., Hollinshead, A., McCredie, K. B., Mavligit, G. M., and Gutterman, J. U. 1978. Active specific immunization with allogeneic leukemia associated antigens or irradiated allogeneic leukemia cells in acute leukemia. Cancer (in press).

Farquhar, D., Loo, T. L., Gutterman, J. U., Hersh, E. M., and Luna, M. A. 1976. Inhibition of drug-metabolizing enzymes in the rat after bacillus Calmette-Guerin treatment. Biochem. Pharmacol., 25:1529–1535.

Granatek, C. H., Hersh, E. M., Gutterman, J. U., and Mavligit, G. M. 1978. Tumor-related blocking of anti-fetal immunity. Eur. J. Cancer (in press).

Gutterman, J. U., Rossen, R. D., Butler, W. T., McCredie, K. B., Bodey, G. P., Sr., Freireich, E. J, and Hersh, E. M. 1973. Immunoglobulin on tumor cells and tumor-induced lymphocyte blastogenesis in human acute leukemia. N. Engl. J. Med., 288:169–173.

Hellström, I., Warner, G. A., Hellström, K. E., and Sjögren, H. O. 1973. Sequential studies of cell mediated tumor immunity and blocking serum activity in ten patients with malignant melanoma. Int. J. Cancer, 11:280.

Hersh, E. M. 1974. Immunosuppressive agents. In Sartorelli, A. C., and Johns, D. G. (eds.): Antineoplastic and Immunosuppressive Agents I. Berlin, Springer-Verlag, pp. 577–617.

Hersh, E. M., Gutterman, J. U., and Mavligit, G. M. 1975. Cancer and host defense mechanisms. In Ioachim, H. L. (ed.): Pathobiology Annual. New York, Appleton-Century-Crofts, pp. 133–167.

Hersh, E. M., Gutterman, J. U., and Mavligit, G. M. 1976a. Immunotherapy of human cancer. Adv. Intern. Med., 22:145–185.

Hersh, E. M., Gutterman, J. U., Mavligit, G. M., McCredie, K. B., Burgess, M. A., Matthews, A., and Freireich, E. J. 1974. Serial studies of immunocompetence in patients undergoing chemotherapy for acute leukemia. J. Clin. Invest., 54:401–408.

Hersh, E. M., Gutterman, J. U., Mavligit, G. M., Mountain, C., McBride, C. M., and Burgess, M. A. 1976b. Immunocompetence and immunodeficiency and prognosis in cancer. Ann. NY Acad. Sci., 276:386–406.

Hollinshead, A. C., Chretien, P. B., Obong, I., Tarpley, J. L., Kerney, S. E., Silverman, N. A., and Alexander, J. C. 1976. In vivo and in vitro measurements of the relationship of human carcinomas to herpes simplex virus tumor associated antigens. Cancer Res., 36:821–828.

Jubert, A. V., Lee, E. T., Hersh, E. M., and McBride, C. M. 1973. Effects of surgery anesthesia and intraoperative blood loss on immunocompetence. J. Surg. Res., 15:399–403.

Lewinski, U., Mavligit, G. M., Gutterman, J. U., and Hersh, E. M. 1977. Administration of a single dose of levamisole to carcinoma patients: In vivo and in vitro enhancement of cellular immune response. In Chirigos, M. (ed.): Control of Neoplasia by Modulation of the Immune System. New York, Raven Press, pp. 183–196.

Mathé, G., Kamel, M., Dezfulian, M., Halle-Pannenko, O., and Bourut, C. 1973. An experimental screening for systemic adjuvants of immunity applicable in cancer immunotherapy. Cancer Res., 33:1987.

Patt, Y. Z., Hersh, E. M., Schafer, L. A., Heilbrun, L. K., Washington, M. L., Gutterman, J. U., Mavligit, G. M., and Goldstein, A. I. 1978. Clinical and immunological evaluation of the use of thymosin plus BCG ± DTIC in the adjuvant treatment of stage 3B melanoma. In Chirigos, M. (ed.): Immune Modulation and Control of Neoplasia by Adjuvant Therapy. New York, Raven Press, pp. 357–371.

Rossen, R. D., Reisberg, M. A., Hersh, E. M., and Gutterman, J. U. 1977. The C1q binding test for soluble immune complexes. Clinical correlations obtained in patients with cancer. J. Natl. Cancer Inst., 58:1205–1215.

Sample, W. F., Gertner, H. R., and Chretien, P. B. 1971. Inhibition of phytohemagglutinin induced in vitro lymphocyte transformation by serum from patients with carcinoma. J. Natl. Cancer Inst., 46:1291–1297.

Schafer, L. A., Gutterman, J. U., Hersh, E. M., Mavligit, G. M., Dandridge, K., Cohen, G., and Goldstein, A. L. 1976. Partial restoration by in vivo thymosin of E-rosettes and delayed-type hypersensitivity reactions in immunodeficient cancer patients. Cancer Immunol. Immunother., 1:259–264.

Schafer, L. A., Gutterman, J. U., Mavligit, G. M., Reed, R. C., and Hersh, E. M. 1975. Permanent slide preparation of T lymphocyte sheep red blood cell rosettes. J. Immunol. Methods, 8:241–251.

Twomey, D. L., Catalona, W. J., and Chretien, P. B. 1974. Cellular immunity in cured cancer patients. Cancer, 33:435–440.

APPROACHES TO IMMUNOTHERAPY

Immunotherapy of Human Cancer,
The University of Texas System Cancer Center
M. D. Anderson Hospital and Tumor Institute.
Raven Press, New York © 1978.

Chairman's Introduction

Animal Models of Cancer Immunotherapy: Some Considerations

David W. Weiss, Ph.D., D.Phil.Med.

Lautenberg Center for General and Tumor Immunology, Hebrew University-Hadassah Medical School, Jerusalem

This section is devoted entirely to a presentation of laboratory animal studies, and precedes the discussions of results of trials of immunotherapy in the clinic. This sequence of topics is not, of course, coincidental, but rather reflects what most of us believe to be the necessary, rational progression of steps in our search for effective modalities of immunologic intervention in human malignant disease: to elaborate and test ideas in animal tumor models, and then to apply the information gathered to the clinical situation. The vast efforts that have gone into the immunologic study of neoplasia in laboratory animals have been predicated on, and justified by, the tacit assumption that experimental animal tumors serve *de facto* and *de jure* as valid examples of malignant growths in man.

As is so often the case for tacit assumptions, however, the distance between supposition and reality may be considerable and tends to lengthen with time and habituation. In fact, the relevance to human neoplasia of the experimental tumor systems to which most of us commonly resort must be questioned seriously today; further progress toward the delineation of more categorically efficacious avenues of clinical immunotherapy seems heavily dependent on the replies advanced, that is, on a reasoned formulation of the nature, implications, and contributions of test models in animals. These must be made realistic.

That a wide gap exists between the clinical circumstances of progressive neoplasia and the conditions that pertain to our usual laboratory models is epitomized by a question that overshadows the field of tumor immunology: Why have there been such definitive successes in the immunoprophylaxis and immunotherapy for many experimental neoplasms of mice, rats, guinea pigs, and other animals when there has been such a paucity of clear and appreciable reward to the large, similar attempts in man? In affording opportunities to the immunologist not matched in the clinic, our stock-in-trade animal models may be largely unrealistic. Is neoplasia of animals characterized, then, by fundamental biologic parameters and determinants that do not apply to the circumstances of human disease?

This suggestion appears untenable if applied to animal neoplasia inclusively. There is no reason to believe that a hard boundary separates the phenomena of neoplastic growth in the species man on the one hand, and in the remainder of the vertebrate phyla on the other. There are at least as many similarities as dissimilarities between malignant growths of man and the corresponding neoplasms of many different species, morphologically, physiologically, and immunologically. Rather, the irrelevance must lie with the design, conduct, and interpretation of the experiments that we undertake in the laboratory with a circumscribed range of tumors. If it is the investigator, then, rather than inherent distinctions in the natural history of malignant processes in man and in animals, who is responsible for the artifacts that rob many of our animal tumor investigations of complementarity with the human situation, we must expose the artifacts if we are to be more germane to our purposes in the future.

That we are indeed ill at ease with our commonplace animal models has been a recurrent theme in our meetings thus far. I believe that I speak for all of us in expressing my own strong opinion that our animal models must be improved radically if they are to serve as veracious guidelines for clinical approaches. In exposing and then obviating their many patent artificialities, we must reconstruct animal models so that, first of all, they will have pertinence *to themselves.* Only thereby can we hope that they will have pertinence to their supposed human analogues. This is not an easy or cheap task, technically, and it is one that demands basic reexamination of the philosophy of experimentation in this area. It is legitimate to ask, therefore: Is it worth the endeavor? After all, it can be argued, there is always the unavoidable leap from the laboratory to the clinic, with accompanying uncertainties and hazards that never can be resolved wholly in the test tube and test animal. Perhaps the large effort of building meaningful animal test systems is not really a necessity for the future of clinical explorations in tumor prevention and treatment by immunologic means, whatever the basic science interests of the laboratory work may be.

I am aware of the fact that not a few immunologic studies in cancer patients indeed have been mounted from thin and short laboratory springboards; the rush to the patient from the drawing board has sometimes been precipitous to astonishment. Despite these precedents or, more accurately, because of them, I hold that we are unlikely to be able to dispense with animal and in vitro models in our pursuit of a major immunologic contribution to the control of cancer. For all the labor and funding that in recent years have gone into clinical trials of immunotherapy, and despite the high hopes with which these were initiated, the returns so far have been most limited; on the whole, the carefully controlled investigations with sizable patient populations have not confirmed the hopes generated by results of some of the preliminary small trials, and evidence that immunologic intervention in neoplastic disease is of concrete value to the patient remains elusive. Must we conclude accordingly that the assumptions that have motivated so much work and optimism—immunology as a new open door to the control of cancer—are faulty intuition and wishful thinking only? We cannot say at this moment, but the sparse showing of immunology in the cancer ward offers little proof of the invalidity of the premises: More often than not, immunotherapy has been carried out in ignorance, if not in actual defiance, of the recognized principles of immunology and tumor biology; the approach has been taken with a shotgun. Perhaps we should be as much surprised by the fact that any positive results have been obtained as we are by their smallness. Until proved otherwise, the suggestive findings made in the clinic can be taken as indications of far greater possibilities, rather than as statements of limits already reached. Also, there is always the reflection of the attainments with laboratory animals that meets us when we turn in disappointment from the patient, and that preserves the expectation that more could be achieved if only we knew how.

How can we achieve more? By working out the *areas of principle* on which immunologic intervention in cancer must be based if it is to be given a fair chance of succeeding. There is an aphorism in the Mishnah: "It is not incumbent on you to complete the task, neither are you free to desist from it." I, myself, am not prepared to desist unless clinical trials predicated on sound principles of immunology and on the operative recognition that neoplastic diseases constitute dynamic interactions between host and (neoplastic) parasite should truly reveal that stimulation and modulation of immunologic reactivity can do little to alter the course of an evolving neoplastic pathology.

It is surpassingly difficult and dangerous, however, to work out these principles, cold, in patients without at least the major guidelines that can be delineated from exhaustive animal experimentation in appropriate model constellations. I emphasize the latter term. It seems nonsensical to me to strive for the discovery of the ideal animal model. There can be no such thing. Cancer in any one species, and throughout the animal world, comprises a family of diseases, varying greatly from each other despite aspects of relatedness; no one form of malignant disease can be taken to be the model of neoplasia in that species, and certainly not as the model for the entire grouping of such diseases in nature. What we need is a manifold variety of model systems, each one posing distinct questions, each one relevant to itself—the primary condition—and, as much as possible, to the clinical circumstances of analogous types of disease. Only from a broad and variegated spectrum of models can we hope to obtain blocks of principle-information. It is from repeated, overlapping pathways of investigation in diverse model systems that sets of generally applicable axioms can be distinguished.

For example, a hepatoma arising many years ago in an animal exposed to a given carcinogen and passaged scores or hundreds of times cannot offer, as a subcutaneous implant in hosts of substrains long separated from the original breeding nucleus, a measure of the behavior of liver tumors even in that species;

the artifice is multiple and far too formidable. As another instance, the specification of optimum dosage of a particular agent in one or a few tumors cannot be translated heuristically to the clinic. In contrast, the repeated finding that an agent in only small amounts, within a narrow range despite large differences in host body weight or area, can stimulate resistance, and that supraoptimal amounts exert negative effects becomes policy: Phase I and II trials must be based on the assumption that the less, the better, and that larger quantities may be tried only with caution and under constant supervision.

Many provisions must be incorporated in the creation of adequate series of model systems. The following are among the most salient factors that should underly our posture.

(1) The arcs of immunologic responsiveness that mediate, effect, and suppress reactions cytotoxic to tumor cells must be identified in a succession of models, and the parameters of their actions and interactions characterized. At this moment in the development of insight into the maze of positive and negative signals that make up immunologic function, this is a task not only arduous, but probably still beyond our reach. I do not suggest, therefore, that clinical tumor immunology must pause until the basic research in cellular and humoral immunologic responses and their implications for tumor defenses has made a quantum jump in sophistication. What I do argue is that the program of basic immunologic investigations be encouraged and supported not only for its own intrinsic value, but as the development of an infrastructure of knowledge on which future essays in the clinic can be founded with better prospects; and that clinicians currently initiating studies take cognizance of the information that is available, sparse as it may be, on the differential influence of immunologic stimulation, nonspecific and specific, for the heterogenous manifestations of immune function. At least some pitfalls and risks may be avoided by exploiting the clues now accessible.

(2) Immunotherapy must be based on the philosophy and perspectives of immunology, not, as has been the case so often, on those of chemotherapy or any other modality of cancer treatment. For example, it often may be desirable to introduce a chemical cytoreductive drug in the maximum amounts that are tolerated by the patient in order to eliminate the largest possible numbers of pathogenic transformed cells. With immunologic agents, however, the maximum quantities that can be given safely may be far in excess of those that can effect optimal stimulation of the desired facets of responsiveness, and may fall within the range in which the phenomena of tolerance, paralysis, and suppression become increasingly probable. Similar considerations must be invoked in planning the timing of immunologic treatment, especially when it is administered in conjunction with other therapy. We are only beginning to become aware of the complex interactions of chemotherapy and immunotherapy, but it is already apparent that additive and synergistic as well as antagonistic effects can be elicited. Here, again, we require the principle-information that can come only from a concatenation of experiments with a variety of tumors in different hosts. Which regimens of chemotherapy are likely to bring about a selective inhibition

of suppressor lymphocytes and macrophages, and which, on the other hand, are likely to compromise immunocyte effector capacities? Which immunotherapeutic procedures can be anticipated to alter drug metabolism in desired directions and which in inimical directions? Answers to these and many other questions that accrue from mixed-modality treatment must be sought, to begin with, in animal models. If the data obtained cannot provide direct guidance to the clinician, it can serve, nonetheless, to delimit the latitudes of clinical investigation likely to be most productive. Animal models rarely will yield solutions to clinical problems, but they can make for more intelligent and better-focused clinical inquiry.

(3) The extent to which hoary cell lines of tumor origin maintain a semblance to neoplasia in nature after passage for years in animals and tissue culture is highly questionable. Most of us acknowledge the gross artificiality of such "tumor cells," but with an occasional side journey to the Canossa of Authenticity that lies in the study of primary tumors in the autochthonous host, we continue to work with the safe ancestral models. For reasons of logistics and finance, purity of research design may not be possible, but we can do better than delude ourselves that we are truly studying leukemia when we work with EL4 cells, or liver malignancies when we treat subcutaneous implants of the line 10 hepatoma in guinea pigs, or any form of cancer when we publish results of experiments with Ehrlich ascites cells.

We would be one step ahead if we were to confirm the impressions we obtain from such doubtful systems in the occasional, critical experiment with the primary host of a spontaneously occurring neoplasm. Such confirmatory stabs of experiments are practical for any investigator with access to breeding colonies of laboratory animals in which tumors arise as part of the animal's "natural" life history. Certainly, even such growths are a distance removed from spontaneous neoplasia in outbred species in their normal environment, but they may be considered, nevertheless, as an aspect of the biology of the laboratory-maintained animal lines.

There is little excuse for conducting studies with a tumor in the hundredth transplant generation when first- or second-generation tissue can be used. It may be true that even after a single passage, many characteristics of the spontaneous neoplasm change, adaptively or by selection; there are many precedents for such rapid deviations from the natural in regard to pathogenic bacteria. Still, the greater the distance is from the original event of transformation and progressive growth in the primary host, the greater is the likelihood that we shall be dealing with secondary changes of little bearing to the biology of freshly formed tumors. Newer techniques in cryobiology may afford the possibility of preserving original or early-transplant generation tumors for future study, with a reduced risk of antigenic deterioration in the process of freezing and resuscitation.

(4) It is no longer sufficient to describe tumors as merely antigenic or immunogenic. We have come to know that various types of antigens are expressed on

the neoplastic cell surface, singly, in combination, sometimes in competition with each other. These antigens may be embryonic and neonatal markers; determinants specific to a given tissue or organ and "displaced" in the neoplastic variant from its normal localization; antigens associated with the presence, coding, and derepressing activities of oncogenic and passenger viruses; and perhaps even genuine tumor-specific antigens. The role of each category of tumor-associated antigens in evoking immune defenses is uncertain today, but the uncertainty may be resolved by systematic study of resistance against tumors expressing these antigens to known extent. Such insight would contribute appreciably to our ability to direct defensive reactions against human tumors distinguished by the corresponding antigen groupings.

(5) I have already alluded to the need of making each animal model as relevant as possible to itself. This point deserves emphasis. Little can be hoped for from a model that is a grotesque departure from its own circumstances. There seems to be little justification for not working within the known scope of behavior of a given tumor in a given laboratory host, for not taking into account in the planning of experiments such basic variables as the site of tumor origin (in many instances, it *is* feasible to study implanted tumors in the tissues from which they developed), the strain subline in which the tumor occurred, and the tumor's tendencies to metastasize, be invasive, or remain in situ. Similarly, the timing and quantification of treatment must be determined with consideration of the kinetics of progression of the prototype tumors in the host of origin, and of the relative dimensions of host and tumor size and weight in the spontaneous setting.

It is not easy in the creation of models to reconcile relative and absolute standards of comparison. A one-gram mammary carcinoma implant in a mouse may constitute, in absolute mass, a reasonable facsimile of an early growth in the breast of a woman, but it does not mimic incipient mammary neoplasia in the rodent. In some cases, perhaps, information of comparative value can be gained from experiments in which the human situation is copied in absolute terms. Even in that event, the investigator must be aware of the different standards of comparison with which he deals and must test all possibilities before he can know which criteria offer the best copy.

(6) The advent of an immunologic perspective of neoplasia confirmed the role of the host as an involved participant in the biology of malignant diseases. The interaction of the host and neoplastic parasite is not, however, a two-dimensional episode. A third major factor must be included in a total view of neoplastic processes: environment. In the study of infectious diseases, the transition from a monistic apperception of the pathogenic microorganism as the determinant of the events following infection to a discernment of host, potential parasite, and environment as interacting variables that, together, set the picture came about more than 30 years ago, largely under the influence of René Dubos. A parallel evolution of thinking is now mandatory for our subject, the host-parasite

relationship of neoplastic diseases. Without this perspective, we cannot build models pertinent to the case, and we shall miss cues that could further progress in both the clinic and the laboratory.

An environmental perspective subsumes not only the ambient circumstances in which the interactants of an association find themselves, but also the intrinsic makeup of each partner at the time of meeting and the conditions that define the microenvironment of the field of interaction. Age, sex, nutritional status, intercurrent disease, and every factor that influences the anatomic and physio logic individuality of an organism when progressively growing neoplastic variants appear in its tissues represent one category of environmental determinants. The genetic variations of neoplastic cells and their phenotypic expression are another, and must be defined for each separate aggregate of tumor cells in host tissues and be fixed in time, because the stepwise progressions of neoplasia and the secondary mutations that become expressed in transformed cell populations make for a great lability of tumor cell characteristics. The characteristics of the intimate milieu in which a neoplastic growth develops and is confronted by host defense factors constitute a third category. This grouping of environmental determinants must be stressed today, for its decisive importance has been largely overlooked. We now know, however, that the properties of primary and metastatic tumor foci, including cell surface antigenicities, can differ substantially; that immunocyte populations within a tumor focus may be of composition or adaptive behavior different from those distributed systemically or in removed tissue localities; that tumor cells can mount reactions that evade or neutralize host defenses in situ but that may not be detectable throughout the host organism; and that there are distinctive features of the biochemical environments of different tissues, and even of diverse zones in the same organ, that can act to modulate the realization of host-defensive and tumor-aggressive potentials. It is the entire array of variables that must be considered in portraying the ground of ongoing confrontation between host and neoplastic parasite in the evolution of a neoplastic disease, and this picture must be set into the larger one of the surrounding environs in which the host exists. Only such a total, comprehensive purview is biologically admissible in the description of cancer in nature and in the construct of heuristic model systems.

(7) Not infrequently, the results of preliminary small trials of immunotherapy in humans are far more impressive (and even statistically significant) than are those attained in subsequent larger studies. Whatever may be the reasons for this circumstance, it places a constraint on overenthusiastic evaluations of animal data as well. Impressive findings with immunologic intervention in animal tumors, in fact, are more often evident from early explorative experiments than from larger investigations. The fact that a comparison between an experimental and a control group has reached the point of "statistical significance" by one protocol may have little biologic importance if the finding cannot be confirmed in repeated and extended experiments in which the immunologic variable is

seen to stand out from the background of other variant factors, controlled and uncontrolled. (This is especially true, as every statistician but not every immunologist knows, when a number of experimental groups in any one experiment are compared with one control: A single "significant" comparison can then be a random event in itself.) On the other hand, repeated assessments that reveal a consistent trend in the activities of an immunotherapeutic agent may become biologically meaningful and statistically significant as well, even though the p value of comparison in any one experiment falls short of the critical point.

It is most important, therefore, that the planning of animal as well as human studies be the joint effort of immunologist and biostatistician. Too many of us, myself included, sometimes tend to seek statistical blessing *a posteriori* and are forced into a tortuous belaboring of data that is not always evident to the casual reader who searches for pearls of mathematical respectability; such exercises can strengthen hopeful expectations but also can seriously mislead.

In the reporting of animal investigations, it is not uncommon, moreover, to ignore experiments with negative results, even when these make up an appreciable proportion of the total study. It may be correct to ascribe the failures to inadequate foreknowledge of the optimum conditions for efficacy, but unless the range and frequency of all observations are reported fairly, the appearance is given of a more prevalent expression of desired activity than is actually the case. Such bias of accentuation can be found in series of experiments conducted with the same tumor model, and also with regard to the spectrum of available test systems: We prefer to give our attention to those that lend themselves to the achievement of our goals, and frequently deprecate their remoteness from the natural prototype. In the same light, there is commonly a glossing over of the injurious side effects of therapy in laboratory explorations. Animals in many instances are more resistant to severe manipulations and treatments than are patients; they are often killed after only short periods, before toxicity becomes obvious; they cannot complain, and all but the grossest damage may go undetected; and they are expendable.

Adequate statistical design at the onset, and clarity and honesty in the presentation of findings thus demand far more emphasis than they have been given in animal experimentation, and may well shrink the gap between experimental and clinical impressions of the efficacy of immunologic treatment.

(8) The last of the propositions I wish to make is a call for more investigations in domestic animals. Tumors arise spontaneously in dogs, cats, and some farm animals with not inconsiderable frequency, and there is the great advantage that the hosts have a greater resemblance to life in nature than do laboratory species highly inbred or long raised under pronouncedly artificial conditions. Because of their greater size, domestic animals permit procedures, such as repeated plasma exchange (described in these proceedings by Lucien Israël), that are not practical in small subjects. The design of investigations in domestic animals obviously must be different from that of studies in inbred strains, where

the supply of syngeneic hosts is unlimited; the forced restriction of working with the autochthonous organism, however, is the clinical standard. The recommendation for broadening the range of tumor models is not an argument for numerical promiscuity, but rather one for the diversification of tumors and hosts studied. This opportunity is provided by domestic animals, with greater relevance to the human situation than by the now pedestrian small-animal models to which we have become accustomed.

Immunotherapy of Human Cancer,
The University of Texas System Cancer Center
M. D. Anderson Hospital and Tumor Institute.
Raven Press, New York © 1978.

BCG Immunotherapy: Efficacy of BCG-Induced Tumor Immunity in Guinea Pigs with Regional Tumor and/or Visceral Micrometastases

M. G. Hanna, Jr., Ph.D., and Leona C. Peters, B.S.

Cancer Biology Program, NCI Frederick Cancer Research Center, Frederick, Maryland

Although several studies suggest that patients may possess tumor immunity while tumor burden is minimal (Morton and Malmgren, 1969; Lewis *et al.,* 1969; Black *et al.,* 1974), spontaneous tumor regression is rare (Everson and Cole, 1966). Thus, in the untreated patient, the balance between host responses and tumor proliferation favors progressive tumor growth. Among the strategies of immunotherapy for localized and/or disseminated minimal residual tumor, immune potentiation by microbial agents has received the greatest attention. The most encouraging experimental and clinical data to date have resulted from protocols with bacterial vaccines or nonspecific immunostimulants, primarily *Mycobacterium bovis* strain bacillus Calmette-Guérin (BCG), administered intralesionally (Morton *et al.,* 1970; Pinsky *et al.,* 1973; Seigler *et al.,* 1973) or systemically, either alone (Gutterman *et al.,* 1973a,b; McKneally *et al.,* 1976) or admixed with tumor cells in the form of a vaccine (Sokal *et al.,* 1972, 1973). The clinical procedures have been carried out with limited guidance from experimental animal models and thus, for the most part, have been problematic. Improvement of immunotherapeutic procedures requires more information on the complex interactions among tumor, host response, and therapy. Such investigations should be performed in experimental animal models that can be manipulated. If the experimental models approximate clinical reality, then insights that can contribute to the treatment of cancer in humans may be gained.

One impetus for the use of BCG in immunotherapy was the development of an experimental system that meets some of the requirements of a model to study an established tumor with regional lymph node metastasis (Rapp *et al.,* 1968). The line 10 hepatocarcinoma of strain 2 guinea pigs has several features that make it pertinent to the study of human cancer. It is weakly antigenic, syngeneic with its host, and following intradermal injection, metastasizes spontaneously to draining lymph nodes. It has been demonstrated that regression of transplanted syngeneic hepatocarcinoma (line 10) growing in the skin of strain

2 guinea pigs and elimination of regional lymph node metastases are achieved in most animals after intralesional injection of viable BCG (Zbar and Tanaka, 1971; Hanna *et al.,* 1972). This particular aspect of immunotherapy in the guinea pig model, although intriguing, is limited with respect to the type, stage, and location of the tumor, as well as the route of administration of BCG. Nevertheless, the initial studies established one fact that has broad implications: During BCG-mediated tumor regression and elimination of regional lymph node metastases, there is a development of systemic, cell-mediated tumor immunity, demonstrated by rapid rejection of a second tumor challenge in the skin several weeks after BCG treatment (Zbar *et al.,* 1972; Hanna *et al.,* 1973). This is an important aspect of the model because it is known that at the tumor stage when BCG administration is optimally effective, surgical excision of the tumor and regional lymph nodes would also be curative. However, no significant development of tumor immunity is achieved with surgery alone.

Thus, the BCG immunotherapy model of inbred guinea pigs is particularly appropriate. If metastasis occurs beyond the draining chain of nodes, it might be controlled by the induced systemic tumor immunity (Hanna and Peters, 1975; Hanna *et al.,* 1976). This aspect of the BCG therapy model is important when one considers that adjuvant immunotherapy has been tested mostly in cancers in which control of primary tumor is available with surgery, radiotherapy, and/or chemotherapy, but which have substantial late-relapse rates. (For review of recent clinical immunotherapy trials, see Salmon, 1977.) Recurrence is thought to be due to a few residual tumor cells. Adjuvant immunotherapy is intended to eradicate these residual tumor cells by stimulating immunologic mechanisms. A modification of the BCG immunotherapy model for established dermal tumors in inbred guinea pigs has permitted us to investigate the control of disseminated visceral micrometastases. This modification involves hematogenous metastases initiated by intravenous injection of line 10 tumor cells.

MATERIALS AND METHODS

Animals

Inbred male guinea pigs (Sewall-Wright strain 2) were obtained from the Frederick Cancer Research Center's Animal Production Area. These guinea pigs were shown to be histocompatible by skin grafting. They were housed six to ten per cage and fed Wayne guinea pig chow and kale; they weighed 400 to 500 g at the beginning of the experiments.

Tumors

Induction of primary hepatocarcinomas in strain 2 guinea pigs after they were fed the water-soluble carcinogen diethylnitrosamine was described previously (Rapp *et al.,* 1968). The antigenic and biologic properties of the transplantable ascites tumors developed from the primary hepatocarcinomas also have been described (Zbar *et al.,* 1969).

Ascites hepatocarcinoma cells, line 10, were harvested and washed three times in Hanks' balanced salt solution (HBSS) and diluted to desired concentrations to establish dermal tumors. Guinea pigs were inoculated intradermally in the upper right dorsal quadrant with a 0.1-ml volume of 10^6 viable tumor cells. The resultant tumors grew progressively and metastasized to the draining lymph nodes by seven days after intradermal injection. Guinea pigs died of metastases 60 to 90 days after intradermal inoculation with 10^6 cells. One-milliliter doses of ascites line 10, ranging from 10^2 to 10^6 cells per dose, were also injected into the dorsal vein of the penis, producing artificial vascular metastases. Injections of 10^4 cells into normal guinea pigs resulted in the death of approximately 70% to 100% of the animals, whereas 10^5 and 10^6 cells were routinely fatal to all animals. The times of death varied as a function of dose, and all animals died of metastasis to the lung and mediastinal and hilar lymph nodes with concurrent visceral metastases.

BCG

M. bovis strain BCG (Phipps strain TNC 1029) was obtained from the Trudeau Institute (Saranac Lake, New York). Preparations of BCG, stored at $-70°$C, were rapidly thawed in a $37°$C water bath and diluted to proper concentrations. In all studies, BCG was injected intralesionally seven or 12 days after the initial tumor cell injection into the skin. The tumors were approximately 1 cm in diameter at seven days. It has been demonstrated previously that intralesional BCG-mediated regression of line 10 hepatocarcinoma is optimal at six to seven days in this guinea pig therapy model, and the therapeutic advantage of BCG diminishes with an increase of tumor size or time after primary transplantation (Zbar *et al.,* 1972).

Vaccine Preparation

The ascites line 10 cells used in vaccine preparation were either fresh or frozen and thawed. In preparation for freezing, the cells were concentrated and suspended in an equal volume of chilled 15% dimethylsulfoxide plus 10% fetal calf serum-HBSS solution. The final suspension was 2 to 6×10^7 cells/ml. Two-milliliter aliquots of the line 10 cell suspension were frozen at controlled rates in a Linde Biological Freezer (BF4): $-1°$C/min to the critical freezing point, flash-frozen through the heat of fusion, and continued at $-1°$C/min to a final temperature of $-60°$ C. The rate of freezing was monitored on a Honeywell Electronic III. The vials were stored in liquid nitrogen. The rationale for this method of freezing has been described in detail elsewhere (Leibo *et al.,* 1970;

Mazur *et al.,* 1970). The vials were rapidly thawed in a 37°C water bath. Frozen-thawed cells were slowly diluted to 50 ml in HBSS, washed once, and resuspended in preparation for X-irradiation. Suspensions of fresh and frozen-thawed cells were X-irradiated in 50-ml beakers on ice. X-irradiation was performed with a Phillips MG 301 X-irradiation unit at 500 R/min, for a total dose of 20,000 R. Cell viability counts were performed with the trypan blue dye exclusion test. Viability after irradiation of either fresh or frozen-thawed cells was generally 90%, with less than 10% variation between the fresh and frozen-thawed cells.

BCG (10^9 organisms/ml) was added, in equal volume, to viable line 10 (10^8 cells/ml) for a vaccine ratio of 10:1. A vaccination consisted of an intradermal injection of 0.2 ml. For ratios of 1:10, BCG (10^9 organisms/ml) was diluted 1:100 in HBSS, and aliquots were mixed with 10^8 viable line 10 cells/ml. These vaccinations also consisted of an intradermal injection of 0.2 ml. All vaccinations were performed less than one hour after the BCG-tumor cell mixtures were prepared.

In preliminary vaccination experiments, the line 10 cells were X-irradiated with 12,000 R; however, we noticed that although this irradiated cell preparation was not tumorigenic when admixed with BCG, it was tumorigenic when administered intradermally in the absence of BCG. We were concerned that any growth of 12,000 R X-irradiated line 10 cells in the skin might preempt developing tumor immunity, and thus render the treatment ineffective against disseminated tumor. Therefore, in the majority of the experiments, 20,000 R X-irradiation was used for line 10 cells in BCG-tumor cell vaccines. A comparative study with the 12,000 R and 20,000 R X-irradiation doses also was performed. All vaccinations were given intradermally, beginning in different sites, or intralesionally in the previous vaccination site. Animals were vaccinated either one and seven days or four and ten days after intravenous injection of line 10 cells.

RESULTS

Effect of Intratumoral BCG Therapy on Disseminated Tumor

The purpose of this study was to determine the relative efficacy of BCG-mediated tumor immunity to control or eliminate disseminated tumor. The protocol of this study is shown in Figure 1A. Intradermal tumors were initiated with 10^6 line 10 cells on day 0. Six days later, 10^2 to 10^6 line 10 cells were injected intravenously. The next day, or seven days after dermal tumor initiation, BCG was injected into the tumor site; thus, this protocol simulates an in vivo competition assay in which serial dilutions of disseminated tumor are used. The results were evaluated by three parameters: BCG-mediated regression of skin tumor, tumor immunity as measured by contralateral tumor challenge, and long-term survival.

In this study, skin tumor progression was determined by measuring two per-

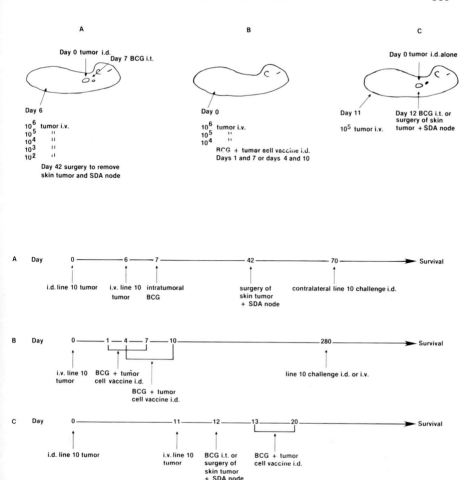

Figure 1. Protocols used for experimental immunotherapy in guinea pigs with regional and/ or disseminated tumor.

pendicular diameters once a week for six weeks after intralesional BCG injection (Fig. 2). BCG injection had a minimal effect in producing tumor regression in animals receiving between 10^3 and 10^6 tumor cells intravenously. No difference in tumor regression between animals receiving 10^2 tumor cells injected intravenously and animals receiving no injection was observed; in both of these groups, the skin tumors were eliminated, and residual scar tissue remained at the tumor site at five weeks after BCG intralesional injection.

Five weeks after intralesional BCG injection, the tumor site and regional lymph nodes were excised from all animals in this experiment. Two weeks after surgery, animals in each group were rechallenged with 10^6 tumor cells to evaluate systemic tumor immunity. The percentages of animals treated with BCG that rejected contralateral challenge two weeks after surgery are shown

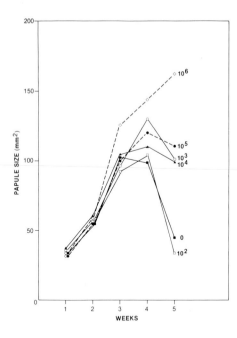

Figure 2. Size changes of line 10 skin tumors after intralesional injection of BCG. Tumor growth calculated from mean papule size (r^2) after various treatments. Guinea pigs were injected intradermally with 10^6 line 10 cells; six days later, groups of nine to ten animals each were injected intravenously with line 10 cells. Intravenous line 10 cell doses were as indicated in figure. One day after intravenous line 10 injection, all animals were injected intralesionally with BCG. Skin tumors were measured with a micrometer caliper at weekly intervals after BCG injection; two diameters were measured on each papule, and sizes are expressed as squares of average radius of each lesion. (Reproduced from Hanna *et al.,* 1976, with permission of Springer-Verlag.)

in Table 1. There was an inverse correlation between rejection of contralateral challenge and initial systemic tumor burden. Thus, in this BCG therapy model, an initial, intravenous, systemic tumor burden of 10^3 cells or more is capable of interfering with or preempting the developing tumor immunity so that skin tumor regression as well as capability of rejecting contralateral challenge is impaired.

In a second experiment, animals were given the same treatments, but in this

Table 1. *Percentage of Intratumoral BCG-Treated Animals Capable of Rejecting Contralateral Challenge After Surgery**

Treated Animals† (no.)	IV Tumor Cells (no.)	Animals Rejecting Challenge (%)		
		Day 7	14	21
9	10^6	11	11	11
10	10^5	20	20	30
9	10^4	33	44	44
9	10^3	44	67	67
10	10^2	80	80	90
10	...	80	80	80

* Modified from Hanna *et al.,* 1976.

† Guinea pigs were injected intradermally with 10^6 line 10 cells, and six days later, intravenously with line 10 cells. On day 7, all animals were injected intralesionally with BCG. Six weeks later, tumor and regional superficial distal axillary lymph node were surgically excised. Two weeks after surgery, animals were challenged in a contralateral skin site with 10^6 line 10 cells.

case, we evaluated the effects of combined BCG immunotherapy and surgery in animals injected either intra-arterially or intravenously with various doses of line 10 tumor cells. The results are shown in Figure 3. Among animals receiving 10^4 line 10 cells intra-arterially, there was a 43-day increase in median survival time for the treated group compared with the control group. Furthermore, 17% of the treated group survived as long as 210 days after tumor cell injection. Among animals receiving 10^3 line 10 cells intra-arterially, there was a 50-day increase in median survival time for the treated group. More importantly, whereas all control animals had died by 150 days after tumor challenge, 34% of the experimental group was still alive at 210 days. The greatest difference in survival rate was achieved in control and treated animals receiving 10^2 tumor cells injected intra-arterially: an 88% mortality for the control group compared with 28% mortality for the experimental group.

In general, death from intravenously induced line 10 artificial metastases occurred later than death from the intra-arterially induced metastases. Furthermore, the limiting fatal dose of line 10 tumor cells was higher for intravenous than for intra-arterial artificial metastases. When 10^2 line 10 cells were injected intravenously into normal strain 2 guinea pigs, there was no mortality, but when injected intra-arterially, there was an 88% mortality. An injection of 10^4 line 10 cells in this particular experiment resulted in 100% mortality and a median survival time of 82 days. Although there was no significant difference in median survival time with the same intravenous tumor cell dose for the treated animals, there was a 25% difference in mortality. Intravenous injection

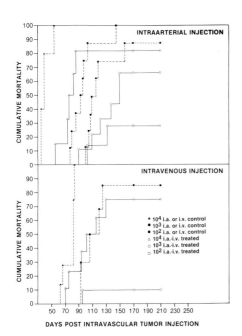

Figure 3. Percentage cumulative mortality for guinea pigs with regional and disseminated micrometastases treated with intralesional BCG injection, followed by surgical excision of the primary skin tumor and superficial distal axillary lymph node. Animals (nine to ten per group) were injected intradermally with 10^6 line 10 tumor cells and six days later, received line 10 cells either intra-arterially in the femoral artery or intravenously in the dorsal vein of the penis. One day later, experimental animals received BCG intradermally, and tumors were surgically excised six weeks later. Control animals received no treatment subsequent to intravascular injections.

of 10^3 line 10 cells into normal animals was fatal to 85%. Only 10% mortality occurred, however, among animals receiving 10^3 line 10 cells intravenously prior to BCG therapy and surgery. As can be seen in other competition assays, the greatest differences are achieved at doses just below the maximum threshold (100% mortality), such as the 10^2 intra-arterial cell dose and the 10^3 intravenous dose.

All animals that died during the course of this study had widespread visceral metastases, and the majority had distinct tumor foci in the lungs. The most convincing evidence that systemic tumor immunity was effective in controlling and eliminating pulmonary metastases came from the gross and histologic measurements of pulmonary metastases in the animals that died during the course of the study. Among the control groups injected intra-arterially with line 10 tumor cells (10^4, 10^3, or 10^2), 67% of the animals that died had pulmonary metastases. Only 22% of the experimental animals that died had pulmonary metastases. Among the control groups injected intravenously with line 10 cells (10^4 or 10^3), 100% of the animals had pulmonary metastases. Only 27% of the treated animals that died had gross pulmonary metastases. Thus, although the line 10 tumor burden was fatal to 73% of the treated animals, pulmonary metastases were prevented or eliminated. Histologic examination of the pulmonary hepatocarcinoma metastases indicated that in those animals that had BCG therapy and surgery and died during the course of the study, there was a mononuclear cell infiltration in and around the pulmonary tumors. However, no such mononuclear cell infiltration was detected in the control animals.

In general, these results demonstrate that there is a direct causal relationship between the distant tumor burden and the escape of skin tumor and regional lymph node metastases from BCG-induced regression. A major consideration was whether the development of tumor immunity was blocked or whether tumor immunity indeed did develop and was then preempted by this systemic tumor burden. By surgically excising the regional tumor and following the survival time of the animals, we could determine the efficacy of tumor immunity in controlling or eliminating the systemic tumor burden. Thus, these studies show that BCG injected intralesionally in guinea pigs with regional tumor results in the stimulation of tumor immunity that is effective against metastasis. However, the efficacy of tumor immunity is dependent on total systemic tumor burden. There is no evidence of lack of development of tumor immunity, but rather that tumor immunity is preempted at distant sites to a degree that there is a dilution effect, which is a function of increased tumor burden (Hanna *et al.,* 1973). To a certain extent, this effect can be abrogated in the guinea pig model by strategic surgery.

It would appear from these results that a therapeutic modality involving injection of BCG into the localized tumor mass, followed by surgery, may be beneficial to systemic tumor in patients with limited regional tumor and possible systemic metastases. However, based on all that we have learned, the translation of the results of intralesional BCG injection in the guinea pig model to humans would require careful attention to certain aspects of the treatment. These include tumor stage, and dose, injection route, regimen, and source of BCG. It is not always possible to translate these considerations to human cancer, as immunotherapy is often used for advanced cancer after other forms of treatment have failed. In addition, this model is inappropriate for cases in which intralesional injections are not possible.

An important advance in immunotherapy would be to achieve effective systemic tumor immunity without the intervention of intralesional injection of BCG. We have approached this problem by systematically evaluating the ability of vaccines composed of BCG admixed with tumor cells to protect against disseminated tumor burden.

Immunotherapy for Established Micrometastases with BCG-Tumor Cell Vaccine

Previous attempts at BCG-tumor cell vaccine immunotherapy in both inbred guinea pigs (Bartlett and Zbar, 1972; Bartlett *et al.,* 1976) and man (Sokal *et al.,* 1972, 1973) have been limited and somewhat discouraging, and relatively little has been done to determine the optimal conditions for vaccination. With the protocol shown in Figure 1B, we investigated several variables, such as the ratio of viable BCG organisms to tumor cells, the freezing procedures, X-ray treatment of cells, and vaccination regimen. Although these factors cannot possibly be investigated systematically in man for ethical reasons, they can be studied in the guinea pig model. Our studies demonstrate that under defined conditions, nontumorigenic vaccines of BCG and tumor cells can cure the majority of animals with lethal, disseminated tumor established as visceral micrometastases.

An intravenous dose of 10^4 line 10 tumor cells does not routinely lead to the death of all guinea pigs. Approximately 25% of the animals may survive clean injections, i.e., whereby leakage to the regional site does not occur. This inoculum is the optimal dose for assessing both the influence of the nonspecific side effects of vaccination on tumor cell arrest, extravasation, and establishment in organs, and the immunologically specific effects of the vaccine. Thus, animals were vaccinated at either one and seven or four and ten days after intravenous injection of 10^4 line 10 tumor cells.

Several modes of vaccination as well as two ratios of viable BCG to tumor cells were tested in guinea pigs injected intravenously with line 10 cells. The BCG-tumor cell ratios were 10^8 or 10^6 BCG admixed with 10^7 line 10 cells. These were administered as either a single vaccination, a single injection of BCG-line 10 vaccine followed six days later by an intralesional injection of line 10 cells into the previous vaccination site, a single injection of BCG-line 10 vaccine followed six days later by line 10 cells alone on the opposite side, or two separate injections of BCG-line 10 vaccine. Also, the efficacy of frozen line 10 cells was compared with that of fresh line 10 cells. The results are shown in Table 2.

Table 2. *Survival of Guinea Pigs Injected Intravenously with Syngeneic Line 10 Hepatocarcinoma Cells**

| | | No. of Survivors/No. of Animals IV Tumor Cell Dose/Vaccination Time† | | | |
| | | 10^4 | | 10^5 | 10^6 |
Treatment	Day	1 & 7	4 & 10	1 & 7	1 & 7
None		3/12	...	0/10	0/10
Single vaccination					
(10^8 BCG)(10^8 BCG)		3/12	3/10	0/10	0/10
(10^7 L10)(10^7 L10)		2/10	...	0/10	0/10
(10^6 BCG + 10^7 L10)‡		4/10	4/10	1/10	0/10
(10^8 BCG + 10^7 L10)‡		2/10	...	2/10	0/10
Single vaccination + line 10 intralesionally					
(10^6 BCG + 10^7 L10)(10^7 L10)		8/10	8/10	1/10	0/10
(10^8 BCG + 10^7 L10)(10^7 L10)		9/10	9/10	5/10	1/10
(10^8 BCG + 10^7 FL10§)(10^8 BCG + 10^7 FL10)		8/10	...	5/10	...
Single vaccination + line 10 contralateral					
(10^6 BCG + 10^7 L10)(10^7 L10)		10/10	10/10	1/10	0/10
(10^8 BCG + 10^7 L10)(10^7 L10)		10/10	9/10	8/10	5/10
Two sequential vaccinations					
(10^6 BCG + 10^7 L10)(10^6 BCG + 10^7 L10)		10/10	10/10	1/10	1/10
(10^8 BCG + 10^7 L10)(10^8 BCG + 10^7 L10)		9/10	10/10	9/10	6/10
(10^8 BCG + 10^7 FL10)(10^8 BCG + 10^7 FL10)		...	...	9/10	...

* Experiments were evaluated 240 days after intravenous tumor cell injection. All animals in nontreated and single-vaccination control groups died: those that received 10^4 intravenous tumor cell dose, at 120 days; 10^5, at 95 days; and 10^6, at 77 days. Significance of difference in survival was calculated by the Fisher exact test (two-tailed).

† Days after intravenous injection of tumor.

‡ Administered as single injections. All other treatments administered six days apart.

§ Frozen line 10 cells.

Compared with the untreated tumor-bearing guinea pigs, no significant difference in survival was detected in animals treated with two intradermal injections of BCG or tumor cells alone, regardless of whether the first treatment was performed one or four days after intravenous injection of line 10 cells. Single BCG plus line 10 vaccinations at ratios of 1:10 or 10:1 did not confer significantly greater protection than vaccinations of BCG alone, tumor cells alone, or no treatment. Compared with the survival rates for animals that received single vaccinations of BCG plus tumor cells, BCG alone, or tumor cells alone, or no treatment, survival rates were significantly better for tumor-bearing guinea pigs that received second vaccinations of either tumor cells administered intralesionally ($p < .03$) or on the opposite side ($p < .01$), or BCG-line 10 mixture ($p < .01$). From 80% to 100% of the animals in these treatment groups survived, regardless of whether the first vaccine was administered one or four days after tumor cell injection. Also, no significant differences in efficacy between fresh and frozen line 10 cells were detected.

At 280 days, representative animals from the groups that received 10^4 line 10 cells intravenously were either tested for tumor immunity, measured by ability to reject intradermal challenge of 10^6 line 10 cells, or killed for gross and histologic examination of residual tumor. In none of the animals did autopsy results indicate evidence of residual tumor. Tumor challenge groups varied in their abilities to reject contralateral challenge. All nontreated controls and the groups that had been treated with BCG or tumor cells alone failed to reject contralateral challenge, indicating that these animals were not tumor-immune at 280 days after treatment. Seventy percent to 90% of the survivors in the various multiple-vaccination groups rejected contralateral challenge; however, no significant difference in tumor immunity, as measured by contralateral challenge, could be detected among these treatment groups. These data demonstrate that animals that survived after treatment with ineffective modes of vaccination were not tumor-immune, whereas significant protection as well as long-term tumor immunity was conferred on those animals that received efficacious modes of vaccination.

Intravenous injections of 10^5 or 10^6 syngeneic line 10 cells are routinely fatal to strain 2 guinea pigs. Survival is a function of the BCG-line 10 cell ratio (Table 2). However, without exception, in guinea pigs given 10^5 or 10^6 cells intravenously, a vaccine containing BCG and line 10 cells in a ratio of 10:1 yielded significant protection, whereas a ratio of 1:10 was ineffective. Thus, the ratio of viable BCG organisms to tumor cells is a critical factor in the efficacy of the vaccine. No significant difference in protection could be detected when the group that received a single BCG plus line 10 (10:1) injection was compared with a similar treatment group that received a second line 10 injection intralesionally. In contrast, the survival rate was improved for those animals that received a second injection of line 10 alone or BCG plus line 10 on the opposite side ($p < .02$ or $< .01$, respectively). In two groups of animals injected intravenously with 10^5 line 10 cells, no significant difference in protection was detected when frozen-thawed line 10 cells were used in the vaccine in place of the fresh cells.

We next investigated whether multiple BCG plus line 10 vaccinations at either the 10:1 or 1:10 ratio would increase the number of survivors in comparison with single or two sequential vaccinations. Guinea pigs were injected intravenously with 10^6 line 10 cells and vaccinated either 1 day, 1 and 7 days, or 1, 7, and 14 days after intravenous tumor cell inoculation. The treatments consisted of (1) a single vaccination of BCG plus line 10, followed by injection of line 10 alone or combined with BCG; (2) two simultaneous vaccinations of BCG plus line 10, followed by two simultaneous injections of line 10 alone or combined with BCG; or (3) three sequential vaccinations of BCG plus line 10. The results are shown in Table 3.

Initial BCG plus line 10 vaccinations at a ratio of 1:10 were ineffective, regard-

Table 3. *Survival of Guinea Pigs Injected Intravenously with 10^6 Syngeneic Line 10 Hepatocarcinoma Cells: Effect of Multiple Vaccinations**

Treatment	Survival†
None	0/13
(10^6 BCG + 10^7 L10)‡	0/10
(10^8 BCG + 10^7 L10)‡	0/10
(10^6 BCG + 10^7 L10)(10^7 L10)	0/10
2(10^6 BCG + 10^7 L10) 2(10^7 L10)	3/9
(10^8 BCG + 10^7 L10)(10^7 L10)	3/10
2(10^8 BCG + 10^7 L10) 2(10^7 L10)	6/10
(10^6 BCG + 10^7 L10)(10^6 BCG + 10^7 L10)	1/10
2(10^6 BCG + 10^7 L10) 2(10^6 BCG + 10^7 L10)	1/10
(10^8 BCG + 10^7 L10)(10^8 BCG + 10^7 L10)	5/10
2(10^8 BCG + 10^7 L10) 2(10^8 BCG + 10^7 L10)	6/10
(10^8 BCG + 10^7 L10)(10^8 BCG + 10^7 L10)(10^8 BCG + 10^7 L10)	4/9

* Experiment was evaluated 120 days after intravenous tumor injection. All animals in non-treated and single-vaccination control groups died by 80 days. Significance of differences in survival calculated by Fisher exact test (two-tailed).

† No. of survivors/total no. of animals.

‡ Administered as single injections. All other treatments administered six days apart.

less of the vaccination schedule. Significant protection ($p < .01$) was achieved with all initial vaccinations at ratios of 10:1, but no significant increase in survival rate was achieved with multiple or sequential vaccinations.

One important consideration was whether BCG-immune guinea pigs could generate effective tumor immunity after BCG plus line 10 vaccination. Normal guinea pigs as well as guinea pigs previously immunized to BCG and shown to be reactive to purified protein derivative (PPD) by skin testing were injected intravenously with 10^5 line 10 cells. In this particular experiment, vaccinations were performed four and ten days after intravenous tumor cell inoculation. Two modes of vaccination, BCG plus line 10 (10:1) at days 4 and 10, and BCG plus line 10 (10:1) at day 4 followed by intralesional injection of line 10 at day 10, were compared in PPD-reactive and PPD-anergic guinea pigs. Regardless of whether the animals were PPD-reactive, the two modes of vaccination conferred significant protection ($p < .01$) and did not differ significantly from each other (Table 4).

Another important question was whether the treatment would be effective in animals that have tumor immunity. In one experiment, this question was approached by an attempt to use the BCG plus line 10 (10:1) vaccine to boost immunity in guinea pigs previously cured of 10^5 or 10^6 intravenously injected line 10. Animals were rechallenged eight months after the first treatment. The results demonstrated that whereas tumor-immune guinea pigs cannot reject an intravenous challenge of 4×10^6 line 10 cells, 50% will survive this challenge if boosted with BCG plus line 10 vaccine (administered on days 1 and 7 after tumor challenge). Fifty percent can reject an intravenous challenge of 10^6 line 10 cells, but 70% of those boosted with the vaccine can reject the challenge. All animals can reject intradermal challenge of 10^6 line 10 cells.

Table 4. *Survival of Guinea Pigs Injected Intravenously with 10^5 Line 10 Hepatocarcinoma Cells: Effectiveness of Vaccination in BCG-Immune Guinea Pigs**

Treatment at 4 and 10 Days	PPD[†] Sensitivity	Survival[‡]
None	−	0/10
	+	0/10
(10^8 BCG + 10^7 L10) (10^8 BCG + 10^7 L10)	−	5/10
	+	6/10
(10^8 BCG + 10^7 L10) (10^7 L10 intralesionally)	−	2/10
	+	6/10

* Guinea pigs were injected intradermally with 10^8 BCG and were skin tested with PPD 21 days after immunization. Two weeks later, animals were injected intravenously with 10^5 line 10 cells. Experiment was terminated 270 days after tumor injection. All nontreated control animals died by 128 days after tumor injection. Significance of differences in survival calculated by Fisher exact test (two-tailed).
† Purified protein derivative.
‡ No. of survivors/no. of animals.

To determine if the therapeutic effect of BCG plus line 10 treatment is associated with specific tumor immunity, animals injected intravenously with 10^5 line 10 cells were treated with a vaccine of BCG and syngeneic line 1 hepatocarcinoma. This tumor, although syngeneic in strain 2 guinea pigs, will regress upon intradermal transplantation of 10^6 cells in contrast to the progressive growth of line 10. In some respects, it would be analogous to an allogeneic tumor of similar histologic type in man. The results of this treatment (Table 5) demonstrate that no therapeutic effect on line 10 can be achieved with vaccines containing line 1 tumor cells. This experiment also demonstrates that tissue culture-maintained or frozen-thawed line 10 cells are equally as effective as ascites form

Table 5. *Survival of Guinea Pigs Injected Intravenously with 10^5 Syngeneic Line 10 Hepatocarcinoma Cells: Comparison of Various Preparations and Radiation Doses*

Treatment	Tumor Cell Irradiation Dose (R)	Survival* Vaccination Days[†] 1 & 7	Survival* Vaccination Days[†] 4 & 10
None	. . .	0/10	. . .
(10^8 BCG + 10^7 L1[‡])(10^8 BCG + 10^7 L1)	20,000	0/10	. . .
(10^8 BCG + 10^7 TC§ L10)(10^8 BCG + 10^7 TC L10)	20,000	10/10	. . .
(10^8 BCG + 10^7 L10)(10^8 BCG + 10^7 L10)	12,000	10/10	10/10
	20,000	10/10	8/10
(10^8 BCG + 10^7 FL10 #)(10^8 BCG + 10^7 FL10)	12,000	7/8	9/10
	20,000	10/10	9/10

* No. of survivors/total no. of animals.
† After intravenous injection of tumor cells.
‡ Line 1 hepatocarcinoma, a regressor syngeneic hepatocarcinoma with weak antigenic cross-reactivity with line 10 progressor hepatocarcinoma.
§ Tissue culture-maintained cells, which are tumorigenic in strain 2 guinea pigs.
# Frozen line 10 cells.

line 10 cells, and that there is no appreciable difference in the efficacy of the BCG plus line 10 vaccine if the tumor cells are irradiated with 12,000 R or 20,000 R.

Immunotherapy with BCG plus Tumor Cell Vaccine after Surgery

The most critical evaluation of therapy with BCG plus line 10 vaccine would be in guinea pigs with both regional and disseminated tumor. By the protocol shown in Figure 1C, guinea pigs were injected intradermally with 10^6 line 10 cells (day 0) and intravenously with 10^5 line 10 cells on day 11. Treatment was started on day 12. One group of animals was injected intralesionally with BCG; the skin tumor and superficial distal axillary node were surgically excised in a second group; and the remaining animals were treated with BCG-ascites form line 10 vaccine after the skin tumor and superficial distal axillary node were excised. All animals treated with intralesional BCG or surgery alone died (Fig. 4); however, the median survival was longer for the surgery treatment group. Approximately 30% of the animals treated with the combination of surgery and BCG plus line 10 vaccine survived. Preliminary results of another experiment using this same protocol, but with 10^4 tumor cells injected intravenously, suggest that 60% to 70% of the animals will survive after surgery and vaccine treatment, whereas no animals will survive after surgery alone.

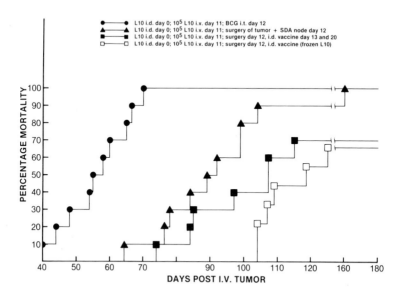

Figure 4. Percentage cumulative mortality for guinea pigs with regional and disseminated micrometastases, injected intradermally with 10^6 line 10 cells and on day 11, intravenously with 10^5 line 10 cells. On day 12, animals received either intralesional BCG injection, surgery, or surgery and BCG plus line 10 vaccine on days 13 and 20. Nine to ten animals per group. SDA, superficial distal axillary.

This indicates that surgery plus vaccine treatment (protocol, Fig. 1C) compared with intralesional BCG followed by surgery (protocol, Fig. 1A) is therapeutic at a greater (tenfold) minimal tumor burden.

Many of the animals that died in the surgery and vaccine treatment groups had tumor growth in the proximal axillary lymph nodes and cervical nodes as well as pulmonary metastases. This suggests that an even better survival rate may have been achieved for this treatment group if surgical excision of draining lymph nodes had been more extensive.

A second study was done to compare intralesional BCG, surgery, and surgery plus vaccine treatment in animals with only regional skin tumor and lymph node metastases. The results are shown in Figure 5. One of nine animals survived after intralesional BCG treatment. Six of nine animals survived after surgery of the skin tumor and the regional, superficial distal axillary node. The remaining animals died of metastases beyond the superficial distal axillary node. Long-term survival of all animals occurred when treatment consisted of surgery and subsequent immunotherapy with BCG plus line 10 vaccine. This, again, strongly supports the possibility that vaccine treatment can be effective against minimal lymph node metastases, both in the region of a primary tumor as well as in pulmonary lymph nodes. These points need to be more thoroughly evaluated in animals in which skin tumors have been present longer than 12 days, and in which surgery alone is a less effective treatment.

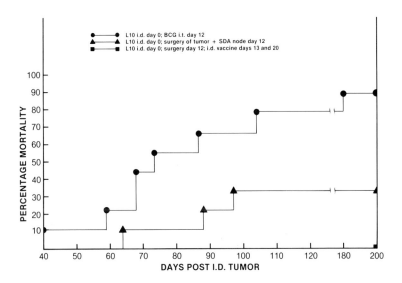

Figure 5. Percentage cumulative mortality for guinea pigs with regional line 10 tumor in the skin and limited lymph node metastases, injected intradermally with 10^6 line 10 cells and on day 11, intravenously with 10^5 line 10 cells. On day 12, animals received either intralesional BCG injection, surgery, or surgery and BCG plus tumor cell vaccine on days 13 and 20. Nine to ten animals per group. SDA, superficial distal axillary.

DISCUSSION

In this study, we have shown that visceral and lymph node micrometastases can be eliminated by induced tumor immunity, whether elicited through an intralesional injection of BCG or by the systemic effect of a tumor cell-BCG vaccine. Furthermore, it is clear from these data that the nontumorigenic vaccine, under certain defined conditions, is effective in controlling and eliminating micrometastases in this syngeneic guinea pig tumor system, regardless of whether the animals exhibit prior immunity to BCG or tumor antigens. At the outset, it should be stated that this experimental model has a major limitation in that it employs a transplantable tumor established for a short time in normal guinea pigs, and the system, of necessity, does not take into account such factors as variations in the biologic behavior of tumors of other histologic types and individual variations in the hosts. Thus, the model can be used to answer only specific questions about the immunotherapy for micrometastases.

Under natural conditions, the development of metastases is dependent on an interplay of the host and the tumor cells. The process is highly selective and represents the end point of a host-tumor interaction that few tumor cells survive. Only a few tumor cells within the primary neoplasm may actually invade blood vessels, and of those, even fewer will survive in the circulation. Similarly, not all malignant cells that survive transport are successfully arrested and undergo extravasation and so on. Also, tumor cells, in principle, could be susceptible to host immune and nonimmune defense mechanisms, which could destroy malignant cells during any of the steps described above (Fidler, 1976; Fidler and Nicolson, 1976).

Metastases were artificially induced in guinea pigs by intravenous injection of line 10 tumor cells, and treatment was not started until adequate time had elapsed to ensure extravasation and localization of tumor cells into the parenchyma of visceral organs. No significant differences in the effectiveness of vaccines were found when the treatment was started one or four days after tumor cell transplantation. It has been demonstrated previously with intravenous injection of B16 melanoma in mice (Fidler, 1970) that, between one and four hours after intravenous transplantation, there is a 50% reduction in the number of arrested tumor cells in the lung, and at 24 hours, only 2% of the cells are retained in the lung as a stable metastatic population. Thus, the results of any treatment administered prior to 24 hours after transplantation are impossible to interpret because beneficial effects could be due to prevention of metastases rather than treatment. In the present study, the lack of difference between various effective vaccines when treatment was administered one or four days after transplantation suggests that a therapeutic effect indeed was achieved with these vaccinations.

Of the two basic BCG-tumor cell vaccines used in this study, the preparation consisting of 10^8 viable BCG organisms admixed with 10^7 tumor cells was more effective for a broad range of increasing initial tumor burdens. Whether this 10:1 BCG-tumor cell ratio is critical or simply a function of total BCG cannot be determined from the study. It is interesting to note, however, that in the study of effectiveness of BCG-tumor cell mixtures as vaccines against LSTRA murine leukemia (Bartlett *et al.,* 1976), the proportion of immune mice was high (100%) if the BCG:LSTRA ratio was low (either $5 \times 10^4{:}10^3$ or $5 \times 10^6{:}10^5$), and the proportion was low (8%) if the ratio was high ($5 \times 10^6{:}10^3$).

Tumor cells that were frozen by an established procedure used for preservation of bone marrow in transplantation studies, and assessed as an optimal procedure in several low-temperature biology studies were as effective as fresh tumor cells in the vaccines. Tissue culture-maintained line 10 cells also were effective in the vaccines. Although in one study, there was no significant difference between vaccine tumor cells X-irradiated with 12,000 R and those with 20,000 R, the selected irradiation dose used in all of the therapy studies was 20,000 R. It is interesting to note that in a limited study with another syngeneic tumor (line 1), we have a suggestion that the immunity induced by the vaccine is tumor-specific. The fact that the line 1 tumor in this tumor model may be analogous in some respects to allogeneic tumors in humans questions the appropriateness of some of the clinical vaccination procedures in which allogeneic tumor cells are used.

Of the basic vaccination schedules tested, the two that were consistently effective for all tumor burdens were injection of 10^8 BCG admixed with 10^7 line 10 cells, followed by injection of 10^7 line 10 alone on the opposite side, and two separate injections of 10^8 BCG admixed with 10^7 line 10. The fact that BCG was not required in the second injection of the former schedule and the fact that multiple vaccinations did not improve therapy with respect to the latter schedule or with a less effective vaccine (10^6 BCG plus 10^7 line 10) suggest that the critical aspect of all the vaccination schedules is the initial dose of BCG.

We have demonstrated that a nontumorigenic vaccine, either alone or in combination with surgery, can effect immunotherapy. Furthermore, the induced tumor immunity, which can cure the majority of guinea pigs with micrometastatic disease, is achieved by two vaccinations administered during a period of one week, requiring a total of 2×10^7 tumor cells. This is equivalent to approximately 20 mg of tumor. Also, the tumor cells, when frozen under established optimal conditions or when maintained in tissue culture, possess the degree of immunogenicity required for efficacious vaccines.

Of the three experimental models investigated, the systems that provided localized tumor with regional lymph node metastases as well as visceral micrometastases most closely approximate the clinical reality. In these experimental systems, intralesional BCG injection followed by surgical excision of localized tumor and regional lymph nodes (protocol, Fig. 1A) and surgery followed by BCG-tumor cell vaccine treatment (protocol, Fig. 1C) both induced effective tumor immunity. It is interesting to compare these two treatment modalities with respect to initial tumor burdens and difference in survival time compared with untreated control animals. Among guinea pigs treated with intralesional BCG and surgery, the differences in survival rate between untreated control animals and animals receiving 10^5, 10^4, or 10^3 tumor cells intravenously were 0%, 25%, and 75%, respectively. Among guinea pigs treated with surgery and two vaccinations, the differences in survival rate between untreated animals and animals receiving 10^5 or 10^4 tumor cells intravenously were 30% and approximately 60%, respectively (preliminary data). These results suggest that limited surgery and vaccination is therapeutic in animals with greater disseminated tumor burdens. Additional studies are needed to test this point further, and future approaches will include more extensive surgical excision of the lymph node chain and variation of the vaccination schedules.

ACKNOWLEDGMENT

This research was sponsored by the National Cancer Institute, contract NO1-CO-25423, with Litton Bionetics, Inc.

REFERENCES

Bartlett, G. L., Purnell, D. M., and Kreider, J. W. 1976. BCG inhibition of murine leukemia: Local suppression and systemic tumor immunity require different doses. Science, 191:229–301.

Bartlett, G. L., and Zbar, B. 1972. Tumor-specific vaccine containing *Mycobacterium bovis* and tumor cells: Safety and efficacy. J. Natl. Cancer Inst., 48:1709–1726.

Black, M. M., Leis, H. P., Shore, B., and Zachrau, R. E. 1974. Cellular hypersensitivity to breast cancer. Assessment by a leukocyte migration procedure. Cancer, 33:952–958.

Everson, T. C., and Cole, H. W. (eds.). 1966. Spontaneous Regression of Cancer. Philadelphia, W. B. Saunders Co.

Fidler, I. J. 1970. Metastasis: Quantitative analysis of distribution and fate of tumor emboli labeled with ^{125}I-5-iodo-2'-deoxyuridine. J. Natl. Cancer Inst., 45:773–782.

Fidler, I. J. 1976. Patterns of tumor cell arrest and development. In Weiss, L. (ed.): Fundamental Aspects of Metastasis. New York, American Elsevier, pp. 276–289.

Fidler, I. J., and Nicolson, G. L. 1976. Organ selectivity for implantation and growth of B16 melanoma variant tumor lines. J. Natl. Cancer Inst., 57:1199–1202.

Gutterman, J. U., Mavligit, G., McBride, C., Frei, E., and Hersh, E. M. 1973a. Immunoprophylaxis of malignant melanoma with systemic BCG: Study of strain, dose and schedule. Natl. Cancer Inst. Monogr., 39:205–212.

Gutterman, J. U., McBride, C., Freireich, E. J, Mavligit, G., Frei, E., and Hersh, E. M. 1973b. Active immunotherapy with BCG for recurrent malignant melanoma. Lancet, 1:1208–1212.

Hanna, M. G., Jr., and Peters, L. C. 1975. Efficacy of intralesional BCG therapy in guinea pigs with disseminated tumor. Cancer, 36:1298–1304.

Hanna, M. G., Jr., Peters, L. C., and Fidler, I. J. 1976. The efficacy of BCG-induced tumor immunity in guinea pigs with regional and systemic malignancy cancer. Cancer Immunol. Immunother., 1:171–177.

Hanna, M. G., Jr., Snodgrass, M. J., Zbar, B., and Rapp, H. 1973. Histopathology of tumor regression after intralesional injection of *Mycobacterium bovis*. IV. Development of immunity to tumor cells and BCG. J. Natl. Cancer Inst., 51:1897–1908.

Hanna, M. G., Jr., Zbar, B., and Rapp, H. J. 1972. Histopathology of tumor regression after intralesional injection of *Mycobacterium bovis*. I. Tumor growth and metastasis. J. Natl. Cancer Inst., 48:1441–1455.

Leibo, S. P., Farrant, J., Mazur, P., Hanna, M. G., Jr., and Smith, L. H. 1970. Effects of freezing on marrow-stem cell suspensions: Interactions of cooling and warming rates in the presence of PUP, sucrose and glycerol. Cryobiology, 6:315–332.

Lewis, M. G., Ikonopisov, R. L., Nairn, R. C., Phillips, T. M., Fairley, G. H., Bodenbam, D. C., and Alexander, P. 1969. Tumour-specific antibodies in human malignant melanoma and their relationship to the extent of the disease. Br. Med. J., 3:547–552.

Mazur, P., Leibo, S. P., Farrant, J., Chu, E. H. Y., Hanna, M. G., Jr., and Smith, L. H. 1970. Interactions of cooling rate, warming rate, and protective additive on the survival of frozen mammalian cells. In Wolstenholme, G. E. W., and O'Connor, M. (eds.): The Frozen Cell. London, Churchill, pp. 69–85.

McKneally, M. F., Maver, C., and Kausel, H. W. 1976. Regional immunotherapy of lung cancer with intrapleural BCG. Lancet, 1:377–379.

Morton, D. L., Eilber, E. R., Joseph, W. L., Trahan, E., and Ketcham, A. S. 1970. Immunological factors in human sarcomas and melanomas: A rational basis for immunotherapy. Ann. Surg., 172:740–749.

Morton, D. L., and Malmgren, R. A. 1969. Human osteosarcomas—Immunologic evidence suggesting an associated infectious agent. Science, 162:1279–1281.

Pinsky, C., Hirshaut, Y., and Oettgen, H. 1973. Treatment of malignant melanoma by intratumoral injection of BCG. Natl. Cancer Inst. Monogr., 39:225–228.

Rapp, H. J., Churchill, W. H., Jr., Kronman, B. S., Rolley, R. T., Hammond, W. G., and Borsos, T. 1968. Antigenicity of a new diethylnitrosamine-induced transplantable guinea pig hepatoma: Pathology and formation of ascites variant. J. Natl. Cancer Inst., 41:1–11.

Salmon, S. E. 1977. Immunotherapy of cancer: Present status of trials in man. Cancer Res., 37:1245–1248.

Seigler, H. F., Shingleton, W. W., Metzgar, R. S., Buckley, C. E., III, and Bergoc, T. M. 1973. Immunotherapy in patients with melanoma. Ann. Surg., 178:352–359.

Sokal, J. E., Aungst, C. W., and Grace, J. T., Jr. 1973. Immunotherapy of chronic myelocytic leukemia. Natl. Cancer Inst. Monogr., 39:195–198.

Sokal, J. E., Aungst, C. W., and Han, T. 1972. Use of bacillus Calmette-Guérin as adjuvant in human cell vaccines. Cancer Res., 32:1584–1589.

Zbar, B., Bernstein, I. D., Bartlett, G. L., Hanna, M. G., Jr., and Rapp, H. J. 1972. Immunotherapy of cancer: Regression of intradermal tumors and prevention of growth of lymph node metastases after intralesional injection of living *Mycobacterium bovis* (bacillus Calmette-Guérin). J. Natl. Cancer Inst., 49:119–130.

Zbar, B., and Tanaka, T. 1971. Immunotherapy of cancer: Regression of tumors after intralesional injection of *Mycobacterium bovis*. Science, 172:271–273.

Zbar, B., Wépsic, H. T., Rapp, H. J., Borsos, T., Kronman, B. S., and Churchill, W. H., Jr. 1969. Antigenic specificity of hepatomas induced in strain-2 guinea pigs by diethylnitrosamine. J. Natl. Cancer Inst., 43:833–841.

Immunotherapy of Human Cancer,
The University of Texas System Cancer Center
M. D. Anderson Hospital and Tumor Institute.
Raven Press, New York © 1978.

Immunotherapy for Tumors with Microbial Constituents or Their Synthetic Analogues. A Review

Edgar Ribi, Ph.D., Charles A. McLaughlin, D.V.M., Ph.D.,
John L. Cantrell, Ph.D., Werner Brehmer, M.D.,*
Ichiro Azuma, Ph.D.,† Yuichi Yamamura, M.D.,†
S. Michael Strain, B.S.,‡ Kou M. Hwang, Ph.D.,§
and Raoul Toubiana, Ph.D.#

*National Institutes of Health, National Institute of Allergy and Infectious Diseases, Rocky Mountain Laboratory, Hamilton, Montana; * Robert Koch Institute, Berlin, West Germany; † The Third Department of Internal Medicine, Osaka University Hospital, Osaka, Japan; ‡ Hamilton Biochemical Research Laboratory, Hamilton, Montana; § Department of Developmental Therapeutics, The University of Texas System Cancer Center M. D. Anderson Hospital and Tumor Institute, Houston, Texas; # CNRS Institute de Chimie des Substances Naturelles, Gif sur Yvette, France*

Inoculation of living bacillus Calmette-Guérin (BCG) in doses recommended for the prevention of tuberculosis causes relatively few side effects, and millions of BCG vaccinations have been given without incident. However, occasional, severe reactions have occurred in young children (Brehmer *et al.,* 1977). The use of BCG as a therapeutic agent differs in several respects from its prophylactic use. Effective BCG immunotherapy for cancer requires repeated administrations and relatively large doses, and to be most effective, BCG must be inoculated directly into the tumor masses (Zbar *et al.,* 1976). Complications observed include persistent BCG infection, which can disseminate widely; activation of old, dormant, acid-fast infections; and hypersensitivity reactions (Holmes *et al.,* 1975; Aungst *et al.,* 1975).

Because of the need for more potent, nonviable immunotherapeutic agents that can be given locally and/or systemically without harmful side effects, a major objective of our research effort is to identify and evaluate chemically defined microbial components that are effective antitumor agents. The goals of our research are to (1) circumvent the use of infectious agents, (2) separate active components from potentially antagonistic substances, (3) remove or chemically modify components producing undesirable biologic responses, (4) develop and supply such preparations in a stable and standardized form, and (5) delineate at the cellular and molecular levels the mechanisms of action of microbial components in immunopotentiation.

In experimental models, we found that cell walls from *Mycobacterium tuberculosis* and *M. bovis,* associated with minute droplets of mineral oil in an oil-in-water emulsion, were as effective as viable BCG in protecting mice and monkeys against airborne infection with H37Rv (Ribi *et al.,* 1966b, 1971; Anacker *et al.,* 1967). Cell walls were obtained by disrupting whole cells with a refrigerated pressure cell specially designed for this purpose (Ribi *et al.,* 1959). Physical adherence of microbial components to the oil droplets was an essential feature of active prophylactic preparations (Barclay *et al.,* 1967). BCG cell wall-oil droplet preparations were also at least as effective as viable BCG in inducing regression of established, palpable skin tumors (line 10) of inbred guinea pigs and in eliminating lymph node metastases upon intralesional injection (Zbar *et al.,* 1973): Immunotherapy with 6×10^6 viable units of BCG for six- to seven-day-old line 10 tumors gave a cure rate of 59% (30/51), compared with a 58% (31/53) cure rate obtained with 300 μg of BCG cell-wall oil droplet vaccine for six- to eight-day-old tumors. The line 10 tumor is weakly immunogenic and causes distant metastases, and it is for such tumors that clinically useful immunotherapy must be developed. Doses of viable BCG that cured about half of the line 10 tumors in guinea pigs produced large, ulcerating lesions. Little reaction was produced by doses of BCG cell walls that brought about similar cure rates (Ribi *et al.,* 1973). Tumors also regressed more rapidly with the cell wall preparations than with viable BCG (Zbar *et al.,* 1974). Recently, BCG cell walls in an oil emulsion were used successfully to treat spontaneous ocular squamous cell carcinoma in cattle (Rapp *et al.,* 1975; Kleinschuster *et al.,* 1977).

By fractionating the BCG cell wall, we have obtained components that retain antitumor activity and have the potential advantages of increased potency and reduced allergenicity. To isolate and define mycobacterial cell wall components required for tumor regression, we first digested the cell walls with proteolytic enzymes to remove most of the protein and then exhaustively extracted them with organic solvents to liberate free lipids (Fig. 1). The resulting cell wall skeleton, an insoluble, polymeric mycolic acid-arabinogalactan-mucopeptide, had reduced antitumor activity compared with cell walls. The activity was restored when the cell wall skeleton was combined with trehalose dimycolate (P3), which was obtained from the free lipids of the cell wall (Azuma *et al.,* 1974; Meyer *et al.,* 1974; Ribi *et al.,* 1976a). The fraction P3, which was not active alone, corresponded to cord factor, from which components other than trehalose mycolates have been removed by microparticulate gel chromatography (Ribi *et al.,* 1974). Data from representative experiments are presented in Table 1. Accordingly, 300-μg quantities of untreated cell walls (CW), Lot 182, which contained about 10% protein as determined by the method of Lowry, afforded cures of one half of the animals (group 1). The cell wall skeleton (CWS) prepared from this lot of CW contained only 0.45% protein and cured one third of the animals (group 3). This reduction in antitumor activity was more than offset by adding P3 to the CWS (group 4; 73% cures). The efficacy of the original CW also

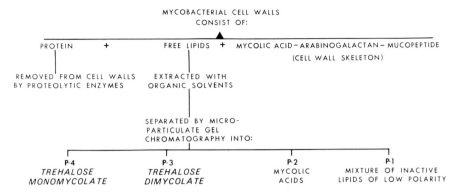

Figure 1. Mycobacterial cell wall fractionation scheme showing origin of cell wall skeleton and P3. (Adapted from Ribi *et al.*, 1976a.)

was improved by combining the CW with P3 (group 2; 75% cures). Another CWS preparation, Lot 176, was inactive alone but upon addition of P3, provided a cure rate of 50% (groups 5 and 6, respectively).

The oil-in-water emulsions for these experiments were prepared by adding a minimal amount of medicinal mineral oil to a mixture of CW or CWS plus P3. This mixture was ground to a paste which, when emulsified with a relatively large volume of saline containing 0.2% Tween 80, formed a stable suspension. In our experience, the minimal effective quantity of oil amounted to 5 μl per milligram of microbial fraction or 0.75 μl of oil per therapeutic dose of 0.4 ml. This volume was sufficient to infiltrate a six-day-old line 10 tumor. Yarkoni (personal communication) found that a dose of 200 μg of CWS, Lot 176, produced 100% (6/6) regression of seven-day-old line 10 tumors in guinea pigs when the quantity of oil used to prepare the emulsion was 60 μl/mg or 12 μl of oil per therapeutic dose. In a repeated test under the same conditions, however, he scored only 6/12 cures (group 7). We confirmed this result: A 300-μg dose of CWS, Lot 182, prepared with a sixfold larger quantity of oil than that used in the emulsion for group 2 (33% cures) led to the cure of all tumor-bearing animals treated (group 8). This larger quantity of oil, however, did not provide a similar high cure rate when used with a tenfold lower dose of CWS, 30 μg (group 9; 56%). It was difficult to prepare stable homogeneous emulsions with large doses of CWS, e.g., 3,000 μg contained in the standard volume of 0.4 ml with as much as 15 μl of oil per dose. The cure rate obtained with the resulting emulsion was poor (group 10; 11% cures). In summary, maximal antitumor activity of CWS is attained by combining CWS with P3 in emulsions containing small quantities of mineral oil (5 to 10 μl/mg or 1.5 to 3 μl of oil per dose of microbial fractions). Combinations of 300 μg of CWS and 300 μg of P3 have been well tolerated by humans in phase I trials (Richman *et al.*, 1977).

We first reported that in the line 10 tumor system, a combination of CWS

Table 1. *Immunotherapy for Line 10 Tumors with Oil Droplet-BCG Cell Wall (CW) and BCG Cell Wall Skeleton (CWS) Emulsions Alone or Combined with Trehalose Dimycolate (P3)*

| Group | Mycobacterial Fraction | Material Associated with Oil Droplets* | | | | No. Cured‡/Total (%) |
		Protein (%)†	Dose (µg)	µl Oil/ mg CW or CWS + P3	µl Oil/Dose/ Animal	
1	CW (Lot 182)	10.00	300	2.5	0.75	11/22 (50)
2	CW (Lot 182) + P3		150 + 150	2.5	0.75	6/8 (75)
3	CWS (Lot 182)	0.45	300	2.5	0.75	5/15 (33)
4	CWS (Lot 182) + P3		150 + 150	2.5	0.75	11/15 (73)§
5	CWS (Lot 176)	1.31	150	2.5	0.75	0/6 (0)
6	CWS (Lot 176) + P3		150 + 150	2.5	0.75	3/6 (50)
7	CWS (Lot 176)		200	60.0	12.00	6/6 (100) # 6/12 (50) #
8	CWS (Lot 182)	0.45	300	20.0	6.00	9/9 (100)
9			30	200.0	6.00	5/9 (56)
10			3,000	15.0	15.0	1/9 (11)
	Oil droplets in Tween-saline		⋯	⋯	0.75	0/44 (0)
			⋯	⋯	6.00	0/9 (0)
			⋯	⋯	15.00	0/9 (0)

* Suspended in 0.4 ml saline containing 0.2% Tween 80 and injected into six-day-old intradermal tumors (10 mm in diameter).
† Determined by Lowry method.
‡ Tumor regression three months after treatment.
§ Difference between groups 3 and 4, $p < 0.05$.
# Yarkoni, personal communication.

and P3 was immunotherapeutically more active than either of the two fractions alone (Ribi *et al.*, 1973); this was confirmed by Bekierkunst *et al.* (1974). At that time, we and these authors prepared the oil-in-water emulsions containing cell walls attached to oil droplets with the aid of a tissue grinder equipped with a Teflon pestle (Ribi *et al.*, 1966a). Recently, Yarkoni *et al.* (1977) described the advantageous use of ultrasonic waves for preparing cell wall-oil droplet vaccines. Whereas ultrasonication is useful for processing untreated cell walls, we found it to be deleterious for preparing vaccines consisting of CWS alone or combined with P3, presumably because of the distinctly different physical properties of CW and CWS. For example, for a given CWS sample (Lot 112274) and P3 sample (Lot D17) tested in parallel, the results (cured/total) with vaccines prepared by grinding were: CWS, 12/28 (45%), and CWS plus P3, 14/18 (78%); and with vaccines prepared by sonication were: CWS, 0/9 (0%), and CWS plus P3, 2/9 (22%). We also noted that the aqueous phase of phenol-water extract from the Re mutant (G30/C21) strain of *Salmonella typhimurium* (Re glycolipid) plus P3 (150 μg and 15 μg, respectively), which consistently provided high cure rates when prepared by the grinding method (see Table 3), was completely inactive when prepared by ultrasonication. We therefore concluded that at present, the standard grinding method is more reliable.

Table 2 lists results of a single experiment designed to compare the tumor-regressive efficacy of CW with that of CWS preparations having different amounts of protein and to determine the skin-reactive properties of these preparations. Again, it was evident that removal of essentially all of the protein from CW did not impair tumor-regressive potency and was paralleled by a reduction of the CW's capacity to sensitize. Only animals whose tumors had been treated with either CW (group 1) or CWS with 1% or more protein (groups 2 and 3) showed necrotic reactions at sites of skin tests performed with the homologous samples. Skin indurations observed 24 hours after injection of the antigens were approximately the same size as the reactions observed seven days after injection (data not shown). The reactions to the CWS preparations containing less than 1% protein are thought to be delayed-type hypersensitivity reactions produced against the peptides of the peptidoglycan portion of the CWS. The reactions to all CW or CWS preparations in normal and treated animals of groups 4 through 7 lacked the necrosis seen in groups 1, 2, and 3. The results of these experiments show the possible benefit of the removal of tuberculoprotein from the cell wall.

We found that P3 combined with CW of *Escherichia coli,* but not CW alone, induced regression of line 10 tumors (about 40%). This led to a reinvestigation of the value of endotoxins known to be powerful microbial adjuvants (Ribi *et al.*, 1975). When endotoxin is used alone, whether injected into the tumor or given intraperitoneally or intravenously, there is a prompt, Shwartzman-like reaction in the tumor, leading to partial regression. The tumor is rarely eliminated, however, and shortly resumes its growth. Thus, as a result of the extensive investigations that followed the early reports, endotoxin has come to be regarded

Table 2. Results of Skin Tests in Strain 2 Guinea Pigs after Treatment of Established Line 10 Tumors with BCG Cell Walls (CWI), or BCG Cell Wall Skeleton (CWS) Alone or Combined with Trehalose Dimycolate (P3)

Group	Mycobacterial Fraction†	Protein (%)‡	Skin Reactions* (diameter of induration, mm)		Cures (%)§
			PPD (1 µg), 24-hr Reaction	Homologous Fractions (100 µg), 7-day Reaction	
1	CW	11.80	5.7	9.2 (necrosis)	56
2	CWS	1.40	3.0	7.5 (necrosis)	33
3	CWS + P3		5.0	8.0 (necrosis)	56
4	CWS	0.51	±	7.0	56
5	CWS + P3		±	8.0	89
6	CWS	0.45	±	7.7	56
7	CWS + P3		±	6.3	67

* Seven-day skin reactions in normal guinea pigs (fraction, protein, induration): CW, 11:80%, 7.6 mm; CWS, 1.40%, 6.0 mm; CWS, 0.51%, 5.3 mm; CWS, 0.45%, 5.3 mm; PPD, negative.
† Mycobacterial fractions associated with oil droplets suspended in 0.4 ml saline containing 0.2% Tween 80 and injected into six-day-old intradermal tumors. 10 µl/mg of microbial fraction or 1.5 µl/dose of 300 µg CW or CWS, and 2.3 µl/dose of 300 µg CWS + 150 µg P3, respectively. The diluent control (0.2% Tween 80 in saline containing oil droplets) at 24 hours produced 5 mm induration without redness, which essentially disappeared at day 7.
‡ Determined by Lowry method.
§ Tumor regression. Nine animals per group.

as essentially worthless for the treatment of tumors (Milner *et al.,* 1971). Work in our laboratory showed that when certain preparations of endotoxin, in combination with P3 and oil droplets, are injected into established malignant tumors, a high rate of cures concomitant with development of specific tumor immunity is obtained. Also, regression occurs much more rapidly than when the tumors are treated with either viable BCG, BCG cell walls, or CWS plus P3, and longer-established tumors may be treated successfully (Ribi *et al.,* 1975, 1976b). In our studies, the tumors treated with the endotoxin preparations disappeared within two weeks, whereas tumors treated with viable BCG ulcerated and needed six weeks to regress and heal. The most powerful endotoxin adjuvants are phenol-water or chloroform-methanol (4:1) extracts from Re (heptoseless) mutant gram-negative bacteria (Ribi *et al.,* 1975, 1976a,b,c; Ribi and Nowotny, unpublished data). These extracts contain endotoxic glycolipids (Re glycolipids).

In recent experiments, the minimal amount of each of these components required for maximal tumor regression was established (Table 3) (McLaughlin *et al.,* 1978d in press). At least 90% of the tumors disappeared when 150 μg Re glycolipid was combined with 15 μg of P3. However, a tenfold reduction of the Re glycolipid to 15 μg in combination with an excess of P3 (150 μg) resulted in total loss of antitumor activity. With 50 μg of Re glycolipid combined with 150 μg of P3, a respectable rate of 65% regression was obtained. Granger *et al.* (1976b) found that P3 caused bovine serum albumin to adhere to oil droplets in our oil-in-water emulsions. McLaughlin *et al.* (1978c in press) have found that the P3 or natural or synthetic cord factor analogues having tumor-regressive activity all have this property, whereas ineffective ones, such as trehalose dipalmitate and trehalose dibehenate, lack it (see also Toubiana *et al.,* 1977).

Table 3. *Regression of Line 10 Tumors in Strain 2 Guinea Pigs: Titration of Dose of Phenol-Water Extract from Re Mutant* Salmonella typhimurium *(Re Glycolipid) and of Trehalose Dimycolate (P3)**

Group	Material Associated with Oil Droplets and Injected into Tumor		No. Cured/No. Treated (%)	p†
	ReGl (μg)	P3 (μg)		
1	150	150	37/40 (93)	< 0.0005 (vs. 7)
2	150	15	37/40 (93)	< 0.0005 (vs. 7)
3	150	5	4/10 (40)	< 0.001 (vs. 7)
4	150	1.5	2/10 (20)	> 0.05 (vs. 7)
5	50	150	13/20 (65)	< 0.0005 (vs. 8)
6	15	150	0/10 (0)	> 0.05 (vs. 8)
7	150	0	5/78 (6.4)	< 0.0005 (vs. 9)
8	0	150	1/217 (0.5)	> 0.05 (vs. 9)
9	Oil droplets in Tween-saline		0/239 (0)	. . .

* Adapted from McLaughlin *et al.,* 1978d in press.
† Determined by two-tailed chi-square contingency table analysis.

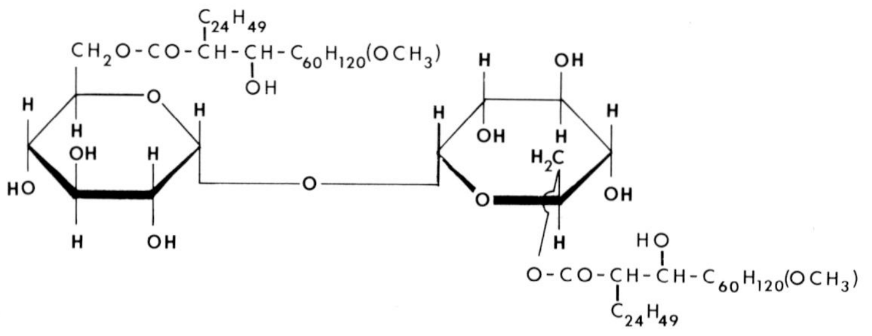

Figure 2. Structure of 6,6-dimycolate of α-D-trehalose ("cord factor").

Purified cord factor (P3) consists of two molecules of mycolic acid esterified to the 6 and 6' positions of α, α-D-trehalose (Noll *et al.,* 1956) (Fig. 2). Mycolic acids are α-branched, β-hydroxy fatty acids of approximately 88 carbon atoms. P3 from all mycobacterial species studied contained a mixture of different mycolic acids that could be liberated by saponification and then chromatographically separated as methyl esters (Ribi *et al.,* 1974; Toubiana *et al.,* 1977). Figure 3 illustrates that, based primarily on results of mass spectrometric analysis, the individual types of mycolic acid vary according to functional groups substituted along the $C_{60}H_{120}$ hydrocarbon chain. These results indicate that P3 is a mixture of components consisting of trehalose molecules to which different pairs of mycolic acids are esterified. P3 isolated from stains of *M. tuberculosis, M. bovis, M. avium,* or *M. phlei* was subjected to trimethylsilylation to permit chromatographic resolution of trehalose dimycolates. Figure 4 shows that samples of trimethylsilylated P3 from virulent strains of human and bovine tubercle bacilli were resolved into six different components based on pairs of α-, β-, and γ-mycolic acids, whereas P3 from avirulent or attenuated strains contained fewer components because of the absence of detectable, β-mycolic, acid-containing diesters (Strain *et al.,* 1977). The lipid composition of mycobacteria might

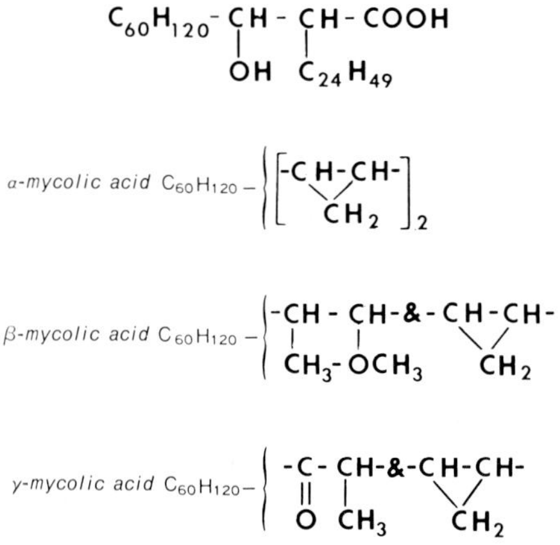

Figure 3. Structure of individual types of mycolic acids (general formula, top) from *M. tuberculosis,* strain Brevannes, varies according to functional groups substituted along the $C_{60}H_{120}$ hydrocarbon chain. (Reproduced from Toubiana *et al.,* 1977, with permission of Springer-Verlag.)

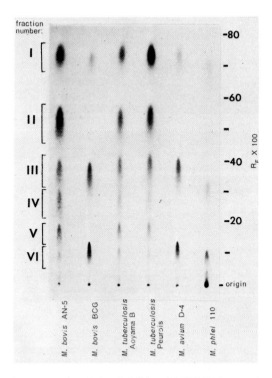

Figure 4. Thin-layer chromatograms of trimethylsilylated (TMS) P3 from various strains of mycobacteria, showing the resolved trehalose dimycolate constituents. Developing solvent, petro-
leum ether-benzene (1:1, v/v). Single components from *M. bovis,* strains AN-5 (fractions I-
VI) and BCG (fractions I, III, and IV), were isolated by preparative thin-layer chromatography.
Components I through VI of *M. bovis* AN-5 were found to contain α , α + β , α + γ , β ,
β + γ, and γ-mycolic acids, respectively; components I, III, and IV of BCG strain contained
α, α + γ, and γ-mycolic acids, respectively. (Reproduced from Strain *et al.,* 1977, with
permission of Academic Press, Inc.).

be important in the pathogenesis of tuberculosis. Conceivably, the variation in
virulence of different mycobacteria may be due to variation in lipid composition
of the mycobacterial cell wall.

The first step in our efforts to learn more about the structural attributes of
mycobacterial trehalose mycolates that play a role in bringing about tumor
immune responses was to determine if a trehalose mycolate containing only
one type of mycolic acid would possess the same high activity displayed by
the naturally occurring, heterogeneous P3 samples. To circumvent the tedious
task of isolating and testing each type of trehalose mycolate from P3, we prepared
semisynthetic trehalose mycolates by condensation of trehalose with individual
mycolic acids isolated from mycobacteria (Toubiana *et al.,* 1977).

Data in Table 4 show the high degree of activity obtained with these partially
synthetic products when combined with Re glycolipid. Cure rates of 85% and
90% were obtained with Re glycolipid combined with 6,6′-trehalose dimycolate

Table 4. *Tumor Regression and Re Glycolipid Binding to Oil Droplets**

Compound Tested	Tumor Regression (%)	^{51}Cr-ReGl in Oil (%)
Naturally occurring		
6,6'-Trehalose dimycolate	90	16
6-Trehalose monomycolate	90	17
Arabinomycolate	80	8
Mycolic acid	90	11
Trehalose	0	1
Synthetic		
6,6'-Trehalose dimycolate (γ-mycolic acid)	85†	19
6-Trehalose monomycolate (γ-mycolic acid)	90†	17
6,6'-Trehalose dibehenylbehenate	60†	16
6,6'-Trehalose dibehenate	35†	3
6-Trehalose monobehenate	15†	0
6,6'-Trehalose dipalmitate	25†	3

* Adapted from McLaughlin *et al.,* 1978c in press.
† Data from Toubiana *et al.,* 1977.

and monomycolate, respectively, containing only γ-mycolic acid. This presented evidence that heterogeneity per se is not important and that activity is not critically dependent on a particular type of mycolic acid (Toubiana *et al.,* 1977). Subsequently, we found arabinose mycolate and free mycolic acid as effective as trehalose mycolates; in combination with Re glycolipid, these compounds cured 80% and 90%, respectively, of the tumors (McLaughlin *et al.,* 1978c in press).

In addition, we tested the synthetic 6,6'-trehalose ester of the 44-carbon behenylbehenic acid prepared by condensation of two molecules of 22-carbon behenic acid. This ester structurally resembles mycolic acid, which is an α-branched, β-hydroxy acid, but contains a shorter hydrocarbon chain and fewer functional groups. Data in Table 4 show that this compound possessed significant activity (cure rate, 60%), but less than that of trehalose mycolates. Synthetic trehalose esters of the shorter, straight chain C_{22} behenic acid and C_{18} palmitic acid displayed only barely significant activity (Toubiana *et al.,* 1977).

Using radiolabeled Re glycolipid, McLaughlin *et al.* (1978c in press) observed that synthetic and naturally occurring trehalose dimycolate and monomycolate, arabinomycolate, mycolic acid, and trehalose dibehenylbehenate enhanced the binding of the Re glycolipid to oil droplets of the oil-in-water emulsions (Table 4). In contrast, the smaller fatty acid esters, which are barely active in the tumor regression assay, did not enhance the binding of the Re glycolipid to oil droplets. It is concluded that for an adjuvant to produce tumor regression when combined with Re glycolipid and for it to enhance binding of Re glycolipid with the oil droplets, the acyl mass of the fatty acid must contain at least 44 carbon atoms and/or have a branched configuration. As envisioned, the acyl

Table 5. *Antitumor Effects of Extracts from Various Sources**

Preparation	No. of Curest/Total (%)	
	Extract Alone, 300 μg	Extract + P3, 300 + 300 μg
S. enteritidis, wild-type, aqueous ether extract (lipopolysaccharide)	0/27 (0)	0/27 (0)
S. minnesota, wild-type, phenol-water extract (lipopolysaccharide)	0/9 (0)	2/9 (22)
S. minnesota, Re mutant, phenol-water extract (glycolipid)	1/15 (7)	13/15 (87)
S. typhimurium, Re mutant, phenol-water extract (glycolipid)	3/23 (13)	26/28 (93)
E. coli, wild-type, phenol-water extract (lipopolysaccharide)	0/40 (0)	7/22 (32)
C. burnetii, wild-type, phenol-water extract (lipopolysaccharide)‡	0/10 (0)	18/30 (60)

* Adapted from Ribi *et al.,* 1976b.
† Line 10 tumor regression.
‡ Nontoxic and weakly pyrogenic (Kelly *et al.,* 1976).

nonpolar region of the fatty acid or fatty acid ester is buried in the oil, with the polar portion projecting into the water to thereby interact with the polar portion of the Re glycolipid. This complex was proposed to serve as a biologically active depot of immunopotentiating microbial substances in vivo.

We have noted consistently that antitumor properties of an endotoxin do not correlate with its toxicity, as measured by lethality in mice and pyrogenicity in rabbits. The lack of correlation between toxicity and antitumor activity is supported by data shown in Table 5. Phenol-water extracts without P3 were almost valueless for tumor therapy, and there was great variability among preparations when combined with P3. A highly toxic material tested, namely a lipopolysaccharide- and protein-rich aqueous ether extract from wild-type *S. enteritidis,* was incapable of causing regression of line 10 tumors (Ribi *et al.,* 1975, 1976a,b). Lipopolysaccharides extracted from wild-type, gram-negative bacteria with aqueous phenol were moderately effective; however, less toxic, lipid-rich glycolipids extracted with aqueous phenol from Re mutant strains of gram-negative bacteria were highly effective in inducing tumor regression. A phenol-water extract of the Q-fever rickettsia, *Coxiella burnetii,* was described by Baca and Paretsky (1974) as a weak endotoxin. However, the sample prepared in our laboratory was not lethal for chick embryos (a sensitive toxicity assay) and was of low pyrogenicity in rabbits (Kelly *et al.,* 1976), but it was markedly effective against tumors when mixed with P3 (cure rate, 60%; Table 5).

One possibly important reason for the inactivity of *S. enteritidis* extract is that it contains the complete O-antigen in a highly immunogenic form, which stimulates rapid antibody production rather than delayed-type hypersensitivity and cell-mediated immunity. The other preparations from wild-type bacteria were obtained by extraction with phenol-water, a rather drastic procedure that is known to degrade the products and result in impaired immunogenicity (Milner *et al.,* unpublished data; Ribi *et al.,* 1976b). The phenol-water-extracted Re glycolipids from Re mutant bacteria, which are deficient in polysaccharide and are poor immunogens (Milner *et al.,* 1971) but are lipid-rich and contain a small amount of firmly bound peptide or denatured protein, would lend themselves to the induction of delayed-type hypersensitivity, as discussed later.

Intraperitoneal doses of glycolipid-containing phenol-water extract from Re mutants of *S. typhimurium* as high as 3,000 μg dissolved in saline were not lethal for mice (Table 6; also see McLaughlin *et al.,* 1978d in press). A potent endotoxin, such as the *S. enteritidis* aqueous ether extract (Fukushi *et al.,* 1964), given in this manner will kill 50% of the mice at a dose level of a few hundred micrograms.

When Re glycolipid was administered in combination with a dose of 50 μg of P3 and incorporated into oil droplets, i.e., in the form in which it is used as an immunotherapeutic agent, a dose of 1,000 μg was not lethal. A dose of 3,000 μg was needed to kill mice. As shown in Table 3, the optimal dose of Re glycolipid plus P3 to induce regression of one-week-old line 10 tumors was 150 μg and 15 μg, respectively.

Even though guinea pigs and mice tolerate doses of Re glycolipid required to induce regression of line 10 tumors, we are continuing to explore the possibility of reducing the toxicity and pyrogenicity of Re glycolipid by means of chemical

Table 6. *Toxicity of Glycolipid-Containing Phenol-Water Extract from Re Mutants of* Salmonella typhimurium *Injected Intraperitoneally into 21-Day-Old RML Mice*

Preparation[†]	Dose (μg)	Oil (μl)	Avg. Body Weight (g) of Mice After Inoculation*		
			Day 1	5	12
S. typhimurium, Re mutant,	100	. . .	12	21	26
phenol-water	300	. . .	12	21	27
extract (ReGl)	1,000	. . .	12	20	25
	3,000	. . .	12	20	25
S. typhimurium, Re mutant,	100 + 50	10	12	22	26
phenol-water extract	300 + 50	12	12	21	26
(ReGl) + P3	1,000 + 50	40	12	17	24
	3,000 + 50	120	12	21‡	25‡
Diluent control	. . .	. . .	16	22	25
	. . .	120	13	21	24

* Six mice per group.
† 0.5-ml volumes containing graded doses of Re glycolipid in aqueous suspension or admixed with P3 and incorporated into oil droplets.
‡ Three mice per group (three died).

and physicochemical modifications while retaining its tumor-regressive properties. Alkaline hydrolysis in aqueous or organic solvents (Niwa *et al.,* 1969) or acetylation with acetic acid anhydride reduced the toxicity of Re glycolipid extracts, as determined by lethality in chick embryos and pyrogenicity in rabbits, but also impaired the tumor-regressive potency. Transesterification of Re glycolipid with sodium methoxide reduced antitumor activity by about one half (50% cures), whereas the toxicity and pyrogenicity were reduced tenfold or more. However, therapy for line 10 tumors with double or quadruple the usual dosage of this modified product did not improve the cure rate. Tentatively at least, we conclude that although there was no direct correlation between endotoxic potency and tumor-regressive activity, a certain level of toxicity may be necessary for antitumor activity.

In all cases tested to date, recovered animals that were immune to rechallenge with a lethal dose of line 10 tumor cells have been found to be hypersensitive to some antigen thought to be nitrogenous in the therapeutic agent (Ribi *et al.,* 1975, 1976a,b). The tuberculoprotein-free mycobacterial cell wall skeleton contains a mucopeptide moiety. Peptides are known to be present also in endotoxic Re glycolipid extracts, against which delayed hypersensitivity might develop. It may be significant that the most prolonged state of pure delayed-type hypersensitivity with associated stimulation of cell-mediated immunity has been induced by either small amounts of native proteins (Salvin, 1958) or denatured proteins or peptides (Gell and Benacerraf, 1959). We suggested that these lipid-rich Re glycolipid extracts to which small amounts of partly denatured protein or peptide are firmly bound, when further associated with P3 or structurally related compounds and oil droplets, should be ideal inducers of delayed hypersensitivity (Ribi *et al.,* 1975). Inasmuch as it takes delayed-type hypersensitivity five days to develop (Granger *et al.,* 1976a), this mechanism probably could not come into play until a few days after intralesional therapy. Early antitumor activity elicited by Re glycolipid may be caused by microvascular damage by the endotoxin. Perhaps Re glycolipid is effective mainly because of its structural similarity to the tumor cell surface (see discussion in Ribi *et al.,* 1976b) and/or because it contains a small amount of proteinaceous antigen most suitable for stimulation of delayed-type hypersensitivity and cell-mediated immunity. Also, endotoxin can directly activate macrophages (Wilton *et al.,* 1975), which could mediate early tumor cell destruction. Consequently, the early and sustained antitumor activity of endotoxin-P3-oil droplet emulsions might be due to a combination of various biologic properties. Presentation of immunopotentiators on oil droplets is thought to result in a persistent source of antigenic stimulation, which produces an influx of the effector cells, resulting in tumor cell destruction and development of tumor-specific immunity.

We shall digress at this point to emphasize the important distinction between suppression and regression of tumors. We showed earlier (Ribi *et al.,* 1973) that P3 alone would produce a marked *suppression* of tumor growth if injected with the tumor cells. However, we are concerned in recent work with *regression,* by which we mean complete and permanent cures of established tumors and lymph node metastases and concomitant development of specific antitumor immunity. P3 alone, which is nonsensitizing and nonimmunogenic, cannot produce regression of line 10 hepatocellular carcinomas in strain 2 guinea pigs, and neither can trehalose dipalmitate nor any of the other synthetic or naturally occurring analogues of cord factor so far examined.

Trehalose dimycolate, including both P3 and cord factor, is granulomatogenic when dissolved and administered in mineral oil to mice (Saito *et al.*, 1976; McLaughlin *et al.*, 1978b in press). The same is true for the simple compound, trehalose dipalmitate (Kato, personal communication; Yarkoni *et al.*, 1973), which did not meet the structural requirements to be successful in the line 10 tumor regression assay (Table 5). Perhaps an intense, nonallergic granuloma is all that is required for tumor suppression, however. Thus, several suppressive and prophylactic phenomena have been attributed to cord factor or trehalose dipalmitate alone. These include resistance to challenge with tubercle bacilli (Bekierkunst *et al.*, 1969) or *Salmonella* (Yarkoni and Bekierkunst, 1976) in mice, suppression of urethan-induced lung adenomas (Bekierkunst *et al.*, 1971) and Ehrlich ascites tumors in mice (Yarkoni *et al.*, 1973), and prevention of tumor growth by cord factor administered alone for L1210 leukemia in mice (Leclerc *et al.*, 1976). We presume, therefore, that the combinations P3 plus Re glycolipid and P3 plus CWS, and CWS alone for that matter, operate by a mechanism similar to that proposed by Hanna and collaborators (Hanna *et al.*, 1972a,b; Snodgrass and Hanna, 1973) when BCG is injected into line 10 tumors. However, in the case with the mentioned microbial fractions, the hypersensitivity granuloma or the related cell-mediated immunity is directed to antigens other than tuberculin, namely, to extracts of lipid-rich compounds to which peptides are firmly attached, as in the case of mycobacterial CWS or Re glycolipids.

We have shown that the nonimmunogenic mixture of trehalose mycolates (P3) can be replaced by a synthetic analogue of simpler structure and lower molecular weight, trehalose dibehenylbehenate, and still retain the tumor-regressive potency (Toubiana *et al.*, 1977). We now report that the immunogenic, adjuvant-active portion of our "complex," the mycobacterial cell wall skeleton or Re glycolipid, also can be replaced by a simple synthetic analogue that consists of bacterial peptidoglycan units, N-acetylmuramyldipeptide, to which either mycolic acid, nocardomycolic acid, or corynomycolic acid is covalently linked (Kusumoto *et al.*, 1976a,b) (see Fig. 5). These lipid-rich compounds enhance cellular immune responses, such as induction of cell-mediated cytotoxicity to mastocytoma P815-X2 in allogeneic mice in vivo, but are less effective in enhancing humoral immunity or helper T cell functions (Yamamura *et al.*, 1976a).

Data in Table 7 show that some of these synthetic "lipopeptides," when mixed with P3 and incorporated into oil droplets, provide a significant cure rate, in some cases up to 70%, when injected into line 10 tumors. It is noteworthy that the tumors regressed at a rate faster than that observed when the animals

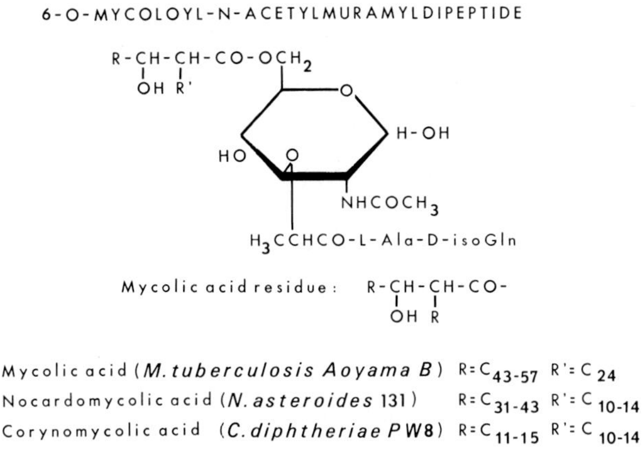
6-O-MYCOLOYL-N-ACETYLMURAMYLDIPEPTIDE
R-CH-CH-CO-OCH2
OH R'
H-OH
HO
NHCOCH3
H3CCHCO-L-Ala-D-isoGln
Mycolic acid residue: R-CH-CH-CO-
OH R
Mycolic acid (M. tuberculosis Aoyama B) R=C43-57 R'=C24
Nocardomycolic acid (N. asteroides 131) R=C31-43 R'=C10-14
Corynomycolic acid (C. diphtheriae PW8) R=C11-15 R'=C10-14

Figure 5. Structure of fatty-acid esters of *N*-acetylmuramyldipeptide. (Reproduced from Azuma *et al.*, 1977.)

were treated with CWS plus P3; the rate of regression compared favorably with that provided by the P3-Re glycolipid combinations.

The smallest adjuvant-active molecule that so far has been found capable of replacing whole mycobacterial cells in Freund's complete adjuvant (killed mycobacterial cells in a water-in-oil emulsion containing an antigen in the water phase) is a synthetic *N*-acetylmuramyldipeptide, prepared first by Mercer *et al.* (1975), and tested by Ellouz *et al.* (1974) and later by Kotani *et al.* (1975). [For more details, see the recent review by Lederer (1977) on natural and synthetic immunostimulants related to the mycobacterial cell wall.] The synthetic

Table 7. *Antitumor Effect of Fatty Acid Esters of Synthetic* N-*Acetylmuramyldipeptides Combined with P3**

Material Associated with Oil Droplets, Injected into Line 10 Tumors	Dose (μg)	No. Cured†/ Total (%)
6-*O*-mycoloyl-*N*-acetylmuramyl-L-alanyl-D-isoglutamine	300	0/9 (0)
6-*O*-mycoloyl-*N*-acetylmuramyl-L-alanyl-D-isoglutamine + P3	300 + 150	2/18 (11)
6-*O*-mycoloyl-*N*-acetylmuramyl-L-seryl-D-isoglutamine + P3	300 + 150	5/10 (50)
6-*O*-nocardomycoloyl-*N*-acetylmuramyl-L-seryl-D-isoglutamine + P3	300 + 150	4/9 (44)
6-*O*-corynomycoloyl-*N*-acetylmuramyl-L-seryl-D-isoglutamine + P3	300 + 150	7/10 (70)
Oil droplets in Tween-saline	...	0/18 (0)

* From Azuma *et al.*, unpublished data. Adjuvant active synthetic fatty acid *N*-acetylmuramyldipeptides were prepared by Azuma *et al.* according to the method described by Kusumoto *et al.*, 1976a.

† Tumor regression two months after treatment.

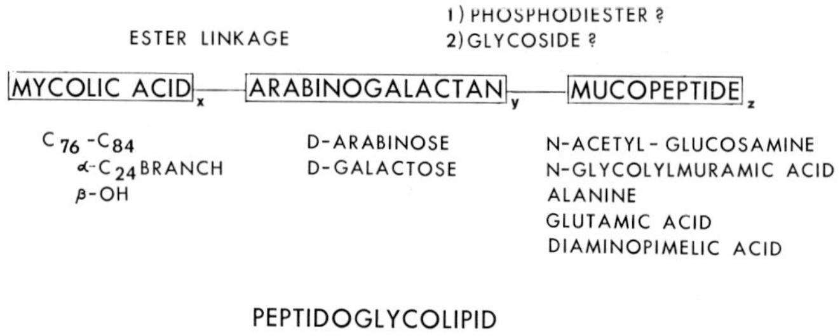

                                                    1) PHOSPHODIESTER ?
                        ESTER LINKAGE   2) GLYCOSIDE ?

MYCOLIC ACID$_x$	ARABINOGALACTAN$_y$	MUCOPEPTIDE$_z$

C_{76}-C_{84}	D-ARABINOSE	N-ACETYL-GLUCOSAMINE
α-C_{24} BRANCH	D-GALACTOSE	N-GLYCOLYLMURAMIC ACID
β-OH		ALANINE
		GLUTAMIC ACID
		DIAMINOPIMELIC ACID

PEPTIDOGLYCOLIPID

Figure 6. Structure of cell wall skeleton existing in the intact cell wall of the tubercle bacillus as an insoluble, complex polymer. (Reproduced from Azuma *et al.,* 1974.)

N-acetylmuramyldipeptide augmented the production of antibodies as well as delayed hypersensitivity to the antigen used. However, it was inactive as an adjuvant for cell-mediated cytotoxicity in allogeneic mice (Azuma *et al.,* 1976a), and it did not enhance in vivo antitumor activity in transplantable tumor systems in syngeneic mice (Juÿ and Chedid, 1975; Azuma *et al.,* 1976a).

N-Acetylmuramyldipeptides replaced the defined, water-soluble, adjuvant-active, mycobacterial cell wall fragments (WSA), which are obtained by lysozyme digestion of cell walls (Adam *et al.,* 1972, 1973; Chedid *et al.,* 1972). A similar product was obtained by autolysis of mycobacteria (Migliore and Jollès, 1972). These products consisted of arabinogalactan linked to peptidoglycan (Fig. 6). Apparently, because of the lack of covalently bound fatty acid of a certain molecular size and/or a particular molecular conformation, WSA did not meet the requirements to qualify as a cancer immunotherapeutic agent. In our experience, WSA (prepared by Pierre Jollès, Ph.D.) or Neo-WSA (prepared and supplied by Wallace Laboratories) alone or in combination with P3, when incorporated into oil droplets, failed to induce regression of line 10 tumors. The same was true for lipid-free peptidoglycan isolated from *Staphylococcus aureus* (Schleifer, 1975).

Subsequent experiments were done to evaluate cell-mediated immunity in guinea pigs cured of tumors by treatment with Re glycolipid admixed with mycobacterial glycolipid (P3) (Cantrell *et al.,* in press). Spleen cells taken from these animals were tested for antitumor activity by means of an adoptive neutralization test in vivo (Winn test). Various concentrations of spleen cells admixed with 10^5 viable line 10 cells were implanted subcutaneously. Control animals were given normal spleen cells admixed with tumor cells or tumor cells only. Passive transfer of spleen cells from animals cured by combinations of P3 with either BCG or Re mutant phenol-water extracts prevented line 10 tumor growth (Table 8). As few as 10^7 immune spleen cells completely prevented the growth of 10^5 tumor cells in about 43% of the animals. The best inhibition of tumor growth (approximately 77%) was observed in animals give 5×10^7 immune cells admixed with 10^5 tumor cells. No inhibition of tumor growth was observed in animals given spleen cells from normal or untreated tumor-bearing guinea

Table 8. *Transfer of Antitumor Activity with Spleen Cells from Line 10 Tumor-Bearing Guinea Pigs Following Immunotherapy**

Source of Spleen Cells	Spleen Cell to Tumor Cell Ratio	No. Without Tumor/Total No. (%) 84 Days after Transfer	*p*†
Normal strain 2 animals	10:1	0/6 (0)	...
	100:1	0/10 (0)	...
	500:1	0/20 (0)	...
Tumor-bearing animals given oil-Tween-saline	500:1	0/18 (0)	...
Tumor-bearing animals given Re ET + P3	10:1	0/5 (0)	...
	100:1	6/13 (43)	< 0.02
	500:1	10/13 (77)	< 0.001
Animals immunized with Re ET + P3 only	500:1	0/5 (0)	...
Challenged controls (10^5 tumor cells only)	...	0/14 (0)	...

* Pooled results from three experiments. Various numbers of spleen cells were admixed with 10^5 line 10 cells and injected subcutaneously into untreated syngeneic animals. Adapted from Cantrell *et al.*, in press.

† Obtained from 2×2 contingency tables; test groups were compared with animals given normal spleen cells admixed with 10^5 line 10 cells.

pigs. Moreover, spleen cells obtained from normal guinea pigs immunized only with Re glycolipid plus P3 and admixed with line 10 tumor cells failed to transfer tumor immunity to normal animals.

In addition, the antitumor activity of spleen cells from immune donors, as measured by adoptive transfer, was abolished following pretreatment with T cell-specific antiserum. Conversely, no significant reduction in antitumor activity was observed when immune spleen cells were treated with B cell-specific antiserum. Preliminary lymphocyte assays in vitro also have demonstrated the presence of cytotoxic lymphocytes in the spleens of animals cured by Re glycolipid plus P3. Hence, cell-mediated tumor immunity is elicited in treated animals cured of line 10 tumors, and immune lymphocytes can effectively transfer systemic tumor immunity to normal recipients. In addition, the transfer of tumor immunity is dependent mainly on the presence of sensitized T cells (Cantrell *et al.*, in press).

To improve the tumor-regressive activity of microbial fractions, it seemed rational to combine the immunopotentiating properties of the microbial extracts with the antitumor toxicity of chemotherapeutic drugs. Such combinations conceivably could be designed to minimize the adverse side effects of each treatment and yet take full advantage of the complementary qualities of both. In collaboration with Eugene Goldberg, Ph.D., we have utilized oil-in-water emulsions of trehalose dimycolates combined with delipidated, deproteinized cell walls from *M. bovis* strain BCG given in conjunction with intralesional chemotherapy with mitomycin C (Table 9). Immunotherapy used in combination with intralesional chemotherapy was statistically more effective than either treatment modality

Table 9. *Regression of Line 10 Tumors in Guinea Pigs Treated with Mitomycin and Cell Wall Skeleton (CWS)**

Dose of Mitomycin Given Day 6 (μg)	Quantity of CWS Combined with 50 μg P3 Given Day 7 (μg)	Tumor Regression (%)
250	0	80
	300	100
100	0	50
	300	80
50	0	17
	300	90
0	300	30
Controls	. . .	0

* From McLaughlin *et al.*, 1978a.

alone ($p < 0.01$). Combined treatment permitted a fivefold reduction of the dose of chemotherapy required for maximal antitumor activities (McLaughlin *et al.*, 1978a). No tissue necrosis was observed with the reduced dose of mitomycin C; thus, a major disadvantage of intralesional chemotherapy was circumvented.

Immunotherapy in the guinea pig model was augmented not only when P3 was combined with Re glycolipid, but also when Re glycolipid was combined with CWS. The latter combination was highly active (cure rate, 93%; Table 10). In consideration of the efficacy of synthetic mycoloyl acetylmuramyldipeptide-P3 described above (Table 7), it was not unexpected that combinations of such synthetic cell wall skeleton analogues combined with Re glycolipid would fare as well (cure rate, 78%). Moreover, because the peptide moiety of the CWS prepared from *Corynebacterium parvum* is identical to that of the mycobacterial CWS and also contains a large amount of covalently bound lipid (Azuma

Table 10. *Immunotherapy for Line 10 Tumors: Effects of Preparations of Cell Wall Skeleton (CWS) from Mycobacteria or Propionibacteria and Glycolipids from Re Mutant Salmonella (ReGl)*

Material Attached to Oil Droplets, Injected into 6-Day-Old Tumors	Dose (μg)	No. Animals Treated	Cured (%)
BCG CWS (Lot 112274)	300	28	29
+ ReGl	150 + 150	27	93
Mycolic acid-*N*-acetylmuramyldipeptide (synthetic)	300	9	0
+ ReGl	300 + 150	9	78
C. parvum CWS* (Lot 313)	300	9	11
+ ReGl	150 + 150	9	55
ReGl (Lot Stm-12)	150	28	0
Vehicle control	. . .	25	0

* Prepared from *C. parvum*, Pasteur Institute strain 4182.

Table 11. *Eradication of Line 10 Tumor Lymph Node Metastases in Strain 2 Guinea Pigs by Immunotherapy at Time of or After Surgery**

Material Injected†	Interval Between Surgery and Immuno- therapy (days)	No. of Tumor Free/ Total Animals	Cured (%)‡	*p*§
Oil droplets	0 #	2/23	9	
P3 + CWS + ReGI	0	9/11	63	< 0.001
		4/10**		
Oil droplets	2††	0/12	0	
P3 + CWS + ReGI	2	10/12	83	< 0.001

* Adapted from Kelly *et al.,* in press.

† Doses containing 300 μg of each microbial component were administered as four 0.1-ml injections intradermally between tumors and draining lymph nodes.

‡ Animals free of detectable tumor 90 days after treatment.

§ Statistical significance determined from 2 × 2 contingency tables and chi-square analysis. Pooled results of two experiments.

Surgery and immunotherapy given day 6.

** Three of the four tumor-free animals did not reject challenge with 10^6 line 10 tumor cells. However, the fourth animal of this group and all other cured animals listed in the table rejected this challenge.

†† Surgery, day 4; immunotherapy, day 6.

et al., 1976b), it was not surprising that, when combined with Re glycolipid, it was markedly effective in inducing regression of line 10 tumors (cure rate, 55%).

A combination of CWS, P3, and Re mutant glycolipid was the most powerful adjuvant-antigen system in the treatment of line 10 tumors. This triple combination not only led to rapid destruction of tumors, but also was successful in treating older, well-metastasized tumors (Ribi *et al.,* 1976b). Data listed in Table 11 show that intracutaneous inoculation of this combination adjacent to the site of the primary line 10 tumors at the time or two days after they were surgically removed retarded or, in some experiments, eliminated metastatic tumor growth (Kelly *et al.,* in press). In similarly performed experiments, these results had not been observed when viable BCG or BCG cell walls were used (Zbar *et al.,* 1976). Based on previous findings by others, it was believed that a microbial immunostimulant, to be effective, had to be injected directly into the tumor or, as we reported recently, injected intradermally between the primary tumor and the draining lymph node prior to surgical excision of the primary tumor (Zbar *et al.,* 1976).

The studies with guinea pigs demonstrating the antitumor efficacy of CWS combined with the Re glycolipid and P3 were extended to a clinical trial in cattle. In collaboration with Ray Woodward, Ph.D. (USDA Livestock Experiment Station, Miles City, Montana), we treated spontaneous carcinomas of the eye with intralesional injections of the triple combination of microbial components. These studies appear promising, but the final results are as yet unavailable. This clinical trial was initiated after preliminary results were obtained from studies wherein three bovines with squamous cell carcinomas of the eye and two horses with equine sarcoids were successfully treated (complete regressions) with either BCG CW or CWS in combination with Re glycolipid (McLaughlin, unpublished data).

We recently have obtained an Investigational New Drug permit for Re glycolipid plus P3 or Re glycolipid plus CWS plus P3. These combinations will be used for phase I trials in humans at M. D. Anderson Hospital and Tumor Institute, Houston, and the University of Minnesota, Minneapolis.

Meanwhile, during the development of more effective microbial immunotherapeutic reagents, clinical trials with CWS in Japan and with the combination of CWS plus P3 in the United States have had encouraging results. Yamamura and co-workers (1975) reported that intralesional therapy with CWS for malignant melanoma nodules was effective in causing tumor regression. In an extensive series of studies on lung cancer, the use of intradermal, intrapleural, and intralesional therapy with CWS, depending on the stage of disease, was reported to have improved the remission and survival durations for patients with stage I to stage IV lung cancer (Yamamura *et al.,* 1976b,c; Yasumoto *et al.,* 1976). In phase I and early phase II trials, BCG CWS or *M. smegmatis* CWS has been combined with P3 in intralesional therapy for metastatic nodules, in intrapleural therapy for patients with pleural effusions from breast cancer, and in intradermal therapy in conjunction with chemotherapy for patients with metastatic breast cancer. Maximally tolerated doses of CWS plus P3 have been established for these three routes of administration, and preliminary analysis of the data indicates that this therapy is effective (Richman *et al.,* 1977; Vosika *et al.,* 1977). Thus, a number of clinical assay systems by which the purified microbial subcomponents can be evaluated are available. Furthermore, if man responds in a manner similar to the guinea pig, as in the case of treatment with CWS plus P3, treatment of human tumors with Re glycolipid plus CWS plus P3 might also be superior.

REFERENCES

Adam, A., Ciorbaru, R., Petit, J.-F., and Lederer, E. 1972. Isolation and properties of a macromolecular, water-soluble, immuno-adjuvant fraction from the cell wall of *Mycobacterium smegmatis.* Proc. Natl. Acad. Sci. USA, 69:851–854.

Adam, A., Ciorbaru, R., Petit, J., Lederer, E., Chedid, L., Lamensans, A., Parant, F., Parant, M., Rosselet, J., and Berger, F. M. 1973. Preparation and biological properties of water-soluble adjuvant fractions from delipidated cells of *Mycobacterium smegmatis* and *Nocardia opaca.* Infect. Immun., 7:855–861.

Anacker, R. L., Barclay, W. R., Brehmer, W., Larson, C. L., and Ribi, E. 1967. Duration of immunity to tuberculosis in mice vaccinated intravenously with oil-treated cell walls of *Mycobacterium bovis* strain BCG. J. Immunol., 98:1265–1273.

Asselineau, J. 1966. The Bacterial Lipids. Paris, Hermann, p. 174.

Aungst, C. W., Sokal, J. E., and Jager, B. V. 1975. Complications of BCG vaccination in neoplastic disease. Ann. Intern. Med., 82:666–669.

Azuma, I., Ribi, E. E., Meyer, T. J., and Zbar, B. 1974. Biologically active components from mycobacterial cell walls. I. Isolation and composition of cell wall skeleton and P3. J. Natl. Cancer Inst., 52:95–101.

Azuma, I., Sugimura, K., Taniyama, T., Yamawaki, M., Yamamura, Y., Kusumoto, S., Okada, S., and Shiba, T. 1976a. Adjuvant activity of mycobacterial fractions: Adjuvant activity of synthetic N-acetylmuramyldipeptide and the related compounds. Infect. Immun., 14:18–27.

Azuma, I., Sugimura, K., Yamawaki, M., Uemiya, M., Yoshimoto, T., Yamamura, Y., Kusumoto, S., Okada, S., and Shiba, T. 1977. Adjuvant and antitumor activities of synthetic 6-0-"mycoloyl"-N-acetyl-L-alanyl-D-isoglutamine. In: Proceedings, Twelfth US-Japan Tuberculosis Research Conference. NIH, NIAID, US-Japan Cooperative Medical Science Program, pp. 398–424.

Azuma, I., Taniyama, T., Sugimura, K., Aladin, A., and Yamamura, Y. 1976b. Mitogenic activity of the cell walls of mycobacteria, nocardia, corynebacteria and anaerobic coryneforms. Jpn. J. Microbiol., 20:263–271.

Baca, O. G., and Paretsky, D. 1974. Partial chemical characterization of a toxic lipopolysaccharide from *Coxiella burnetii.* Infect. Immun., 9:959–961.

Barclay, W. R., Anacker, R. L., Brehmer, W., and Ribi, E. 1967. Effects of oil-treated mycobacterial cell walls on the organs of mice. J. Bacteriol., 94:1736–1745.

Bekierkunst, A., Levij, I. S., Yarkoni, E., Vilkas, E., Adam, A., and Lederer, E. 1969. Granuloma formation induced in mice by chemically defined mycobacterial fractions. J. Bacteriol., 100:95–102.

Bekierkunst, A., Levij, I. S., Yarkoni, E., Vilkas, E., and Lederer, E. 1971. Suppression of urethan-induced lung adenomas in mice treated with trehalose-6,6-dimycolate (cord factor) and living bacillus Calmette Guérin. Science, 174:1240–1242.

Bekierkunst, A., Wang, L., Toubiana, R., and Lederer, E. 1974. Immunotherapy of cancer with non-living BCG and fractions derived from mycobacteria: Role of cord factor (trehalose-6,6'-dimycolate) in tumor regression. Infect. Immun., 10:1044–1050.

Brehmer, W., Falkenberg, N., Hussels, H., Otto, H.-S., Preussler, H., and Waldschmidt, J. 1977. Regional suppurative lymphadenitis after BCG vaccination. Dtsch. Med. Wochenschr., 102:89–92.

Cantrell, J. L., Ribi, E., and McLaughlin, C. A. 1978. Passive transfer of tumor immunity with spleen cells from guinea pigs cured of hepatocarcinoma by nonspecific immunotherapy. Cancer Immunol. Immunother. (in press).

Chedid, L., Parant, M., Parant, F., Gustafson, R. H., and Berger, F. M. 1972. Biological study of a nontoxic, water-soluble immunoadjuvant from mycobacterial cell walls. Proc. Natl. Acad. Sci. USA, 69:855–858.

Ellouz, F., Adam, A., Ciorbaru, R., and Lederer, E. 1974. Minimal structural requirements for adjuvant activity of bacterial peptidoglycan derivatives. Biochem. Biophys. Res. Commun., 59:1317–1325.

Fukushi, K., Anacker, R. L., Haskins, W. T., Landy, M., Milner, K. C., and Ribi, E. 1964. Extraction and purification of endotoxin from Enterobacteriaceae: A comparison of selected methods and sources. J. Bacteriol., 87:391–400.

Gell, P. G., and Benacerraf, B. 1959. Studies on hypersensitivity. II. Delayed hypersensitivity to denatured proteins in guinea pigs. Immunology, 2:64–70.

Granger, D. L., Brehmer, W., Yamamoto, K., and Ribi, E. 1976a. Cutaneous granulomatous response to BCG cell walls with reference to cancer immunotherapy. Infect. Immun., 13:543–553.

Granger, D. L., Yamamoto, K., and Ribi, E. 1976b. Delayed hypersensitivity and granulomatous response after immunization with protein antigens associated with a mycobacterial glycolipid and oil droplets. J. Immunol., 116:482–488.

Hanna, M. G., Zbar, B., and Rapp, H. J. 1972a. Histopathology of tumor regression after intralesional injection of *Mycobacterium bovis.* I. Tumor growth and metastasis. J. Natl. Cancer Inst., 48:1441–1455.

Hanna, M. G., Zbar, B., and Rapp, H. J. 1972b. Histopathology of tumor regression after intralesional injection of *Mycobacterium bovis.* II. Comparative effects of vaccinia virus, oxazolone, and turpentine. J. Natl. Cancer Inst., 48:1697–1707.

Holmes, E. C., Eilber, F. R., and Morton, D. L. 1975. Immunotherapy of malignancy in humans. JAMA, 232:1052–1055.

Juÿ, D., and Chedid, L. 1975. Comparison between macrophage activation and enhancement of nonspecific resistance to tumors by mycobacterial immunoadjuvants. Proc. Natl. Acad. Sci. USA, 72:4105–5109.

Kelly, M. T., Granger, D. L., Ribi, E., Milner, K. C., Strain, S. M., and Stoenner, H. G. 1976. Tumor regression with Q fever rickettsia and a mycobacterial glycolipid. Cancer Immunol. Immunother., 1:187–191.

Kelly, M. T., McLaughlin, C. A., Ribi, E., and Zbar, B. 1978. Eradication of microscopic lymph node metastases of the guinea pig line 10 tumor after intradermal injection of endotoxin plus mycobacterial components. Cancer Immunol. Immunother. (in press).

Kleinschuster, S. J., Rapp, H. J., Leuker, D. C., and Kainer, R. A. 1977. Regression of bovine ocular carcinoma by treatment with a mycobacterial vaccine. J. Natl. Cancer Inst., 58:1807–1814.

Kotani, S., Watanabe, Y., Kinoshita, F., Shimono, T., Morisaki, T., Shiba, T., Kusumoto, S., Tarumi, Y., and Ikenaka, K. 1975. Immunoadjuvant activities of synthetic N-acetyl-muramylpeptides or amino acids. Biken J., 18:105–111.

Kusumoto, S., Okada, S., Shiba, T., Azuma, I., and Yamamura, Y. 1976a. Synthesis of 6-0-mycoloyl-N-acetylmuramyl-L-alanyl-D-isoglutamine with immunoadjuvant activity. Tetrahedron Lett., 47:4287–4290.

Kusumoto, S., Tarumi, Y., Ikenaka, K., and Shiba, T. 1976b. Chemical synthesis of N-acetyl-muramylpeptides of cell wall partial structure and their analogs in relation to immunoadjuvant activity. Bull. Chem. Soc. Jpn., 19:533–539.

Leclerc, C., Lamensans, A., Chedid, L., Drapier, J. C., Petit, J. F., Wietzerbin, J., and Lederer, E. 1976. Nonspecific immunoprevention of L1210 leukemia by cord factor (6,6'-dimycolate of trehalose) administered in a metabolizable oil. Cancer Immunol. Immunother., 1:227–232.

Lederer, E. 1977. Natural and synthetic immunostimulants related to the mycobacterial cell. In: Medicinal Chemistry V (Proceedings of the Fifth International Symposium on Medicinal Chemistry). Amsterdam, Elsevier Scientific Publishing Co., pp. 257–279.

McLaughlin, C. A., Cantrell, J. L., Ribi, E., and Goldberg, E. 1978a. Intratumor chemotherapy with mitomycin C and components from mycobacteria in regression of line 10 tumors in guinea pigs. Cancer Res., 38:1311–1316.

McLaughlin, C. A., Parker, R., Hadlow, W. J., Toubiana, R., and Ribi, E. 1978b. Structural moieties of mycobacterial lipids required for producing granulomatous reactions. Cell. Immunol. (in press).

McLaughlin, C. A., Ribi, E. E., Goren, M. B., and Toubiana, R. 1978c. Tumor regression induced by defined microbial components in an oil-in-water emulsion is mediated through their binding to oil droplets. Cancer Immunol. Immunother. (in press).

McLaughlin, C. A., Strain, S. M., Bickel, W. D., Goren, M. B., Azuma, I., Milner, K., Cantrell, J. L., and Ribi, E. 1978d. Regression of line 10 hepatocellular carcinomas following treatment with aqueous-soluble microbial extracts combined with trehalose or arabinose mycolates. Cancer Immunol. Immunother. (in press).

Mercer, C., Sinay, P., and Adam, A. 1975. Total synthesis and adjuvant activity of bacterial peptido-glycan derivatives. Biochem. Biophys. Res. Commun., 66:1316–1322.

Meyer, T. J., Ribi, E., Azuma, I., and Zbar, B. 1974. Biologically active components from mycobacter-ial cell walls. II. Suppression and regression of strain-2 guinea pig hepatoma. J. Natl. Cancer Inst., 52:103–111.

Migliore, D., and Jollès, P. 1972. A hydrosoluble, adjuvant-active mycobacterial "polysaccharide-peptidoglycan." Preparation by a simple extraction technique of the bacterial cells (strain peurois). FEBS Lett., 25:301–304.

Milner, K. C., Rudbach, J. A., and Ribi, E. 1971. Microbial toxins. A comprehensive treatise. In Weinbaum, G., Kadis, S., and Ajl, S. J. (eds.): Bacterial Endotoxins. General Characteristics. New York, Academic Press, vol. 4, pp. 1–65.

Niwa, M., Milner, K. C., Ribi, E., and Rudbach, J. A. 1969. Alteration of physical, chemical, and biological properties of endotoxin by treatment with mild alkali. J. Bacteriol., 97:1069–1077.

Noll, H., Bloch, H., Asselineau, J., and Lederer, E. 1956. The chemical structure of the cord factor of *Mycobacterium tuberculosis.* Biochim. Biophys. Acta, 20:299–309.

Rapp, H. H., Kleinschuster, S. J., Lueker, D. C., and Kainer, R. A. 1975. Immunotherapy of experimental cancer as a guide to treatment of human cancer. Ann. NY Acad. Sci., 276:550–556.

Ribi, E., Anacker, R. L., Barclay, W. R., Brehmer, W., Harris, S. C., Leif, W. R., and Simmons, J. 1971. Efficacy of mycobacterial cell walls as a vaccine against airborne tuberculosis in the rhesus monkey. J. Infect. Dis., 123:527–538.

Ribi, E., Anacker, R. L., Brehmer, W., Goode, G., Larson, C. L., List, R. H., Milner, K. C., and Wicht, W. C. 1966a. Factors influencing protection against experimental tuberculosis in mice by heat-stable cell wall vaccines. J. Bacteriol., 92:869–879.

Ribi, E. E., Granger, D. L., Milner, K. C., and Strain, S. M. 1975. Tumor regression caused by endotoxins and mycobacterial fractions (Brief Communication). J. Natl. Cancer Inst., 55:1253–1257.

Ribi, E., Larson, C., Wicht, W., List, R., and Goode, G. 1966b. Effective nonliving vaccine against experimental tuberculosis in mice. J. Bacteriol., 91:975–983.

Ribi, E., Meyer, T. J., Azuma, I., and Zbar, B. 1973. Mycobacterial cell wall components in tumor suppression and regression. Natl. Cancer Inst. Monogr., 39:115–119.

Ribi, E., Milner, K. C., Granger, D. L., Kelly, M. T., Yamamoto, K., Brehmer, W., Parker, R., Smith, R. F., and Strain, S. M. 1976a. Immunotherapy with nonviable microbial components. Ann. NY Acad. Sci., 277:228–238.

Ribi, E., Milner, K., Kelly, M. T., Granger, D., Yamamoto, K., McLaughlin, C. A., Brehmer, W., Strain, S. M., Smith, R. F., and Parker, R. 1976b. Structural requirements of microbial agents for immunotherapy of the guinea pig line-10 tumor. In Lamoureux, G., Turcotte, R., and Portelance, V. (eds): BCG in Cancer Immunotherapy. New York, Grune and Stratton, pp. 51–61.

Ribi, E., Parker, R., and Milner, K. C. 1974. Microparticulate gel chromatography accelerated by centrifugal force and pressure. In Glick, D. (ed.): Methods of Biochemical Analysis. New York, John Wiley and Sons, vol. 22, pp. 355–400.

Ribi, E., Perrine, T., List, R., Brown, W., and Goode, G. 1959. Use of pressure cell to prepare cell walls from mycobacteria. Proc. Soc. Exp. Biol. Med., 100:647–649.

Ribi, E., Takayama, K., Milner, K., Gray, G. R., Goren, M., Parker, R., McLaughlin, C., and Kelly, M. 1976c. Regression of tumors by an endotoxin combined with trehalose mycolates of differing structure. Cancer Immunol. Immunother., 1:265–270.

Richman, S. P., Gutterman, J. U., Hersh, E. M., and Price, H. R. 1977. Phase I study of intratumor immunotherapy with BCG cell wall skeleton plus P3 (Abstract). Proc. Am Assoc. Cancer Res. Am. Soc. Clin. Oncol., 18:351.

Saito, R., Tanaka, A., Sugiyama, K., Azuma, I., Yamamura, Y., Kato, M., and Goren, M. B. 1976. Adjuvant effect of cord factor, a mycobacterial lipid. Infect. Immun., 13:776–781.

Salvin, S. B. 1958. Occurrence of delayed hypersensitivity during the development of Arthus type hypersensitivity. J. Exp. Med., 107:109–124.

Schleifer, K. H. 1975. Chemical structure of the peptidoglycan, its modifiability and relation to the biological activity. Z. Immunitaetsforsch., 149:104–117.

Snodgrass, M. J., and Hanna, M. G., Jr. 1973. Ultrastructural studies of histiocyte-tumor cell interactions during tumor regression after intralesional injection of *Mycobacterium bovis.* Cancer Res., 33:701–716.

Strain, S. M., Toubiana, R., Ribi, E., and Parker, R. 1977. Separation of the mixture of trehalose 6,6′-dimycolates comprising the mycobacterial glycolipid fraction, "P3." Biochem. Biophys. Res. Commun., 77:449–456.

Toubiana, R., Ribi, E., McLaughlin, C., and Strain, S. M. 1977. The effect of synthetic and naturally occurring trehalose fatty acid esters in tumor regression. Cancer Immunol. Immunother., 2:189–193.

Vosika, G., Schmidtke, J., Parker, R., Ribi, E., and Gray, G. 1977. Phase I study of *Mycobacterium smegmatis* cell wall skeleton (CWS) immunotherapy (Abstract). Proc. Am. Assoc. Cancer Res. Am. Soc. Clin. Oncol., 18:318.

Wilton, J. M., Rosenstreich, D. L., and Oppenheim, J. J. 1975. Activation of guinea pig macrophages by bacterial lipopolysaccharide requires bone marrow-derived lymphocytes. J. Immunol., 114:388–393.

Yamamura, Y., Azuma, I., Sugimura, K., Yamawaki, M., Uemiya, M., Kusumoto, S., Okada, S., and Shiba, T. 1976a. Adjuvant activity of 6-0-mycoloyl-N-acetylmuramyl-L-alanyl-D-isoglutamine. Gann, 67:867–877.

Yamamura, Y., Azuma, I., Taniyama, T., Sugimura, K., Hirao, F., Tokuzen, R., Okabe, M., Nakahara, W., Yasumoto, K., and Ohta, M. 1976b. Immunotherapy of cancer with cell wall skeleton of *Mycobacterium bovis*-bacillus Calmette-Guérin: Experimental and clinical results. Ann. NY Acad. Sci., 277:209–227.

Yamamura, Y., Ogura, T., Yoshimoto, T., Nishikawa, H., Sakatani, M., Itoh, M., Masuno, T., Namba, M., Yazaki, H., Hirao, F., and Azuma, I. 1976c. Successful treatment of the patients with malignant pleural effusion with BCG cell-wall skeleton. Gann, 67:669–677.

Yamamura, Y., Yoshizaki, K., Azuma, I., Yagura, T., and Watanabe, T. 1975. Immunotherapy of human malignant melanoma with oil-attached BCG cell wall skeleton (BCG CWS). Gann, 66:355–363.

Yarkoni, E., and Bekierkunst, A. 1976. Nonspecific resistance against infection with *Salmonella typhi* and *Salmonella typhimurium* induced in mice by cord factor (trehalose-6,6′-dimycolate) and its analogues. Infect. Immun., 14:1125–1129.

Yarkoni, E., Bekierkunst, A., Asselineau, J., Toubiana, R., Toubiana, M. J., and Lederer, E. 1973. Suppression of growth of Ehrlich ascites tumor cells in mice pretreated with synthetic analogs of trehalose-6-6′-dimycolate (cord factor). J. Natl. Cancer Inst., 51:717–720.

Yarkoni, E., Rapp, H. J., and Zbar, B. 1977. Immunotherapy of a guinea pig hepatoma with ultrasonically prepared mycobacterial vaccines. Cancer Immunol. Immunother., 2:143–146.

Yasumoto, K., Manabe, H., Ueno, M., Ohta, M., Iida, A., Nomoto, K., Azuma, I., and Yamamura, Y. 1976. Immunotherapy of human lung cancer with BCG cell-wall skeleton. Gann, 67:787–795.

Zbar, B., Ribi, E., Kelly, M., Granger, D., Evans, C., and Rapp, H. J. 1976. Immunologic approaches to the treatment of human cancer based on a guinea pig model. Cancer Immunol. Immunother., 1:127–137.

Zbar, B., Ribi, E., Meyer, T. J., Azuma, I., and Rapp, H. J. 1974. Immunotherapy of cancer. Regression of established intradermal tumors after intralesional injection of mycobacterial cell walls attached to oil droplets. J. Natl. Cancer Inst., 52:1571–1577.

Zbar, B., Ribi, E., and Rapp, H. J. 1973. An experimental model for immunotherapy of cancer. Natl. Cancer Inst. Monogr., 39:3–6.

Immunotherapy of Human Cancer,
The University of Texas System Cancer Center
M. D. Anderson Hospital and Tumor Institute.
Raven Press, New York © 1978.

Actions and Interactions of *Corynebacterium parvum* in Experimental Tumor Systems

Lester J. Peters, M.D.

Section of Experimental Radiotherapy, The University of Texas System Cancer Center M. D. Anderson Hospital and Tumor Institute, Houston, Texas

In 1964, Halpern *et al.* reported that injection of killed vaccines of *Corynebacterium parvum* into mice caused marked reticuloendothelial stimulation; soon afterwards, a tumor-inhibitory effect of the vaccine was demonstrated (Woodruff and Boak, 1966; Halpern *et al.,* 1966). Since then, *C. parvum* and several other closely related anaerobic coryneforms, probably best classified as *Propionibacterium* sp. (Johnson and Cummins, 1972), have been studied in a large variety of experimental protocols, with two basically separate yet overlapping aims: to elucidate the mechanisms of antitumor action of the organisms, and to provide pragmatic information (for possible clinical application) as to their usefulness alone or in combination with other forms of cancer therapy.

In this summary of the important actions and interactions of *C. parvum* in experimental tumor systems, I use the term *C. parvum* to include organisms variously designated *C. granulosum, C. liquefaciens,* or *P. acnes* by the authors of the literature cited. Although differences, especially in potency, among the strains used by different investigators undoubtedly exist, it is unlikely that there are qualitative differences in their antitumor activities (O'Neill *et al.,* 1973).

MODES OF ACTION

C. parvum is an immunostimulant capable of increasing the resistance of animals to a variety of tumors and infective agents in an immunologically nonspecific way (see Halpern, 1975). A large body of evidence points to macrophage "activation" as the mechanism by which nonspecific resistance is exerted. Peritoneal macrophages from mice treated with *C. parvum* have been shown to destroy or inhibit the growth, in vitro, of syngeneic, allogeneic, and xenogeneic tumor cells, but not of normal cultured fibroblasts (Olivotto and Bomford, 1974; Ghaffar *et al.,* 1974; Scott, 1974a; Basic *et al.,* 1975). Recently, in vivo transfer of antitumor activity by *C. parvum*-stimulated peritoneal exudate cells also has been demonstrated (Peters *et al.,* 1977). Activated macrophages appear capable of exerting both cytostatic and cytocidal activity. Lysis of tumor cells has been demonstrated in vitro, but only after direct and intimate contact between the activated macrophage and the target cell (Basic *et al.,* 1975; Puvion *et al.,* 1976). Hibbs (1974) reported that macrophages activated by bacillus Calmette-Guérin (BCG) or *Toxoplasma* appear to kill target cells by direct exocytosis of lysosomal enzymes into their cytoplasm, and a similar mechanism probably holds for macrophages stimulated by *C. parvum.* Corticosteroids have been shown to inhibit this cytocidal action in vitro (Scott, 1975a), probably by stabilizing the plasma membrane and preventing exocytosis. The mechanism by which cytostasis is achieved is unknown, but the possibility of involvement of a soluble factor appears to have been excluded (Ghaffar *et al.,* 1974). Ando *et al.* (in press) found that the cytostatic effect of *C. parvum* in vivo was reflected in a prolongation of mean cell cycle time (especially G_1 phase) accompanied by a reduction in the growth fraction of a murine squamous cell carcinoma.

Activation of macrophages by *C. parvum* in vivo can be inhibited by sublethal, whole body irradiation prior to *C. parvum* administration (Milas *et al.,* 1974c), but activation occurs normally in T cell-depleted (Bomford and Christie, 1975) and athymic (nude) mice (Ghaffar *et al.,* 1975).

In addition to its nonspecific immunostimulant effect, *C. parvum* is capable of modifying specific immunologic reactivity. High doses of *C. parvum,* systemically administered, have been shown to depress a variety of T cell functions, such as the blastogenic response to phytohemagglutinin, mixed lymphocyte reactions, graft versus host reactivity (Scott, 1972), and skin allograft rejection (Castro, 1974b; Milas *et al.,* 1975a), but Scott and Warner (1976) showed that multiple, "clinical sized" doses of approximately 5 mg/m^2 did not cause this depression. Under certain circumstances, *C. parvum* in fact may stimulate T cell-mediated tumor-specific immunity. This subject is considered further in the discussion of interactions of *C. parvum* with tumor-specific immune responses.

The immune response to *C. parvum* itself may result in antitumor activity under some experimental conditions. Tuttle and North (1975) found that the effect of intralesional *C. parvum* was greatly augmented by prior sensitization of the mice to the organism. This effect appears to depend, at least in part, on cross-reacting antigens between the tumor and *C. parvum* (James *et al.,* 1976), as similar experiments have failed to produce an increased antitumor response in other systems (Scott, 1976). *C. parvum,* itself, is not cytotoxic to tumor cells in vitro (Basic and Milas, unpublished data).

When administered intravenously to humans, *C. parvum* causes a marked pyrexial response (Ossorio *et al.,* 1975), and whole-body hyperthermia has been shown to exert antitumor activity in patients with disseminated disease (Pettigrew *et al.,* 1974). No significant pyrexial response to *C. parvum,* however, has been noted in mice (Milas and Hunter, unpublished data) or rabbits (Roumiantzeff *et al.,* 1975), and induction of hyperthermia is unlikely to account for the antitumor activity in experimental systems. This conclusion is strengthened by the duration of protection afforded by a single dose of *C. parvum* in experimental animals (see following section on immunoprophylaxis).

When interactions between *C. parvum* and chemotherapeutic agents are considered, indirect therapeutic gains may result from protection against opportunistic infections provided by *C. parvum* or by increased tolerance to cytotoxic agents resulting from hemopoietic stimulation (Toujas *et al.*, 1975).

IMMUNOPROPHYLAXIS WITII *C. PARVUM*

Immunoprophylaxis is defined as protection against a tumor challenge, conferred by prior administration of the immune adjuvant. This phenomenon (which has no clinical counterpart) was first described by Woodruff and Boak in 1966 and has since been confirmed in many experimental tumor systems (Fisher *et al.*, 1970; Smith and Scott, 1972; Milas *et al.*, 1974d; Bomford and Olivotto, 1974; Castro, 1974a; Scott, 1974a; van Putten *et al.*, 1975; Yuhas *et al.*, 1975; Halpern *et al.*, 1975). The degree of protection induced by different strains of *C. parvum* correlates with the degree of splenomegaly they induce (McBride *et al.*, 1975), but splenectomy prior to *C. parvum* administration does not significantly reduce its effect (Castro, 1974a; Mazurek *et al.*, 1976). Thus, splenomegaly is simply an index of reticuloendothelial stimulation, and systemic administration, which is more efficient in this regard than subcutaneous injection, has been shown to be relatively more protective (Bomford and Olivotto, 1974; Milas *et al.*, 1974d). Protection (and reticuloendothelial stimulation) is also *C. parvum* dose dependent, at least up to single doses of about 80 mg/m^2. However, multiple small doses, individually ineffective, have been shown to exert a cumulative effect (Milas *et al.*, 1975a; Scott and Warner, 1976). Protection is maximal when the route of tumor cell challenge corresponds with that of *C. parvum* administration (Lamensans *et al.*, 1968), but is consistently more pronounced against intravenous or intraperitoneal than against intramuscular or subcutaneous challenges (Milas *et al.*, 1975b; Yuhas and Ullrich, 1976). In general, tumor protection is not absolute and may be overcome by a sufficiently large number of tumor cells. However, the *relative* protection afforded is greatest with large challenges and is less evident with threshold challenges (Stiffel *et al.*, 1971). In some circumstances, the growth of small tumor cell inocula may even be promoted by *C. parvum* pretreatment (Bomford, 1977). The efficacy of prophylactic *C. parvum* treatment correlates well with tumor immunogenicity, as assayed by the ability to immunize animals with injections of lethally irradiated cells (Smith and Scott, 1972). The duration of protection afforded by a single dose of *C. parvum* has been reported to vary from two weeks or less (Yuhas and Ullrich, 1976; Ando *et al.*, 1977) to 130 days (Milas *et al.*, 1975b), again depending on tumor immunogenicity. Yuhas and Ullrich (1976) showed that both duration and magnitude of protection were less in senescent 22-month-old mice, with impaired immunologic responsiveness, than in three-month-old normal control animals.

IMMUNOTHERAPY WITH *C. PARVUM*

Immunotherapy is defined as the treatment of established tumors by immunologic means. *C. parvum* has shown a therapeutic effect of varying degree on a variety of experimental tumors (Woodruff and Boak, 1966; Likhite and Halpern, 1973; Scott, 1974a,b; Milas *et al.*, 1974b; Fisher *et al.*, 1975b; Tuttle and North, 1975; Suit *et al.*, 1976a; Yuhas and Ullrich, 1976; Sadler and Castro, 1976). The therapeutic effect of *C. parvum* depends largely on whether the agent is injected systemically or intralesionally. In general, systemic administration is capable only of inhibiting the time of appearance or growth rate of transplanted tumors, and complete regressions are rare (Woodruff *et al.*, 1972; Scott, 1974a; Fisher *et al.*, 1975b; Sadler and Castro, 1976; Ando *et al.*, 1977). In an experiment that simulates the clinical situation more closely than most, Yuhas and Ullrich (1976) observed temporary partial regression of autochthonous mammary tumors in aged mice following three intraperitoneal injections of approximately 30 mg/ m^2. Complete regressions of growing tumors in response to systemic *C. parvum* have been seen only with highly immunogenic tumors (Milas *et al.*, 1974b), and even then, the tumor response in individual mice was unpredictable. In contrast, local intralesional injection of *C. parvum* not infrequently induces complete regressions, even in tumors of low immunogenicity (Likhite and Halpern, 1974; Scott, 1974b; Woodruff and Dunbar, 1975). Localized injection of *C. parvum* in the region of, but not directly into, the tumor is much less effective.

Induction of complete regressions, whether by systemic or intralesional injections of *C. parvum*, appears to require an intact T cell system, and is associated with the development of specific tumor immunity. This was demonstrated for intralesional injection by Scott (1974b) and Woodruff and Dunbar (1975). Figure 1 presents data from our laboratory illustrating the T cell dependence of the response to systemic *C. parvum* treatment of a methylcholanthrene-induced fibrosarcoma. Whereas complete and long-term regressions were induced in approximately 25% of normal animals and the growth rate of nonregressing tumors was markedly reduced, *C. parvum* treatment of T cell-depleted mice produced only temporary growth delay, and no regressions occurred. In general, growth restraint, as opposed to complete regression of tumors, following systemic administration of *C. parvum* has been found to be relatively independent of T cell function (Woodruff *et al.*, 1973; Castro, 1974a; Scott, 1974a; Woodruff and Warner, 1977) and is probably due to direct macrophage stimulation by *C. parvum*.

Treatment with *C. parvum* alone is usually most effective if given when the tumor burden is small (i.e., soon after transplantation), but with combined treatment, this maxim does not necessarily hold. As with *C. parvum* prophylaxis, tumor enhancement has been demonstrated when *C. parvum* is given soon after small tumor cell challenges (Bomford, 1977) (Table 1). The efficacy of *C. parvum* therapy also appears to depend on the site of tumor growth, with better responses

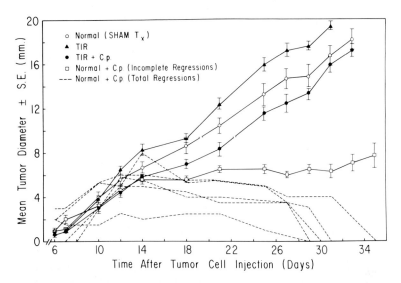

Figure 1. Effect of intravenously administered *C. parvum* on subcutaneous growth of a methyl-cholanthrene-induced fibrosarcoma in normal and T cell-depleted (TIR) mice. *C. parvum* was given at a dose of 0.25 mg (~30 mg/m²) three days after subcutaneous injection of 4 × 10⁵ tumor cells. C.p., *C. parvum* treatment; TIR, thymectomized mice receiving whole-body irradiation and syngeneic bone marrow reconstitution to produce chronic T cell depletion. (Adapted from Peters *et al.*, in press.)

being obtained for the same tumor growing in the lung, skin, or subcutaneous tissue than in the muscle or brain (Milas *et al.*, 1974a; Suit *et al.*, 1976b). As with prophylactic treatment, the therapeutic effect is dose dependent. Whereas multiple small doses can be as effective as a single large dose, multiple high doses have been found to be no more effective but more toxic (Scott, 1974a; Milas *et al.*, 1975b).

Table 1. *Effect of* C. parvum *on Growth of Subcutaneously Transplanted Fibrosarcoma Cells in C₃Hf/Bu Mice: Enhancement with Small Tumor Cell Inocula**

No. of Viable Tumor Cells Injected	Proportion of Mice Accepting Tumor Challenge	
	Untreated	Treated†
125,000	31/32	24/32
25,000	32/32	16/32
5,000	21/32	8/32
1,000	10/32	19/32 ($p < 0.05$)
200	0/16	2/16

* From Peters *et al.*, in press.
† Mice received 0.25 mg *C. parvum* intravenously four days after tumor cell injection.

INTERACTIONS OF C. PARVUM IN EXPERIMENTAL SYSTEMS

Interactions between C. parvum and tumor-specific immune responses, radiation, surgery, chemotherapeutic agents, and heat will be considered. Essentially, two agents may act completely independently, or they may interact with each other in an additive, antagonistic, or synergistic manner. It is sometimes mistakenly inferred that synergism exists whenever the effect of combined treatment with two agents is greater than the sum of the observed effects of the individual agents. However, Figure 2 indicates a hypothetical situation in which two interacting agents individually may produce no tumor cures, but when combined, may produce an appreciable number of cures whether the agents are antagonistic, simply additive in their effects, or truly synergistic. In most systems, it is impossible to resolve which interactive process is occurring without precise information as to the proportion of cells killed by individual treatments (and this information cannot be obtained from gross observations). It is likely on first principles that combinations of immunosuppressive chemotherapy and C. parvum would be antagonistic, and yet these combinations may produce excellent results because the agents have different mechanisms of action and toxicities. From the therapeutic point of view, the usefulness of combinations does not depend fundamentally on whether they are synergistic, simply additive, or even somewhat antagonistic; therefore, these terms have been avoided in the subsequent sections.

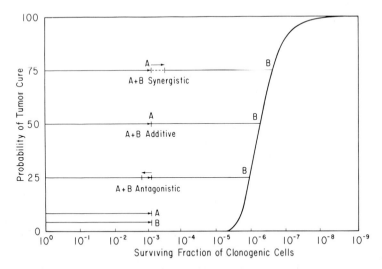

Figure 2. Sigmoid curve indicates probability of local control of a tumor containing 10^6 clonogenic cells as a function of the surviving fraction of these cells after treatment. If two separate treatments, A and B, each reduced the surviving fraction to $10^{-3.08}$, then the effect of A and B interacting additively would be to reduce the surviving fraction to $10^{-6.16}$, giving a mean number of surviving cells per tumor of $10^6 \times 10^{-6.16} = 0.693$, which corresponds to a 50% cure probability. However, the probability of curing a tumor by either treatment alone would be essentially zero, and the clinically desirable end point of curing tumors with combined treatment could occur even if the agents were somewhat antagonistic.

Interactions with Tumor-Specific Immune Responses

Depending on the tumor system studied and possibly on the dose and timing of administration of C. parvum, systemic C. parvum has been shown to augment (Woodruff and Dunbar, 1973; Milas et al., 1975d; Yuhas et al., 1975), depress (Smith and Scott, 1972; Woodruff et al., 1976), or have no effect on (Likhite and Halpern, 1973; Scott, 1975b) the strength of the tumor-specific immune response elicited by injection of inactivated tumor cells, so that no general statement as to the effect of C. parvum by this route is possible. Using the same system in which augmentation of the specific immune response had been demonstrated, Milas et al. (1975d) reported enhancement of concomitant immunity in tumor-bearing animals by systemic C. parvum treatment.

When C. parvum is injected locally admixed with, or in close proximity to, living or killed tumor cells in optimal ratio, it may act as an adjuvant in the generation of tumor-specific immunity (Scott, 1975b; Bomford, 1975; Tuttle and North, 1976), even in systems in which no effect of immunization with tumor cells alone can be demonstrated (Scott, 1975b; Tuttle and North, 1976). Too much C. parvum abrogates this effect, and optimal adjuvant activity has been obtained with low doses (usually less than 0.1 mg). The tumor-specific immunity generated by injection of tumor cells and C. parvum or by intralesional injection of C. parvum generally has been found to be solid (Likhite, 1976). However, Tuttle (personal communication) noted a short, functional life-span of killer T cells in his system, and only memory cells persisted more than 19 days after immunization with C. parvum plus irradiated tumor cells.

As noted already, the therapeutic effect of intralesional C. parvum is almost completely T cell dependent, suggesting that potentiation of specific tumor immunity is its principal mechanism of action by this route. Although systemic C. parvum exerts antitumor activity that is not T cell dependent, its therapeutic effectiveness does correlate with tumor immunogenicity. The reason for this has not been satisfactorily elucidated. Several possibilities exist; e.g., the antitumor action of C. parvum and the specific immune response may be completely independent; the growth-restraining effect of C. parvum may allow the production of immunologically specific killer cells to catch up with the tumor cell burden; or a true interaction between C. parvum and the specific immune response may exist. We have investigated this problem using a strongly immunogenic fibrosarcoma (FSa) which can be made to regress completely by systemic C. parvum administration, but only in T cell-competent animals (Fig. 1). Seemingly paradoxical results have emerged: When evaluated for antitumor activity in a modified Winn assay, separated splenic T cells from tumor-bearing, C. parvum-treated mice were less active than T cells from untreated, tumor-bearing control animals (McBride et al., 1977); but when assayed by adoptive transfer into T cell-depleted, tumor-bearing mice, the T cells showed an increased tumor-inhibitory effect (Peters et al., unpublished data). These findings may be explained by the hypothesis that C. parvum treatment results in augmented production

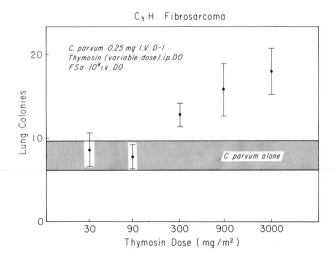

Figure 3. Effect of single doses of thymosin on immunoprophylactic effect of *C. parvum* against intravenously injected fibrosarcoma cells in syngeneic C₃Hf/Bu mice. *C. parvum* was given intravenously at a dose of 0.25 mg (~30 mg/m²) one day before intravenous challenge with 10⁶ fibrosarcoma cells. Thymosin (fraction 5) was given intraperitoneally in varying doses immediately before tumor cell injection. The number of tumor nodules in the lungs 14 days after tumor cell injection was scored. (Peters *et al.*, unpublished data.)

of both killer and suppressor T cells and that the influence of suppressor cells predominates in the Winn assay. Killer T cells, however, may localize more efficiently at the tumor site after adoptive transfer, accounting for the increased antitumor effect observed with this assay.

Because a major part of the response of FSa to systemic *C. parvum* is T cell dependent (see Fig. 1), and because high doses of systemic *C. parvum* lead to thymic atrophy (Castro, 1974b; McBride *et al.*, 1974), Peters *et al.* (unpublished data) investigated the combined effect of treatment with thymosin fraction 5 (Hoffmann-La Roche Inc.) and *C. parvum*. A single injection of thymosin, 600 mg/m² intraperitoneally at times ranging from six days before to five days after *C. parvum* injection (0.25 mg intravenously), did not improve the immunoprophylactic effect of the organism against FSa. Indeed, thymosin given one day after *C. parvum* resulted in a diminution of the protective effect of *C. parvum*. This inhibition was shown to be thymosin dose dependent (Fig. 3), but thymosin doses within the clinical range were not deleterious. Repeated doses of thymosin at 30 mg/m² for seven days beginning one day after *C. parvum* administration resulted in marginal inhibition of the immunoprophylactic effect of *C. parvum* (data not shown).

Interactions with Radiation

Sublethal whole-body irradiation of animals may increase their susceptibility to tumor transplantation, both by suppressing the development of immune resist-

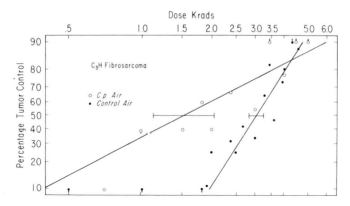

Figure 4. Effect of intravenously administered *C. parvum* on radiocurability of a methyl-cholanthrene-induced fibrosarcoma. *C. parvum* was given intravenously at a dose of 0.25 mg (~30 mg/m²) when tumors reached 6 mm in diameter, and tumors were irradiated with graded doses of gamma rays when 8 mm in diameter. (Adapted from Stone and Milas, 1978.)

ance and, in certain cases, by apparently nonimmunologic means (Peters, 1975). Administration of *C. parvum* prior to, but not after, whole-body irradiation prevents the enhancement of lung colony-forming efficiency resulting from the irradiation (Milas *et al.,* 1974c; Bomford and Olivotto, 1974). A similar effect has been described with respect to local thoracic irradiation (Peters *et al.,* 1978a). The reason for the reduced effectiveness of *C. parvum* when given after irradiation is probably depletion of the pool of stem cells whose proliferation is stimulated by *C. parvum.* Conversely, the effectiveness of *C. parvum* when given before irradiation indicates the radioresistance of *C. parvum*-activated effector cells.

Several investigators have studied the combined effect of *C. parvum* and local-ized tumor irradiation (Milas *et al.,* 1975c; Suit *et al.,* 1976a,b; Stone and Milas, 1978). In general, systemically administered *C. parvum* has been found to produce a major improvement in radiocurability of only immunogenic tumors, and its effect becomes progressively less apparent as the level of tumor control achieved by irradiation alone increases (Suit *et al.,* 1976b). In one study (Fig. 4), *C. parvum* was ineffective in improving the control rate when this reached 80% with radiation alone. This suggests that the actions of *C. parvum* and irradiation are independent, but that the same tumors are resistant to both agents. The timing of *C. parvum* administration with respect to irradiation appears to be important for optimal results: Milas *et al.* (1975c) and Suit *et al.* (1976b) found that *C. parvum* was most effective when given before single radiation doses or early in a course of fractionated irradiation. However, Ullrich and Adams (in press) found that *C. parvum* had an effect only if given after irradiation. It seems likely that the optimal timing of systemic *C. parvum* administration depends on the ability of the tumor to elicit a specific immune rejection response. For tumors capable of eliciting this response, *C. parvum* appears to be most effective when administered in the presence of a sizable antigenic load (i.e., before primary therapy), presumably because it then may stimulate the tumor-specific immune response as well as generate immunologically nonspecific resistance.

Apart from increasing the absolute radiocurability of certain tumors, *C. parvum* has been shown to inhibit the rate of growth of recurrent tumors and to reduce the incidence of metastases in mice with or without local recurrences (Milas *et al.*, 1975c; Suit *et al.*, 1976a). Similarly, using a tumor whose metastasizing ability was increased by local tumor irradiation, Milas *et al.* (1976) found that *C. parvum* treatment prior to irradiation effectively inhibited this enhanced metastatic tumor growth.

Interactions with Surgery

Data concerning interactions of *C. parvum* and surgery are relatively sparse and mainly relate to the incidence of metastasis following surgical removal of transplanted tumors. Systemic *C. parvum* administered before surgical resection has either reduced the incidence of metastases (Sadler and Castro, 1976; Milas *et al.*, 1976) or had no effect (Proctor *et al.*, 1973). Given after surgery, *C. parvum* appears capable of either inhibiting (Proctor *et al.*, 1973) or enhancing (Milas *et al.*, 1976) the incidence of metastases, depending on the tumor system.

Interactions with Chemotherapy

Like irradiation, cancer chemotherapeutic agents may increase the susceptibility of animals to tumor growth, especially when administered before tumor challenge (van Putten *et al.*, 1975). Pretreatment with cyclophosphamide, in particular, has been shown to increase the lung colony-forming efficiency of intravenously injected tumor cells up to 1,000-fold. The ability of *C. parvum* to reverse this enhancement of lung colony-forming efficiency depends on the timing of administration of the two agents (Fig. 5), but at all times, it exerts some protective effect. When *C. parvum* is given in high doses before or concurrently with cyclophosphamide, the toxicity of the drug is increased (Currie and Bagshawe, 1970), probably because the hepatic metabolism of cyclophosphamide is modified. Soyka *et al.* (1976) showed that *C. parvum* inhibits the drug-metabolizing activity of liver microsomes in a time- and dose-dependent fashion. This effect may be of considerable importance in analyzing experimental data because it effectively results in more prolonged exposure of animals to the alkylating metabolites of cyclophosphamide. Peters and Mason (1977) have shown that when liver microsomal enzyme activity is inhibited by chloramphenicol, the enhancement of lung colony-forming efficiency by cyclophosphamide is further increased.

A number of pragmatic experiments have been carried out to investigate the combined effect of *C. parvum* and cyclophosphamide in experimental tumor

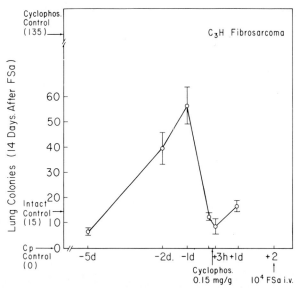

Figure 5. Effect of *C. parvum* on enhancement of lung colony-forming efficiency caused by cyclophosphamide pretreatment of mice. Cyclophosphamide (~450 mg/m²) was given subcutaneously two days before intravenous injection of 10⁴ fibrosarcoma cells. *C. parvum*, 0.25 mg (~30 mg/m²), was given intravenously at varying times with respect to administration of cyclophosphamide. The number of tumor nodules in the lungs 14 days after tumor cell injection was scored. Cp, *C. parvum*; d, day; h, hour.

systems. Most authors have obtained the best results with combined therapy when *C. parvum* was given *after* cyclophosphamide in single-dose experiments (Currie and Bagshawe, 1970; Woodruff and Dunbar, 1973; Pearson *et al.*, 1975) and when given midway between weekly cyclophosphamide doses in multiple-dose experiments (Fisher *et al.*, 1975a; Purnell *et al.*, 1977). The therapeutic effectiveness of cyclical combinations of *C. parvum* and cyclophosphamide was greater than that obtained with a single dose of *C. parvum* plus cyclical cyclophosphamide (Fisher *et al.*, 1975a).

Other chemotherapeutic agents have been less well studied. Houchens *et al.* (1976) reported prolonged survival of mice with transplanted leukemia and solid tumors treated with Adriamycin plus *C. parvum* two days later, compared with Adriamycin alone. Similarly, increased survival of leukemic mice treated with BCNU plus *C. parvum* was reported by Pearson *et al.* (1972, 1974) and with procarbazine plus *C. parvum* by Amiel and Berardet (1970).

Data concerning the combination of corticosteroid therapy and *C. parvum* are conflicting. Scott (1975a) reported impaired antitumor activity in *C. parvum*-stimulated mice treated four days later with a single injection of 2.5 mg cortisone acetate, and Peters *et al.* (unpublished data) found substantial inhibition of

Table 2. *Effect of* C. parvum-*Stimulated Peritoneal Exudate Cells (CpPEC)* on Growth of C₃Hf/Bu Fibrosarcoma in Normal or Cortisol-Treated† Syngeneic Mice‡*

Cell Challenge	Treatment	Proportion of Mice with Tumors	Median Days' Survival Time (Range)
10^4 FSa	None	9/10	35 (23–49)§
	Cortisol	9/9	18 (13–24)
10^4 FSa + 10^6 CpPEC	None	0/10	...§
	Cortisol	10/10	23.5 (17–34)

* Obtained from donors that had received three intraperitoneal injections of 0.25 mg *C. parvum* 16, 12, and 7 days before harvesting.
† 5 mg cortisol injected subcutaneously one hour before intraperitoneal transfer of cell challenge.
‡ From Peters *et al.*, unpublished data.
§ Survival time of mice without tumors is > 150 days.

the antitumor activity of *C. parvum*-stimulated peritoneal exudate cells transferred to recipients treated with hydrocortisone (5 mg) (Table 2). On the other hand, Fisher *et al.* (1976) observed that the growth restraint of a mouse mammary carcinoma produced by weekly injections of *C. parvum* (160 mg/m²) was not adversely affected by biweekly injections of 2.5 mg cortisone acetate. However, in these experiments, cortisone alone produced some tumor-inhibitory effect, and the desirability of ameliorating *C. parvum* toxicity in humans with corticoid hormones is open to question.

Interactions with Heat

Recent experiments conducted by Urano *et al.* (1978) have shown a possibly hazardous complication of combined therapy with *C. parvum* and heat. One of the remarkable attributes of *C. parvum*-stimulated macrophages is their ability to discriminate between normal and malignant cells in cytotoxicity assays. This ability may well be related to membrane differences between normal and malignant cells, such as those involved in contact inhibition. Urano *et al.* (1978) have found that administration of *C. parvum* before heating significantly reduced,

Table 3. *Effect of* C. parvum *on Hyperthermia-Induced Toe Loss in C₃H Mice**

Experiment	Mean Time at 43.5°C to Cause Toe Loss (min)	
	Untreated Mice	Treated Mice†
1	125	82
2	140	96
Pool	133	92

* Adapted from Urano *et al.*, 1978.
† 0.35 mg *C. parvum* injected intravenously three days before hyperthermia.

by about one third, the time of heating at 43.5°C required to produce a given level of damage in the mouse foot (Table 3). When given after heating, *C. parvum* had no effect. Although not proven, it seems possible that hyperthermic injury to the plasma membrane of normal cells makes them vulnerable to attack by *C. parvum*-stimulated macrophages. An even more marked enhancement by *C. parvum* of the thermal response of an immunogenic sarcoma was also noted, but this was not surprising because *C. parvum* alone exerts a significant antitumor effect.

CONCLUSIONS

As mentioned previously, animal tumor models can serve two purposes in experimental oncology: the elucidation of mechanisms, and the pragmatic testing of various methods of application of new cancer therapeutic agents. For the second purpose, an "ideal" animal model would simulate the clinical situation wherein a spontaneous, autochthonous, usually slowly growing tumor is found in a host who is frequently elderly and sometimes immunologically deficient. However, in the laboratory situation, to obtain uniformity of experimental conditions with significant numbers of animals and to keep costs within reasonable bounds, certain features of the ideal model have to be compromised. For example, it is common to use transplanted, rapidly growing tumors in previously healthy, young adult hosts. Furthermore, dose schedules for administration of therapeutic agents usually must be compressed because of rapid tumor growth, and in the case of *C. parvum,* the doses commonly used experimentally greatly exceed those tolerated by human patients. These constraints alone make direct extrapolation from animal experiments to the clinic somewhat hazardous, but when highly immunogenic, chemically or virally induced, or, worse, allogeneic tumors are used, clinical extrapolations are meaningless (Hewitt *et al.,* 1976).

However, in my view, one should not expect to refine the details of treatment in animal models, but rather to derive the principles by which treatment modalities may best be used; the final honing of these principles is the province of the clinical investigator. After reviewing the best experimental data available concerning the use of *C. parvum* as an immunotherapeutic agent, I conclude, therefore, with the following statements of principle: (1) Therapy for most established human tumors with *C. parvum* alone is likely to be relatively ineffective, with, at best, a modest slowing of tumor growth. (2) If *C. parvum* is used in combination with radiotherapy or surgery, it may be advantageous to administer the organism intralesionally before, as well as regionally or systemically after, tumor ablation. For an optimal response, patients should be T cell competent when *C. parvum* is administered. (3) If *C. parvum* is combined with chemotherapy, alternating courses of the chemotherapeutic agents and *C. parvum* should be given. (4) Although the toxicity of systemically administered *C. parvum* may be reduced by corticosteroid therapy, its therapeutic effect also may be impaired. (5) Combined treatment with *C. parvum* and hyperthermia should be approached with extreme caution. (6) In clinical situations in which the tumor burden is minimal, the possibility of growth promotion by *C. parvum* cannot be ignored.

ACKNOWLEDGMENTS

The author gratefully acknowledges the help of Luka Milas and Kathryn Mason in preparing this paper, and the permission of many colleagues to quote from their unpublished data.

This investigation was supported in part by grant number CA-17769 from the National Cancer Institute, Department of Health, Education, and Welfare.

REFERENCES

Amiel, J. L., and Berardet, M. 1970. An experimental model of active immunotherapy preceded by cytoreductive chemotherapy. Eur. J. Cancer, 6:557–559.

Ando, K., Urano, M., and Koike, S. 1978. Cell killing and cytostatic ability of *Corynebacterium liquefaciens* in vivo. Cancer Res. (in press).

Ando, K., Urano, M., Nesumi, N., and Koike, S. 1977. Effect of *Corynebacterium liquefaciens* on C_3Hf mouse squamous carcinoma. Cancer Res., 37:3115–3119.

Basic, I., Milas, L., Grdina, D. J., and Withers, H. R. 1975. *In vitro* destruction of tumor cells by macrophages from mice treated with *C. granulosum*. J. Natl. Cancer Inst., 55:589–596.

Bomford, R. 1975. Active specific immunotherapy of mouse methylcholanthrene induced tumours with *Corynebacterium parvum* and irradiated tumour cells. Br. J. Cancer, 32:551–557.

Bomford, R. 1977. Analysis of the factors allowing promotion (rather than inhibition) of tumour growth by *Corynebacterium parvum*. Int. J. Cancer, 19:673–679.

Bomford, R., and Christie, G. H. 1975. Mechanisms of macrophage activation by *Corynebacterium parvum*. II. *In vivo* experiments. Cell. Immunol., 17:150–155.

Bomford, R., and Olivotto, M. 1974. The mechanism of inhibition by *Corynebacterium parvum* of the growth of lung nodules from intravenously injected tumour cells. Int. J. Cancer, 14:226–235.

Castro, J. E. 1974a. Antitumour effect of *Corynebacterium parvum* in mice. Eur. J. Cancer, 10:121–127.

Castro, J. E. 1974b. The effect of *Corynebacterium parvum* on the structure and function of the lymphoid system in mice. Eur. J. Cancer, 10:115–120.

Currie, G. A., and Bagshawe, K. D. 1970. Active immunotherapy with *Corynebacterium parvum* and chemotherapy in murine fibrosarcomas. Br. Med. J., 1:541–544.

Fisher, B., Rubin, H., Saffer, E., and Wolmark, N. 1976. Further observations on the inhibition of tumor growth by *Corynebacterium parvum* with cyclophosphamide. II. Effect of cortisone acetate. J. Natl. Cancer Inst., 56:571–574.

Fisher, B., Wolmark, N., Rubin, H., and Saffer, E. 1975a. Further observations on the inhibition of tumor growth by *Corynebacterium parvum* with cyclophosphamide. I. Variation in administration of both agents. J. Natl. Cancer Inst., 55:1147–1153.

Fisher, B., Wolmark, N., Saffer, E., and Fisherm, E. R. 1975b. Inhibitory effect of prolonged *Corynebacterium parvum* and cyclophosphamide administration on the growth of established tumors. Cancer, 35:134–143.

Fisher, J. C., Grace, W. R., and Mannick, J. A. 1970. The effect of nonspecific immune stimulation with *Corynebacterium parvum* on patterns of tumor growth. Cancer, 26:1379–1382.

Ghaffar, A., Cullen, R. T., Dunbar, N., and Woodruff, M. F. A. 1974. Anti-tumour effect *in vitro* of lymphocyte and macrophages from mice treated with *Corynebacterium parvum*. Br. J. Cancer, 29:199–205.

Ghaffar, A., Cullen, R. T., and Woodruff, M. F. A. 1975. Further analysis of the anti-tumour effect *in vitro* of peritoneal exudate cells from mice treated with *Corynebacterium parvum*. Br. J. Cancer, 31:15–24.

Halpern, B. (ed.). 1975. *Corynebacterium parvum:* Applications in Experimental and Clinical Oncology. New York, Plenum Press, p. 444.

Halpern, B. N., Biozzi, G., Stiffel, C., and Mouton, D. 1966. Inhibition of tumour growth by administration of killed *Corynebacterium parvum*. Nature, 212:853–854.

Halpern, B., Crepin, Y., and Rabourdin, A. 1975. An analysis of the increase in host resistance to isogenic tumor invasion in mice by treatment with *Corynebacterium parvum*. In Halpern, B. (ed.): *Corynebacterium parvum:* Applications in Experimental and Clinical Oncology. New York, Plenum Press, pp. 191–199.

Halpern, B. N., Prevot, A. R., Biozzi, G., Stiffel, C., Mouton, D., Morard, J. C., Bouthillier, Y., and Decreusefond, C. 1964. Stimulation de l'activite phagocytaire du système reticuloendothelial provoquée par *Corynebacterium parvum*. J. Reticuloendothel. Soc., 1:77–96.

Hewitt, H. B., Blake, E. R., and Walder, A. S. 1976. A critique of the evidence for active host defence against cancer based on personal studies of 27 murine tumors of spontaneous origin. Br. J. Cancer, 33:241–259.

Hibbs, J. B., Jr. 1974. Heterocytolysis by macrophages activated by bacillus Calmette-Guérin: Lysosome exocytosis into tumor cells. Science, 184:468–471.

Houchens, D. P., Johnson, R. K., Ovejera, A., Gaston, M. R., and Goldin, A. 1976. Effects of *Corynebacterium parvum* alone and in combination with Adriamycin in experimental tumor systems. Cancer Treat. Rep., 60:823–828.

James, K., Willmott, N., Milne, I., and McBride, W. H. 1976. Antitumor antibodies and immunoglobulin class and subclass levels in *Corynebacterium parvum*-treated mice. J. Natl. Cancer Inst., 56:1035–1040.

Johnson, J. L., and Cummins, C. S. 1972. Cell wall composition and deoxyribonucleic acid similarities among the anaerobic coryneforms, classical propionibacteria, and strains of *Arachnia propionica*. J. Bacteriol., 109:1047–1066.

Lamensans, A., Stiffel, C., Mollier, M. F., Mouton, D., and Biozzi, G. 1968. Effêt protecteur de *Corynebacterium parvum* contre la leucémie greffee AKR. Rélations avec l'activité catalasique hépatique et la fonction phagocytaire du système reticuloendothelial. Rev. Fr. Etud. Clin. Biol., 13:773–779.

Likhite, V. V. 1976. Suppression of the incidence of death with spontaneous tumours in DBA/2 mice after *Corynebacterium parvum*-mediated rejection of syngeneic tumours. Nature, 259:397–399.

Likhite, V. V., and Halpern, B. N. 1973. The delayed rejection of tumors formed from the administration of tumor cells mixed with killed *Corynebacterium parvum*. Int. J. Cancer, 12:699–704.

Likhite, V. V., and Halpern, B. N. 1974. Lasting rejection of mammary adenocarcinoma cell tumors in DBA-2 mice with intratumor injection of killed *Corynebacterium parvum*. Cancer Res., 34:341–344.

Mazurek, C., Chalvet, H., Stiffel, C., and Biozzi, G. 1976. Study of the mechanism of *Corynebacterium parvum* anti-tumor activity. I. Protective effect on the growth of two syngeneic tumors. Int. J. Cancer, 17:511–517.

McBride, W. H., Barrow, G., Peters, L. J., Mason, K. A., and Milas, L. 1977. *In vivo* antitumour activity of *C. parvum* stimulated peritoneal exudate cells. In James, K., McBride, W., and Stewart, A. (eds.): The Macrophage and Cancer (Proceedings of the EURES Symposium, September 1977). Edinburgh, Scotland, University of Edinburgh, pp. 173–181.

McBride, W. H., Dawes, J., Dunbar, N., Ghaffar, A., and Woodruff, M. F. A. 1975. A comparative study of anaerobic coryneforms. Attempts to correlate their anti-tumour activity with their serological properties and ability to stimulate the lymphoreticular system. Immunology, 28:49–58.

McBride, W. H., Jones, J. T., and Weir, D. M. 1974. Increased phagocytic cell activity and anaemia in *Corynebacterium parvum* treated mice. Br. J. Exp. Pathol., 55:38–46.

Milas, L., Basic, I., Kogelnik, H. D., and Withers, H. R. 1975a. Effects of *C. granulosum* on weight and histology of lymphoid organs, response to mitogens, skin allografts, and a syngeneic fibrosarcoma in mice. Cancer Res., 35:2365–2374.

Milas, L., Gutterman, J. U., Basic, I., Hunter, N., Mavligit, G. M., Hersh, E. M., and Withers, H. R. 1974a. Immunoprophylaxis and immunotherapy for a murine fibrosarcoma with *C. granulosum* and *C. parvum*. Int. J. Cancer, 14:493–503.

Milas, L., Hunter, N., Basic, I., Mason, K., Grdina, D. J., and Withers, H. R. 1975b. Nonspecific immunotherapy of murine solid tumors with *C. granulosum*. J. Natl. Cancer Inst., 54:895–902.

Milas, L., Hunter, N., Basic, I., and Withers, H. R. 1974b. Complete regression of an established murine fibrosarcoma induced by systemic application of *Corynebacterium granulosum*. Cancer Res., 34:2470–2475.

Milas, L., Hunter, N., Basic, I., and Withers, H. R. 1974c. Protection by *Corynebacterium granulosum* against radiation-induced enhancement of artificial pulmonary metastases of a murine fibrosarcoma. J. Natl. Cancer Inst., 52:1875–1880.

Milas, L., Hunter, N., and Withers, H. R. 1974d. Corynebacterium-induced protection against artificial pulmonary metastases of a syngeneic fibrosarcoma in mice. Cancer Res., 34:613–620.

Milas, L., Hunter, N., and Withers, H. R. 1975c. Combination of local irradiation with systemic application of anaerobic corynebacteria in therapy of a murine fibrosarcoma. Cancer Res., 35:1274–1277.

Milas, L., Kogelnik, H. D., Basic, I., Mason, K., Hunter, N., and Withers, H. R. 1975d. Combination of *C. parvum* and specific immunization against artificial pulmonary metastases in mice. Int. J. Cancer, 16:738–746.

Milas, L., Mason, K., and Withers, H. R. 1976. Therapy of spontaneous pulmonary metastases of a murine mammary carcinoma with anaerobic corynebacteria. Cancer Immunol. Immunother., 1:233–237.

Olivotto, M., and Bomford, R. 1974. *In vitro* inhibition of tumour cell growth and DNA synthesis by peritoneal and lung macrophages from mice injected with *Corynebacterium parvum*. Int. J. Cancer, 13:478–488.

O'Neill, G. J., Henderson, D. C., and White, R. G. 1973. The role of anaerobic coryneforms on specific and non-specific immunological reactions. I. Effect on particle clearance and humoral and cell-mediated immunological responses. Immunology, 24:977–995.

Ossorio, R. C., Fahey, J. L., Wilson, W., Plotkin, D., Brossman, S., and Skinner, D. 1975. Toxicity of intravenous *Corynebacterium parvum*. Lancet, 2:1090–1091.

Pearson, J. W., Chirigos, M. A., Charapas, S. D., and Sher, N. A. 1974. Combined drug and immunostimulation therapy against a syngeneic murine leukemia. J. Natl. Cancer Inst., 52:463–468.

Pearson, J. W., Pearson, G. R., Gibson, W. T., Chermann, J. C., and Chirigos, M. A. 1972. Combined chemoimmunostimulation therapy against murine leukemia. Cancer Res., 32:904–907.

Pearson, J. W., Perk, K., Chirigos, M. A., Pryor, J. W., and Fuhrman, F. S. 1975. Histological and combined chemoimmunostimulation therapy studies against a murine leukemia. Int. J. Cancer, 16:142–152.

Peters, L. J. 1975. Enhancement of syngeneic murine tumour transplantability by whole body irradiation—A non-immunological phenomenon. Br. J. Cancer, 31:293–300.

Peters, L. J., and Mason, K. 1977. Enhancement of artificial lung metastases by cyclophosphamide: Pharmacological and mechanistic considerations. In Day, S. B., Laird Myers, W. P., Stansly, P., Garattini, S., and Lewis, M. G. (eds.): Cancer Invasion and Metastasis: Biologic Mechanisms and Therapy. New York, Raven Press, pp. 397–410.

Peters, L. J., Mason, K. A., McBride, W. H., and Patt, Y. Z. 1978a. Enhancement of lung colony-forming efficiency by local thoracic irradiation—Intrepretation of labelled cell studies. Radiology, 126:499–505.

Peters, L. J., McBride, W. H., Mason, K. A., Hunter, N., Basic, I., and Milas, L. 1977. *In vivo* transfer of anti-tumor activity by peritoneal exudate cells from mice treated with *Corynebacterium parvum:* Reduced effect in irradiated recipients. J. Natl. Cancer Inst., 59:881–887.

Peters, L. J., McBride, W. H., Mason, K. A., and Milas, L. 1978b. A role for T lymphocytes in tumor inhibition and enhancement caused by systemic administration of *Corynebacterium parvum*. J. Reticuloendothel. Soc. (in press).

Pettigrew, R. T., Galt, J. M., Ludgate, C. M., and Smith, A. N. 1974. Clinical effects of whole-body hyperthermia in advanced malignancy. Br. Med. J., 4:679–682.

Proctor, J., Rudenstam, C. M., and Alexander, P. 1973. Increased incidence of lung metastases following treatment of rats bearing hepatomas with irradiated tumor cells and the beneficial effect of *Corynebacterium parvum* in this system. Biomedicine, 19:248–252.

Purnell, D. M., Bartlett, G. L., Kreider, J. W., and Biro, T. G. 1977. *Corynebacterium parvum* and cyclophosphamide as combination treatment for a murine mammary adenocarcinoma. Cancer Res., 37:1137–1140.

Puvion, F., Fray, A., and Halpern, B. 1976. A cytochemical study of the *in vitro* interaction between normal and activated mouse peritoneal macrophages and tumor cells. J. Ultrastruct. Res., 54:95–108.

Roumiantzeff, M., Musetescu, M., Ayme, G., and Mynard, M. C. 1975. Effect of inactivated Coryne-bacterium on different experimental tumors in mice. In Halpern, B. (ed.): *Corynebacterium parvum:* Applications in Experimental and Clinical Oncology. New York, Plenum Press, pp. 202–217.

Sadler, T. E., and Castro, J. E. 1976. The effects of *Corynebacterium parvum* and surgery on the Lewis lung carcinoma and its metastases. Br. J. Surg., 63:292-296.

Scott, M. T. 1972. Biological effects of the adjuvant *Corynebacterium parvum*. I. Inhibition of PHA, mixed lymphocyte and GVH reactivity. Cell. Immunol., 5:459–468.

Scott, M. T. 1974a. *Corynebacterium parvum* as a therapeutic anti-tumor agent in mice. I. Systemic effects from intravenous injection. J. Natl. Cancer Inst., 53:855–860.

Scott, M. T. 1974b. *Corynebacterium parvum* as a therapeutic anti-tumor agent in mice. II. Local injection of *C. parvum*. J. Natl. Cancer Inst., 53:861 865.

Scott, M. T. 1975a. In vivo cortisone sensitivity of nonspecific anti-tumor activity of *Corynebacterium parvum*-activated mouse peritoneal macrophages. J. Natl. Cancer Inst., 54:789–792.

Scott, M. T. 1975b. Potentiation of the tumor-specific immune response by *Corynebacterium parvum*. J. Natl. Cancer Inst., 55:65–72.

Scott, M. T. 1976. Failure of *Corynebacterium parvum* presensitization to modify the antitumor effects of systemic and local therapeutic injections of *C. parvum* in mice. J. Natl. Cancer Inst., 56:675–677.

Scott, M. T., and Warner, S. L. 1976. The accumulated effects of repeated systemic or local injections of low doses of *Corynebacterium parvum* in mice. Cancer Res., 36:1335–1338.

Smith, S. E., and Scott, M. T. 1972. Biological effects of *Corynebacterium parvum*. III. Amplification of resistance and impairment of active immunity to murine tumours. Br. J. Cancer, 26:361–367.

Soyka, L. F., Hunt, W. G., Knight, S. E., and Foster, R. S., Jr. 1976. Decreased liver and lung drug-metabolizing activity in mice treated with *Corynebacterium parvum*. Cancer Res., 36:4425–4428.

Stiffel, C., Mouton, D., and Biozzi, G. 1971. Rôle des macrophages dans l'immunité non specifique. Ann. Inst. Pasteur, 120:412–427.

Stone, H. B., and Milas, L. 1978. Modification of radiation response of murine tumors by Misonida-zole (Ro-07-0582), host immune capability and by *Corynebacterium parvum*. J. Natl. Cancer Inst., 60:887–894.

Suit, H. D., Sedlacek, R., Silobrcic, V., and Linggood, R. M. 1976a. Radiation therapy and *Corynebacterium parvum* in the treatment of murine tumors. Cancer, 37:2573–2579.

Suit, H. D., Sedlacek, R., Wagner, M., Orsi, L., Silobrcic, V., and Rothman, J. 1976b. Effect of *Corynebacterium parvum* on the response to irradiation of a C_3H fibrosarcoma. Cancer Res., 36:1305–1314.

Toujas, L., Dazord, L., and Guelfi, J. 1975. Kinetics of proliferation of bone-marrow cell lines after injections of immunostimulant bacteria. In Halpern, B. (ed): *Corynebacterium parvum:* Applications in Experimental and Clinical Oncology. New York, Plenum Press, pp. 117–125.

Tuttle, R. L., and North, R. J. 1975. Mechanisms of antitumor action of *Corynebacterium parvum:* Nonspecific tumor cell destruction at site of immunologically mediated sensitivity reaction to *C. parvum*. J. Natl. Cancer Inst., 55:1403–1411.

Tuttle, R. L., and North, R. J. 1976. Mechanisms of antitumor action of *Corynebacterium parvum:* The generation of cell-mediated tumor specific immunity. J. Reticuloendothel. Soc., 20:197–208.

Ullrich, R. L., and Adams, G. D. 1978. The combined use of local irradiation and *Corynebacterium parvum* in the treatment of line 1 carcinoma. Radiat. Res. (in press).

Urano, M., Overgaard, M., Suit, H., Dunn, P., and Sedlacek, R. 1978. Enhancement by *Corynebacterium parvum* of the normal and tumor tissue response to hyperthermia. Cancer Res., 38:862–864.

van Putten, L. M., Kram, L. K. J., van Dierendonck, H. H. C., Smink, T., and Fuzy, M. 1975. Enhancement by drugs of metastatic lung nodule formation after intravenous tumor cell injection. Int. J. Cancer, 15:588–595.

Woodruff, M. F. A., and Boak, J. L. 1966. Inhibitory effect of injection of *Corynebacterium parvum* on the growth of tumour transplants in isogeneic hosts. Br. J. Cancer, 20:345–355.

Woodruff, M. F. A., and Dunbar, N. 1973. The effect of *Corynebacterium parvum* and other reticu-loendothelial stimulants on transplanted tumors in mice. In Wolstenholme, G. E. W., and Knight, J. (eds.): Immunopotentiation (Ciba Foundation Symposium 18). Amsterdam, Associated Scientific Publishers, pp. 287–300.

Woodruff, M. F. A., and Dunbar, N. 1975. Effect of local injection of *Corynebacterium parvum* on the growth of a murine fibrosarcoma. Br. J. Cancer, 32:34–41.

Woodruff, M. F. A., Dunbar, N., and Ghaffar, A. 1973. The growth of tumours in T-cell deprived mice and their response to treatment with *Corynebacterium parvum*. Proc. R. Soc. Lond. [B], 184:97–102.

Woodruff, M. F. A., Ghaffar, A., Dunbar, N., and Whitehead, V. L. 1976. Effect of *C. parvum* on immunization with irradiated tumour cells. Br. J. Cancer, 33:491-495.

Woodruff, M. F. A., Inchley, M. P., and Dunbar, N. 1972. Further observations on the effect of *C. parvum* and anti-tumour globulin on syngeneically transplanted mouse tumours. Br. J. Cancer, 26:67-76.

Woodruff, M. F. A., and Warner, N. L. 1977. Effect of *Corynebacterium parvum* on tumor growth in normal and athymic (nude) mice. J. Natl. Cancer Inst., 58:111–116.

Yuhas, J. M., Toya, R. E., and Wagner, E. 1975. Specific and nonspecific stimulation of resistance to the growth and metastasis of the line 1 lung carcinoma. Cancer Res., 35:242–244.

Yuhas, J. M., and Ullrich, R. L. 1976. Responsiveness of senescent mice to the antitumor properties of *Corynebacterium parvum*. Cancer Res., 36:161–166.

Immunotherapy of Human Cancer,
The University of Texas System Cancer Center
M. D. Anderson Hospital and Tumor Institute.
Raven Press, New York © 1978.

Thymosin Therapy:
Approach to Immunoreconstitution
in Immunodeficiency Diseases and Cancer

Allan L. Goldstein, Ph.D., Gailen D. Marshall, Jr., M.S., and
Jeffrey L. Rossio, Ph.D.*

*Department of Biochemistry, The George Washington University Medical Center, Washington, D.C.; and *Department of Microbiology and Immunology, Wright State University School of Medicine, Dayton, Ohio*

Proper function of the thymus-dependent component of the immune system is extremely important to the cancer patient in terms of providing (1) endogenous tumor immunity through production of specialized types of T cells, such as "killer cells," which have the capacity to destroy tumor cells; and (2) natural immunity against viruses, fungi, and many other types of pathogens. We now know that a significant portion of the mechanisms through which the T cell immune system functions depend on the production of hormone-like substances that provide signals for maturation and/or migration of the many subpopulations of T cells (Trivers and Goldstein, in press). As illustrated in Figure 1, these thymic factors are directly involved in the maintenance of normal immune balance. Ongoing studies suggest that disruption of the production and/or secretion of thymosin by genetic, viral, chemical, or a number of other agents may result in defects in both T and B cell immune systems. These defects are thought to result ultimately in the appearance of a number of immunologically derived disorders, such as cancer, autoimmune diseases, and a variety of infectious diseases (Goldstein, 1976). Clinical trials with thymosin are being conducted in children with primary immunodeficiency diseases and in cancer patients. Of particular importance to the theme of this monograph are the ongoing studies of thymosin in the treatment of neoplastic disease. Other findings also suggest the usefulness of thymosin in dealing with infections that often occur subsequent to aggressive chemotherapy and/or radiotherapy for cancer patients.

Abbreviations used in this chapter: cyclic GMP—cyclic guanosine monophosphate; pre-T cells—cellular elements that, upon thymic influence, can manifest characteristics of T-lymphocytes; T cells—lymphoid cells "processed" or influenced by the thymus gland or its secretions; TdT—terminal deoxynucleotidyl transferase.

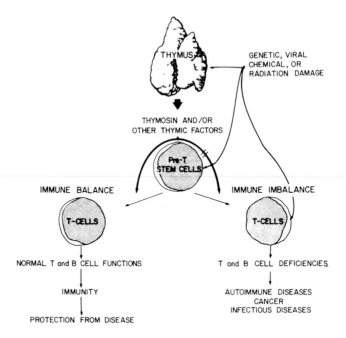

Figure 1. Endocrine thymus and immunity. Ongoing studies suggest that immune imbalance due to deficiencies of thymosin peptide levels may result in functional T and B cell deficiencies, resulting in dyscrasias such as autoimmune diseases, cancer, and infectious diseases.

BASIC PROPERTIES

All thymosin fraction 5 used in our clinical studies was prepared as previously described (Hooper *et al.,* 1975). The first 60 patients in our clinical studies were treated with thymosin fraction 5 prepared in our laboratories. This preparation met FDA standards for safety, sterility, and nonpyrogenicity. Since January 1976, all clinical-quality thymosin has been prepared by Hoffmann-La Roche Inc. (Nutley, New Jersey). Figure 2 indicates that thymosin fraction 5 is a family of primarily small, acidic peptides with molecular weights ranging from 1,000 to 15,000. Current studies suggest that biologic potency of fraction 5 may be due to more than one of these peptides acting either together or individually on various subpopulations of T cells.

To facilitate the identification and comparison of thymic peptides from one laboratory to another, we have suggested a nomenclature for the identification of each of the peptides based on the isoelectric focusing pattern of thymosin fraction 5 in the pH range of 3.5 to 9.5. Peptides are divided into three major regions based on their migration patterns. The regions are identified by the Greek letters alpha (α), beta (β), and gamma (γ). The α region consists of the peptides with isoelectric pH (pI) below 5.0 (highly acidic); the β region consists of peptides with pI between 5.0 and 7.0 (acidic); and the γ region consists of peptides with pI above 7.0 (basic). Sequential numbering is used to

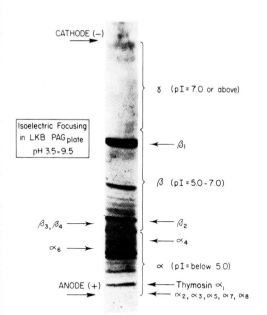

CATHODE (−)

δ (pI = 7.0 or above)

Isoelectric Focusing
in LKB PAG plate
pH 3.5-9.5

← β₁

β (pI = 5.0 - 7.0)

β₃, β₄ →

α₆ →

← β₂

← α₄

α (pI = below 5.0)

ANODE (+)

← Thymosin α₁
← α₂, α₃, α₅, α₇, α₈

Figure 2. Suggested nomenclature for thymosin polypeptides on the basis of an isoelectric focusing gel of thymosin fraction 5 at pH 3.5 to 9.5. Arrows indicate locations of various thymosin peptides, which are numbered in the order of their isolation.

identify peptides from each region in the order of their isolation. As can be seen in Figure 2, we have isolated and purified 12 of the polypeptides to homogeneity or near homogeneity. Eight of the peptides are from the α region, and four are from the β region. Two of the peptides have now been sequenced, and several others are currently being sequenced. Thymosin α_1, the first of the biologically active peptides isolated, is from 10 to 1,000 times as active as fraction 5 in a number of functional in vitro and in vivo T cell assays. Thymosin β_1 is biologically inactive and is probably present as a nonimmunologic biocontaminant. The sequence of β_1 has been found to be homologous to ubiquitin, a degradation product of a nonhistone, acidic, nuclear protein termed A-24.

The amino acid sequence of thymosin α_1 has been determined (Goldstein *et al.,* 1977). The peptide has 28 amino acid residues and a molecular weight of 3,108 (calculated from the established structure). The sequence of this peptide is shown in Figure 3. Recently, Drs. Meienhofer and Wang at Hoffmann-La Roche Inc. have synthesized thymosin α_1 (Meienhofer, personal communication). Preliminary studies indicate that the synthetic peptide has biologic activity. Four other partially purified peptides that have interesting biological properties are thymosin β_3, β_4, α_5, and α_7. Current experimental data indicate that the thymosin peptides can induce the expression of Ly phenotypes and TdT in murine bone marrow cells. Thymosin α_5 may induce helper activity in these cells. Thymosin α_7 induces suppressor activity and the appearance of Ly 1,2,3[+] surface markers. Thymosin α_1 also induces the appearance of the Ly 1,2,3[+] phenotype in Ly[−], immature T cells (murine).

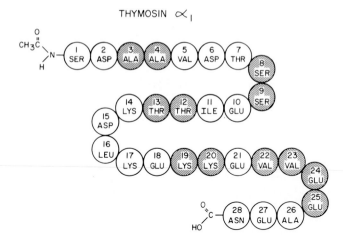

Figure 3. Primary structure of thymosin α_1.

CLINICAL TRIALS AND APPLICATIONS OF THYMOSIN IN IMMUNORECONSTITUTION

More than 50 children with primary immunodeficiency diseases, to date, have been treated with thymosin according to phase I protocols (summarized in Table 1). In addition, more than 150 cancer patients have been treated with thymosin according to phase I and phase II protocols (Table 1). No evidence of central nervous system, liver, kidney, or bone marrow toxicities has been seen. Side effects have been minimal. Eighty percent of the pediatric patients who have responded in vitro to thymosin (as determined by the E-rosette assay) have responded in vivo with increased T cell numbers and function. Significant clinical improvement has been seen in more than 50% of the pediatric patients who have responded in vitro. More than 75% of the cancer patients have shown increases in the number of T cells following thymosin therapy (Rossio and Goldstein, 1977). However, the therapeutic effects of thymosin in decreasing tumor load and increasing survival duration in cancer patients have yet to be determined. Phase II studies in cancer patients to determine the efficacy of thymosin in combination with other modalities of therapy (e.g., chemotherapy, radiotherapy, and/or adjuvant immunotherapy) are in progress at several cancer centers.

POSTULATED MECHANISMS OF THYMOSIN ACTION

Based on accumulating experimental evidence, thymosin appears to trigger maturational progression of several (possibly distinct) early stages of T cell development and perhaps to augment the capacity of certain mature T cells to respond to antigens. Recent studies suggest that thymosin may act through

Table 1. *Thymosin Trials in Pediatric and Cancer Patients*

	Patients	
	Pediatric* (n > 50)	Cancer† (n > 150)
Thymosin treatment		
Dose (mg/m² per injection)	1–400	1–250
Length	7 days–44 mo.	7 days–40 mo.
Side Effects (%)‡		
None	60	70
Mild, local skin reactions	30	20
Moderate skin reactions and/or systemic reactions§	10	10

* Includes unspecified T cell disorders, Nezelof's syndrome, DiGeorge's syndrome, thymic hypoplasia, Wiskott-Aldrich syndrome, severe combined immunodeficiency, ataxia telangiectasia, hypogammaglobulinemia, cartilage hair with short-limbed dwarfism, chronic mucocutaneous candidiasis, and bone marrow transplant.

† Includes leukemia, lymphoma, Hodgkin's disease, multiple myeloma, melanoma and disseminated melanoma, gall bladder cancer, stomach and esophageal cancer, choriocarcinoma, breast cancer, head and neck cancer, pancreatic cancer, leiomyosarcoma, oral cancer, glioma, mycosis fungoides, lung cancer, hypernephroma, and dysgerminoma.

‡ No evidence of liver, central nervous system, kidney, or bone marrow toxicity.

§ Usually low-grade fever, which disappears with continued injections.

a cyclic GMP second messenger (Naylor *et al.,* 1976) and may induce the expression of alloantigens on the surface of T cells as they develop their functional capacity for immunocompetence (Scheid *et al.,* 1973). Thymosin can induce the expression of Ly phenotypes and TdT (a DNA polymerase found primarily in thymocytes) in bone marrow cells (Pazmino *et al.,* 1978). Furthermore, thymosin can regenerate suppressor cells in thymectomized mice, who lose these cells soon after thymectomy (Marshall and Goldstein, unpublished data). This is good evidence on which to base the proposal that thymosin affects the very early stages of T cell development, possibly by acting on pre-T cells. It is this property of thymosin that is thought to induce immune reconstitution in anergic persons (Fig. 5). In addition, it is the ability to induce functionally mature cells from functionally immature cells that may prove thymosin superior to other forms of immunologic therapeutic modalities, such as adjuvant therapy, which requires availability of relatively mature T cells. Thus, the range of thymosin activity (outlined in Fig. 4) points to the usefulness of thymosin in reconstituting severely immunosuppressed patients, provided that they still have the necessary thymosin-sensitive precursor T cell populations. Recent studies (Kenady *et al.,* 1977) provide support for application of this hypothesis to cancer patients. These investigators have observed that even after large doses of radiotherapy or chemotherapy, the peripheral blood of many types of cancer patients still contains thymosin-sensitive lymphocytes.

One of the most important clinical potentials of thymosin is its possible relationship to the management of thymus-dependent diseases. Many such thymus-

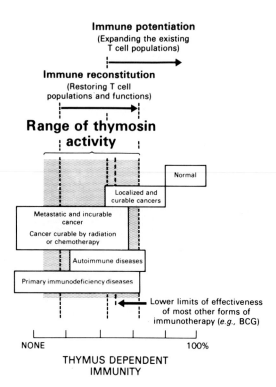

Figure 4. Scheme for possible roles of thymosin in the development or repair of thymus-dependent immunity. Thymosin acts primarily in immune reconstitution.

dependent conditions are known, such as in immunodeficiency diseases and certain autoimmune diseases; other relationships are suspected, such as in cancer. Even though information currently available is limited, the data still provide a continuing hope that thymosin might one day be added to our growing list of agents useful in the treatment of neoplastic disease.

ACKNOWLEDGMENTS

This work was supported, in part, by National Cancer Institute grants CA 16964 and CA 14108; The John A. Hartford Foundation; and Hoffmann-La Roche Inc., Nutley, New Jersey. Gailen Marshall is a James W. McLaughlin Predoctoral Fellow, The University of Texas Medical Branch.

ADDENDUM

The first efficacy trial of thymosin, for nonresectable small cell carcinoma of the lungs, has been completed by Dr. Paul B. Chretien and his associates at the National Cancer Institute (personal communication). In this trial, thymosin fraction 5, when given in conjunction with intensive chemotherapy, was found to significantly prolong the survival of cancer patients. Mean survival time was increased from 225 days with chemotherapy alone to 450 days with chemotherapy plus 60 mg/m² thymosin twice per week for the first six weeks of the chemotherapy induction period.

REFERENCES

Goldstein, A. L. 1976. The history of the development of thymosin: Chemistry, biology and clinical applications. Trans. Am. Clin. Climatol. Soc., 88:79–94.

Goldstein, A. L., Low, T. L. K., McAdoo, M., McClure, J., Thurman, G. B., Rossio, J. L., Lai, C-Y., Chang, D., Wang, S-S., Harvey, C., Ramel, A. H., and Meienhofer, J. 1977. Thymosin α_1: Isolation and sequence analysis of an immunologically active thymic polypeptide. Proc. Natl. Acad. Sci. USA, 74:725–729.

Hooper, J. A., McDaniel, M. C., Thurman, G. B., Cohen, G. H., Schulof, R. S., and Goldstein, A. L. 1975. The purification and properties of bovine thymosin. Ann. NY Acad. Sci., 249:125–144.

Kenady, D. E., Chretien, P. B., Potvin, C., Simon, R. M., Alexander, J. C., and Goldstein, A. L. 1977. Effect of thymosin *in vitro* on T-cell levels during radiation therapy: Correlations with radiation portal and dose, tumor histology, and initial T-cell level. Cancer, 39:642–652.

Naylor, P. H., Sheppard, H., Thurman, G. B., and Goldstein, A. L. 1976. Increase of cyclic GMP induced in murine thymocytes by thymosin fraction 5. Biochem. Biophys. Res. Commun., 73:843–849.

Pazmino, N. H., Ihle, J. N., and Goldstein, A. L. 1978. Induction *in vivo* and *in vitro* of terminal deoxynucleotidyl transferase by thymosin in bone marrow cells from athymic mice. J. Exp. Med., 147:708–715.

Rossio, J. L., and Goldstein, A. L. 1977. Immunotherapy of cancer with thymosin. World J. Surg., 1:605–616.

Scheid, M. P., Hoffman, M. K., Komuro, K., Hammerling, U., Boyse, E. A., Cohen, G. H., Hooper, J. A., Schulof, R. S., and Goldstein, A. L. 1973. Differentiation of T-lymphocytes induced by preparations from thymus and by nonthymic agents. The determined state of the precursor cell. J. Exp. Med., 138:1027–1032.

Trivers, G. E., and Goldstein, A. L. 1978. The endocrine thymus: A role for thymosin and other thymic factors in cancer immunity and therapy. In Hanna, M. (ed.): Basic Immunological Mechanisms in Cancer. New York, Marcel Dekker, Inc. (in press).

Immunotherapy of Human Cancer,
The University of Texas System Cancer Center
M. D. Anderson Hospital and Tumor Institute.
Raven Press, New York © 1978.

Combined Levamisole Therapy: An Overview of Its Protective Effects

Michael A. Chirigos, Ph.D., D.Sc., and William K. Amery, M.D.

Virus and Disease Modification Section, Laboratory of RNA Tumor Viruses, Division of Cancer Cause and Prevention, National Cancer Institute, National Institutes of Health, Bethesda, Maryland; and Janssen Pharmaceutica, Beerse, Belgium

Levamisole, the levoisomer of the synthetic drug tetramisole (tetrahydro-phenylimidazo-thiazole) hydrochloride, was first described as an antihelminthic agent and, as such, has been widely and safely used in Europe (Thienpont *et al.*, 1966, 1969; Seftel and Heinz, 1968). It is a stable powder, highly soluble in aqueous solvents, and has a molecular weight of 240. Its chemical structure is shown in Figure 1. Levamisole has been arousing much interest lately, and the clinical data that have started to emerge strongly suggest its usefulness as an adjuvant to other treatment modalities in clinical cancer therapy.

Several studies of experimentally induced murine malignancies have revealed synergism between levamisole and chemotherapeutic agents, sometimes with augmentation of immunity (Chirigos *et al.*, 1973, 1975, 1977; Perk *et al.*, 1975; Spreafico *et al.*, 1975; Gordon *et al.*, 1977). Levamisole has been shown also to reduce or cure primary tumors and decrease the frequency of pulmonary metastasis in mice and hamsters (Renoux and Renoux, 1972; Sadowski and Rapp, 1975; Sampson *et al.*, 1977; Doller and Rapp, 1977). In contrast to the results of these studies, levamisole has been found to be without effect on a series of tumors, including leukemias, melanoma, adenocarcinomas, and lung tumors (Chirigos *et al.*, 1973; Potter *et al.*, 1974; Fidler and Spitler, 1975; Johnson *et al.*, 1975).

The purpose of this survey is to describe the responses observed in representative tumor models in which levamisole was administered alone or in combination with cytoreductive agents, and to evaluate the available data from all animal tumor experiments in which levamisole was used alone or in combination with cytoreductive therapy to enable us to establish a base line of effect in relation

Abbreviations used in this chapter: BCNU—1,3-bis(2-chloroethyl)-1-nitrosourea; cyclic AMP—cyclic adenosine monophosphate; cyclic GMP—cyclic guanosine monophosphate; DMBA—7,12-dimethylbenz[*a*]anthracene; EAC—erythrocyte antibody complement; LSTRA—transplantable leukemia induced by Moloney leukemia virus; Me-CCNU—1-(2-chloroethyl)-3-(4-methylcyclohexyl)-1-nitrosourea; T cells—thymus-dependent lymphocytes.

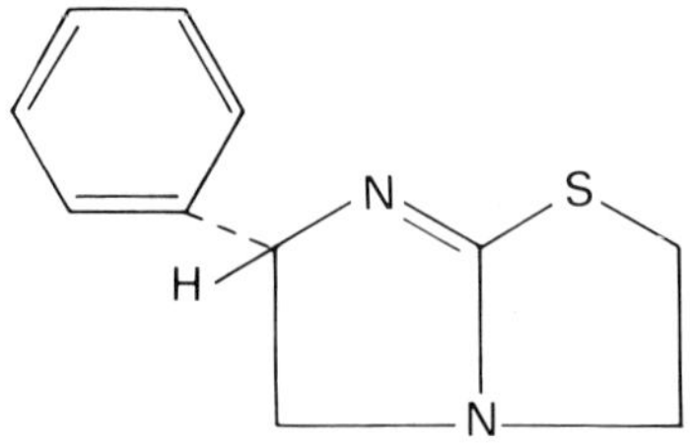

Figure 1. Chemical structure of levamisole (2, 3,5,6-tetrahydro-6-phenylimidazo[2,1-*b*]thiazole).

to the dose of levamisole and the effects on rapidly and slowly growing tumors and metastasis.

The first example of combined therapy with cytoreductive agents and levamisole is shown in Figure 2. Mice with systemic LSTRA leukemia treated with BCNU had a twofold increase in survival time and a 30% survival rate. Levamisole alone was ineffective, but when administered three to ten days after BCNU treatment, a significant number of animals survived. Delaying treatment with levamisole at the 5 mg/kg dose was ineffective and could be attributable to the fact that animals treated with BCNU had begun to relapse. This response seemed to be reversible by a higher dose of levamisole. In a second tumor model, the Lewis lung adenocarcinoma, the effect of Me-CCNU plus levamisole was tested (Fig. 3). Three parameters were evaluated in this study: effect on life-span, effect on primary tumor weight, and the number of metastatic lung lesions occurring. Again, levamisole alone was found to be ineffective in increasing life-span; however, decreases in tumor weight and number of lung lesions were noted. The combined treatment of Me-CCNU and levamisole proved more effective than Me-CCNU alone, resulting in a significant increase in life-span and decreases in primary tumor weight and number of lung lesions.

In a hamster tumor model (Fig. 4), levamisole was examined for its ability to inhibit tumor metastasis to the lung from the subcutaneously inoculated primary tumor. Hamsters were killed ten weeks after tumor inoculation, and the effectiveness of levamisole in reducing pulmonary metastases was evaluated.

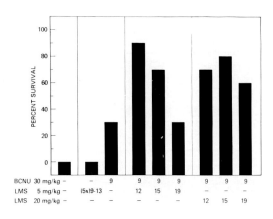

Figure 2. Effect of single or combined drug treatment on survival of mice with MCAs-10 murine leukemia. Mice inoculated with tumor on day 0, and BCNU and/or levamisole (LMS) administered on indicated days. (Adapted from Chirigos *et al.*, 1975.)

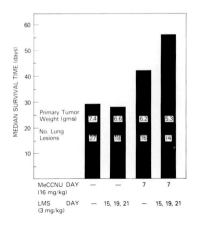

Figure 3. Effect of single or combined treatment with levamisole (LMS) and Me-CCNU on survival of C57BL/6 mice with Lewis lung carcinoma. (Adapted from Spreafico *et al.*, 1975.)

The results indicate that levamisole therapy initiated immediately after tumor inoculation or as late as four weeks after resulted in a significant decrease in the percentage of lung metastases. However, levamisole treatment did not affect the progressive growth of the primary tumor.

Levamisole was tested also in Sprague-Dawley rats with DMBA-induced breast cancers. Following the appearance of tumor, the animals were divided into groups that received various doses of levamisole by mouth. At the end of a six-month period, the tumors were measured and the animals were killed (Fig. 5). The results clearly show a retardation of tumor growth compared with the rapid rate in the untreated control animals. Of particular interest was the dormant condition of tumors in the groups receiving 2 or 4 mg/kg of levamisole; the tumors varied not less than 1 cm nor greater than 2 cm in diameter during the period of observation. The 8 mg/kg dose regimen did not significantly alter the rate of tumor growth. Tumor growth retardation was achieved at doses of levamisole that resulted in immunopotentiation (Table 1), and a signifi-

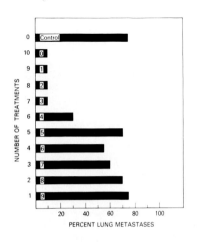

Figure 4. Effect of levamisole on lung metastasis in hamsters inoculated with the HVS-1-transformed hamster tumor. Numbers in boxes indicate week levamisole treatment was started. (Adapted from Doller and Rapp, 1977.)

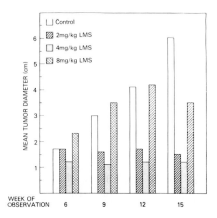

Figure 5. Rate of growth of DMBA-induced tumors in female Sprague-Dawley rats. Treated mice received levamisole (LMS) by mouth daily once they had developed tumors measuring at least 0.5 cm in diameter. (Adapted from Sampson *et al.,* 1977.)

cant correlation between immune competence and tumor inhibition was established. The effect of the different doses of levamisole on cellular immunity was measured by responses of splenic lymphocytes to the mitogens phytohemagglutinin, concanavalin A (ConA), and pokeweed mitogen. Untreated animals with breast cancer had slightly impaired responses compared with normal animals, whereas animals that received doses of levamisole between 2 and 4 mg/kg demonstrated immunopotentiation. The marked response of splenic lymphocytes to ConA suggests activity on a T cell population.

In contrast to the reports of the positive effects of levamisole, several investigators have observed that levamisole is devoid of any demonstrable tumor inhibitory or retarding effect (Potter *et al.,* 1974; Fidler and Spitler, 1975; Johnson *et al.,* 1975). In each case, however, the investigators were testing for a tumoricidal effect; levamisole was administered in various regimens before, simultaneously with, or soon after tumor inoculation. The bulk of experimental reports, however, supports the concept that levamisole acts through a reconstitutive mechanism,

Table 1. *Mitotic Index of DMBA-Induced Tumors in Mice Receiving Levamisole Monotherapy*[*]

| | | Lymphocyte Response to Mitogen[†] | | |
Host[‡]	Levamisole Dose (mg/kg)	PHA	ConA	PWM
Normal	0	12.6	16.6	8.0
Tumor	0	4.6	9.8	4.4
Tumor	2	26.2	37.1	15.3
Tumor	4	15.1	32.4	8.1
Tumor	8	7.5	11.8	5.4

[*] Adapted from Sampson *et al.,* 1977.
[†] PHA, phytohemagglutinin; ConA, conconavalin A; PWM, pokeweed mitogen.
[‡] Rats killed six months after DMBA tumor induction for testing of splenic lymphocytes.

Table 2. *Effect of Levamisole Therapy in Host-Tumor Models*

Neoplasm	Host	Response
P388 leukemia	mouse	−
Moloney LSTRA leukemia	mouse	−
Moloney MCAs-10 leukemia	mouse	−
B16 melanoma	mouse	−
M109 adenocarcinoma	mouse	−
Meth-A fibrosarcoma	mouse	−
Adenocarcinoma 15901	mouse	−
MC-7 sarcoma	rat	−
Walker 256 tumor	rat	−
RD-3 tumor	rat	−
CELO-virus induced tumor	hamster	−
Lewis lung carcinoma	mouse	+
HVS-1 transformed carcinoma	hamster	+
DMBA-induced breast cancer	rat	+

i.e., stimulates a depressed host immunity resulting from tumor burden or cytoreductive therapy.

We attempted to evaluate all in vivo data available to us to determine if a trend could be demonstrated concerning levamisole's beneficial effect. Evaluation was based on whether levamisole was used alone or in combination with other cytoreductive treatment modalities. Each experiment was considered separately and labeled positive or negative according to the presence or absence of a beneficial effect. We considered only those experiments in which the effects on the growth of primary and metastatic tumors in mice were studied synchronously in the same model, and the experiments in which levamisole as adjuvant therapy was compared with its use alone.

Table 2 contains a few examples of the several tumor types with which levamisole alone was tested. Of 14 tumor systems tested, three responded to levamisole treatment. However, when levamisole was combined with chemotherapy, a more beneficial effect was achieved (Table 3). The tumor types listed in Table 3 were

Table 3. *Cytoreductive Therapy for Mouse Neoplasms After Which Levamisole Has Positive Effect*

Neoplasm	Therapy
L1210 leukemia	Me-CCNU
Moloney LSTRA leukemia	BCNU, Cy*
Moloney MCAs-10 leukemia	BCNU, Cy
Graffi leukemia	BCNU, Cy
3-MC induced fibrosarcoma	BCNU, Cy
Meth-A fibrosarcoma	Cy
Lewis lung carcinoma	Me-CCNU
DMBA-induced breast cancer	None

* Cy, cyclophosphamide.

Table 4. *Levamisole Alone Versus Levamisole Adjuvant to Cytoreductive Therapy*

Levamisole Dose (mg/kg)	No. (%) of Positive Responses	
	Levamisole Alone	Levamisole plus Chemotherapy
1–3	0/2 (0)	1/4 (25)
3–5	9/21 (42)	21/34 (61)
5–10	1/8 (12)	5/11 (45)
>10	0/1 (0)	3/3 (100)

selected for representation of the effects of combined chemotherapy and levamisole treatment because they are often used in drug testing; however, results of cytoreductive therapy combined with levamisole for other tumor types also have been reported.

The dose effect of levamisole also was analyzed from all the reports available to us to assess if the dose of levamisole, when used singly or combined with cytoreductive therapy, was an important criterion. The analyses shown in Tables 4, 5, and 6 are based on mouse tumor models because the numbers of experimental animals of other species were considered insufficient. Table 4 shows the results of a comparison between levamisole alone and levamisole adjuvant to chemotherapy. When levamisole alone is employed, the 3 to 5 mg/kg dose appears to be critical: a reasonable number of positive responses were attained (9 of 21 compared with a total of 1 of 11 with the other doses). More positive responses were achieved at all the levamisole doses tested when levamisole was combined with chemotherapy than when used alone. From the results of evaluable tests, levamisole as an adjuvant treatment appears superior to therapy with levamisole alone.

Another analysis was based on the median survival time of animals with slowly and rapidly growing tumors that received levamisole therapy and/or levamisole adjuvant to cytoreductive therapy (Table 5). Positive results were obtained in 77 of 382 experiments with rapidly growing tumors and 59 of 200

Table 5. *Effect of Levamisole on Transplantable Tumors with Different Growth Rates* in Mice*

Levamisole Dose (mg/kg)	No. (%) of Positive Responses		
	Slowly Growing	Rapidly Growing	Both
<1	13/59 (22)	1/35 (2)	14/94 (14)
1–3	13/27 (48)	8/97 (8)	21/124 (16)
3–5	20/63 (31)	39/161 (24)	59/224 (26)
5–10	7/17 (41)	25/80 (31)	32/97 (33)
>10	6/34 (17)	4/9 (40)	10/43 (23)

* Slowly growing tumors, median survival time >20 days; rapidly growing tumors, median survival time < 20 days.

Table 6. *Effect of Levamisole on Metastasizing Transplantable Tumors in Mice*

Levamisole Dose (mg/kg)	No. (%) of Positive Responses	
	Primary Tumor	Metastasis Formation
<1	6/32 (18)	7/32 (21)
1–3	1/7 (14)	4/7 (57)
3–5	5/34 (14)	16/34 (47)
5–10	2/5 (40)	3/5 (60)

experiments with slowly growing tumors. The greater effect on slowly growing tumors represents a highly significant difference. In the overall assessment of levamisole dosage, a dose range of 3 to 10 mg/kg appears favorable for both slowly and rapidly growing tumors. Table 6 contains the evaluation of results reported for the effects of levamisole alone and/or as adjuvant therapy on primary tumor growth and metastasis formation. The evaluation indicates that the primary tumor was influenced only marginally (14 of 78 tests) whereas the concomitant metastatic formation was influenced notably (30 of 78 tests). Because relatively few studies were conducted at the 1 to 3 mg/kg and 5 to 10 mg/kg doses of levamisole, no conclusions concerning a dose-response relationship can be drawn. The evaluation does indicate, however, that a dose less than 1 mg/kg may be ineffective.

One aspect that always must be considered concerning the use of immunostimulators is that of potential, enhanced tumor growth. This paradoxical response has been observed in several animal tumor systems and has been discussed in the literature. In one study, levamisole treatment seemed to be associated with an accelerated growth of Moloney virus-induced primary rhabdomyosarcomas in BALB/c mice (Jedrzejczak, 1976). This association was not considered significant and was even counterbalanced by a greater number of animals that showed inhibited tumor growth when treated with levamisole. In an allogeneic model of an L1210 leukemia transplant in C_3H mice, an increased number of tumor takes was observed with levamisole treatment. This effect was associated with an increase of serum blocking activity (Mantovani and Spreafico, 1975). Levamisole treatment starting before or on the day of tumor inoculation was reported to be without effect on an adenovirus-12 mouse tumor transplanted in hamsters (Potter *et al.*, 1974). The administration of levamisole before transplantation of adenocarcinoma 15901 in syngeneic A mice resulted in earlier appearance of tumors but did not affect the overall incidence or course of tumor growth. In the same study, levamisole treatment was reported to increase or decrease the incidence of pulmonary nodules, depending on the time levamisole was administered (Fidler and Spitler, 1975).

Immunotherapists are often concerned about the concomitant use of immunotherapy and cytotoxic agents. It is well known that many chemotherapeutic

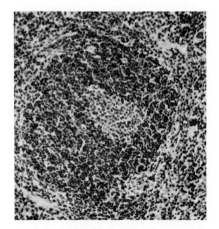 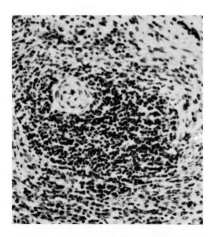

Figure 6. Left, Section of typical splenic lymphoid follicle from mice given BCNU and levamisole and killed on day 15 (×180). Right, Section of typical splenic lymphoid follicle from mice given BCNU alone and killed on day 15 (×180). Compare cellularity of splenic white and red pulp. (Adapted from Perk *et al.,* 1975.)

agents are cytotoxic and indiscriminantly kill normal as well as tumor cells. Most important, however, is that they can depress immunologically competent cells. Based on two tumor models, it was established that the effectiveness of levamisole was maximal when remission was achieved with BCNU treatment, specifically, after the immunosuppressive effect of BCNU had waned (Chirigos *et al.,* 1973, 1975). More direct evidence that the simultaneous use of levamisole and cytostatic drugs may be injurious has been provided by the studies in which splenic cell DNA synthesis was compared with the time levamisole was administered in relation to BCNU treatment (Woods *et al.,* 1975). It was found that levamisole given five to eight days after BCNU treatment resulted in significant recovery of DNA synthetic capacity of spleen cells, whereas treatment with levamisole the first day after BCNU treatment resulted in an additional depression of DNA synthesis. Further evidence of the reconstitutive effect of levamisole on splenic cells was provided by a histologic study (Perk *et al.,* 1975). Levamisole, when administered with an effective remission-inducing drug in leukemic mice, resulted in a high percentage of long-term survivors. Histologic examination of spleens of these treated mice showed that levamisole caused an earlier return of lymphoid cells to the splenic lymphoid follicles and lymphoid elements to the red pulp (Fig. 6). A recent clinical study whereby levamisole was reported to enhance bone marrow reconstitution after cytotoxic treatment supports the latter observation (Lods *et al.,* 1976). Supportive data on the protective effect of levamisole against drug toxicity are presented in Table 7. BCNU, an effective antitumor agent, is known to cause severe marrow hypoplasia and atrophy and/or hemorrhage of lymphoid tissue. Reversible leukopenia and anemia generally occur in animals surviving the initial treatment. Delayed thrombocytopenia

Table 7. *Protective Effect of Levamisole Against Drug Toxicity in Mice**

BCNU‡ (mg/kg)	Day of Levamisole Treatment, 10 mg/kg	Percent Survival†			Spleen Weight (mg)§
		Day 10	20	30	
40	...	80	50	50	50 ± 6.3
	2	70	70	70	76 ± 9.1
	4	80	60	60	51 ± 5.8
	6	90	90	90	83 ± 7.2
50	...	20	10	10	20 ± 2.9
	2	50	30	30	43 ± 5.3
	4	60	50	50	54 ± 10.3
	6	60	40	40	42 ± 12.4
0	0	100	100	100	117 ± 3.2
...	...	100	100	100	106 ± 2.1

* Each group contained 20 mice (CD_2F_1, male, 25 to 27 g).
† On observation day 5, there was 100% survival in all groups.
‡ Injected subcutaneously on day 0.
§ Mean ± standard error.

has also been observed, but is reversible. Results shown in Table 7 indicate that levamisole reverses, in part, the lymphoid cell hyperplasia induced by the BCNU, as evidenced by the enhanced spleen weights of dually treated mice and the higher percentage of survivors.

Based on results of studies with several experimental tumor model systems, the more effective use of levamisole as an adjuvant appears to be following cytoreductive therapy (Fig. 7). Cytoreductive therapy may be in the form of chemotherapy, surgery, irradiation, or a combination of these modalities. Levamisole can be administered soon after the cytoreductive therapy. It is imperative to monitor the immunologic competence of the host. The primary objective of this schema is to reduce the tumor burden as extensively as possible and treat the host with levamisole to restore host immune capacity through early reconstitution of critical lymphoid elements. When chemotherapy is the primary treat-

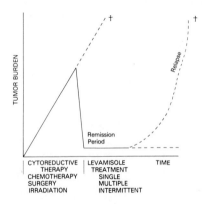

Figure 7. Schema for levamisole adjuvant treatment when combined with cytoreductive therapy.

ment modality, levamisole can be administered intermittently between cycles of chemotherapy.

The indications that levamisole acts as an immunopotentiating agent have stimulated studies to assess the possible mechanism(s) by which levamisole exerts its immunopotentiating and/or reconstitutive activity on lymphoid cellular elements. The following represents an overview of the reported results describing the immunologic profile of levamisole.

Levamisole increases phagocytosis by polymorphonuclear cells or macrophages when added to these cells or when administered to the donor. The effects are most pronounced on hypofunctional cells from cancer patients (Ippen and Qadripur, 1975; Van Huele et al., 1976) and are weak or absent on cells from normal subjects (Schulze and Raettig, 1973; Versijp et al., 1975; Douglas et al., 1976; Al-Ibrahim, in press).

Levamisole has been demonstrated to potentiate antigen-induced stimulation of phagocytosis by macrophages, improved immunophagocytosis (phagocytosis of antibody-coated particles) (Lima et al., 1974), and increased phagocyte adherence and antibody and complement receptor activity (Schreiber et al., 1975). This effect can be reversed by hydrocortisone. Macrophages exposed to levamisole become more hydrophilic, a phenomenon that has been associated with enhanced phagocytosis, and in addition, have increased numbers of lysosomes and cytoplasmic vacuolization. Intracellular killing by macrophages from levamisole-treated mice or rats is reported to be increased (Renoux et al., 1976), but this effect is not seen when levamisole is added to the cells of untreated donors (Versijp et al., 1975). The spontaneous movement of polymorphonuclear cells or monocytes of healthy human donors has been found to be increased when levamisole is added directly to these cells (Douglas et al., 1976; Anderson et al., in press).

Results of studies on the chemotactic response of polymorphonuclear cells and monocytes from cancer patients show an increased response after exposure to levamisole (Gallin and Wolff, 1975; Hill and Quie, 1975; Rabson, unpublished data; Rabson et al., unpublished data). Both the rate of cell migration and the total number of cells capable of responding to chemotactic factors increase (Pike and Snyderman, 1976). Levamisole enhances the in vitro chemotactic activity of human peripheral blood neutrophils as well as rat peritoneal neutrophils and macrophages (Liauw and Stecher, 1977).

When given to anergic patients or when added to their cells, levamisole restores leukocyte migration inhibition in response to antigenic stimulation (Huskisson et al., 1976; Lieberman and Hsu, 1976). The effects are most pronounced when suboptimal concentrations of antigen are used (Lieberman and Hsu, 1976), but levamisole without antigen does not increase migration inhibition. In vitro, levamisole augments the production of the soluble mediators, migration inhibitory factor and macrophage activating factor, by mitogen-stimulated lymphocytes, but has no effect on lymphocyte proliferation (Whitcomb et al., 1976). In the absence of mitogen, levamisole has no effect.

Levamisole increases nucleic acid or protein synthesis by resting lymphocytes, and boosts mitogen, antigen, and allogeneic cell stimulation of T cells. The responsiveness is dependent on several variables, such as lymphocyte type, responsiveness to antigens or mitogens, levamisole concentration, stimulants used, and cell culture technique (Hadden *et al.,* 1975; Lichtenfeld *et al.,* 1977; Sunshine *et al.,* 1977; Al-Ibrahim, in press). Spleen cells from nude mice and mice depressed by pretreatment with antithymocyte serum respond poorly or not at all (Meiluzzi *et al.,* 1975). Lymphocyte responsiveness, when depressed after irradiation therapy in man (Levo *et al.,* 1975) or after cytostatic treatment in mice (Woods *et al.,* 1975; Gordon *et al.,* 1977), is restored if levamisole is given at a critical time. When given too early after cytostatic treatment, levamisole induces a further depression, followed by a delayed restoration. In most of these studies, thymidine has been used as a marker for DNA synthesis, but in some instances, uridine and amino acids also have been used to measure RNA and protein synthesis.

Levamisole activates lymphocytes to become sensitized by allogeneic cells in vitro so that a greater number of target allogeneic cells per lymphocyte are killed. Levamisole exerts its effect before or during sensitization but not thereafter. With a suboptimal lymphocyte-target cell ratio, the effect is most pronounced (Persico and Potter, in press).

In melanoma patients, levamisole increases preexisting specific antitumor lymphocyte cytotoxicity, prolongs lymphocyte cytotoxicity induced by a tumor cell vaccine, and induces lymphocyte cytotoxicity in response to suboptimal and normally ineffective doses of the vaccine (Shibata *et al.,* 1976).

The lysosomal activity of lymphocytes of cancer patients is reported to be increased following levamisole treatment (Thornes, 1975).

Levamisole restores to normal the number of E-rosette-forming cells in patients in whom these cells are depressed. In these patients, the number of Ig-bearing cells, null cells or EAC rosettes, which was found to be increased, could be reduced after levamisole treatment. The increase in T cells and the reduction of B cells or null cells occurs without change in absolute lymphocyte count (Levo *et al.,* 1975; Verhaegen *et al.,* 1975, unpublished data; Bensa *et al.,* 1976; Ramot *et al.,* 1976; Renoux *et al.,* 1977; Ellgaard and Boesen, unpublished data). Levamisole has no effect on the number of human fetal E-rosette-forming cells or immunoglobulin-bearing cells in vitro (Hayward and Graham, 1976), but is reported to increase the number of E-rosette-forming spleen cells of thymectomized mice in vivo (Van Ghinckel and Haebeke, in press).

When the number of E-rosettes or immunoglobulin-bearing cells is normal, levamisole causes no change except at high dose levels (Fenichel *et al.,* 1976). E-rosette formation decreased by azathioprine (Verhaegen *et al.,* unpublished data), histamine, or iodoacetamide can be restored by levamisole. In thymectomized adult mice, levamisole has the reverse effect and makes the rosette-forming spleen cells more sensitive to azathioprine. Because azathioprine is thought to block specific thymic receptors on lymphocytes, sensitization of spleen cells of thymectomized mice to azathioprine might mean that these cells have acquired the specific theta-antigen after levamisole treatment (Van Ghinckel and Haebeke, in press).

A more recent study of the unblocking effect of levamisole on a subpopulation of T-lymphocytes in Hodgkin's disease patients indicates that the substance ferritin is blocking lymphocyte E-rosette formation, and can be removed by incubating the cells with levamisole in vitro and/or by administration of levamisole in vivo (Ramot et al., 1976).

In the great majority of the animal or human models tested, levamisole has had little or no effect on existing serum immune globulin levels or on production of specific antibody to the particular bacterial, viral, or cellular immunogen (Brugmans and Symoens, 1977). Any effect on antibody production is considered most likely to be secondary to T cell or macrophage activation, rather than a direct effect on B cells (Renoux et al., unpublished data).

In recent studies attempting to correlate a cellular biochemical mechanism(s) with levamisole action, levamisole was found to increase cyclic GMP levels in splenic T cells of mice and decrease cyclic AMP levels in these cells in vitro (Hadden et al., 1975). Similar effects were observed in patients' lymphocytes (Ramot et al., 1976) and polymorphonuclear cells (Anderson et al., in press). Fluctuation in levels of both cyclic GMP and cyclic AMP has been observed in lymphocytes of patients with melanoma and squamous cell carcinoma treated with levamisole (Olkowski, in press).

SUMMARY

Levamisole, a dose-dependent agent, is effective in treating slowly growing tumors. It is more effective when used in concert with cytoreductive therapy; the scheduling of treatment with levamisole adjuvant to chemotherapy is critical. Levamisole appears to preferentially affect metastatic formation. It acts as a potentiator of the immune response by enhancing earlier restoration of bone marrow and other lymphoid elements.

REFERENCES

Al-Ibrahim, M. S. 1978. *In vitro* effects of levamisole on human mononuclear phagocytes. In Chirigos, M. A. (ed.): Immune Modulation and Control of Neoplasia by Adjuvant Therapy. New York, Raven Press, vol. 7. (in press).

Anderson, R., Glover, A., Koornhof, H. J., and Rabson, P. 1978. *In vitro* stimulation of neutrophil motility by levamisole. Maintenance of CGP levels in chemotactically stimulated levamisole treated neutrophils. J. Immunol. (in press).

Bensa, J. O., Faure, J., Martin, H., Sotto, J. J., and Schaerer, R. 1976. Levamisole in angio-immuno-blastic lymphadenopathy. Lancet, 1:1081.

Brugmans, J., and Symoens, J. 1977. The effects of levamisole on host defense mechanisms: A review. In Chirigos, M. A. (ed.): Modulation of Host Immune Resistance in the Prevention or Treatment of Induced Neoplasias. Fogarty International Center Proceedings, No. 28, pp. 3–16.

Chirigos, M. A., Fuhrman, F., and Pryor, J. 1975. Prolongation of chemotherapeutically induced remission of a syngeneic murine leukemia by L-2, 3, 5, 6-tetrahydro-6-phenylimidazo [2, 1-b] thiazole hydrochloride. Cancer Res., 35:927–931, 1975.

Chirigos, M. A., Mohr, S. J., and Chaparas, S. D. 1977. Combined modality treatment with levamisole and protective effects against neoplasias. In Chirigos, M. A. (ed.): Modulation of Host Immune Resistance in the Prevention or Treatment of Induced Neoplasias. Fogarty International Center Proceedings, No. 28, pp. 59–63.

Chirigos, M. A., Pearson, J. W., and Pryor, J. 1973. Augmentation of chemotherapeutically induced remission of a murine leukemia by a chemical immunoadjuvant. Cancer Res., 33:2615–2618.

Doller, E. W., and Rapp, F. 1977. Effect of levamisole on metastases by herpesvirus-transformed cells. In Chirigos, M. A. (ed.): Control of Neoplasia by Modulation of the Immune System. New York, Raven Press, vol. 2, pp. 96–106.

Douglas, S. D., Schmidt, M. E., and Daughaday, C. C. 1976. Effects of levamisole on monocyte-macrophage, immunoprotein receptors and *in vitro* function (Abstract). Fed. Proc., 35(3):335.

Fenichel, R. L., Gregory, F. J., and Alburn, H. E. 1976. Anti-tumor and anti-metastatic activity of 3-(p-chlorophenyl)-2, 3-dihydro-3-hydroxythiazolo-3, 2-a-benzimidazole-2-acetic acid (Wy-13, 876). Br. J. Cancer, 33:329–335.

Fidler, I. J., and Spitler, L. E. 1975. Effects of levamisole *in vivo* and *in vitro*. Murine host response to syngeneic transplantable tumor. J. Natl. Cancer Inst., 55:1107-1112.

Gallin, J. I., and Wolff, S. M. 1975. Leucocyte chemotaxis: Physiological considerations and abnormalities. Clin. Haematol., 4(3):567–607.

Gordon, D. S., Hall, L. S., and McDougal, J. S. 1977. Levamisole and Cytoxan in a murine tumor model: *In vivo* and *in vitro* studies. In Chirigos, M. A. (ed.): Control of Neoplasia by Modulation of the Immune System. New York, Raven Press, vol. 2, pp. 121–133.

Hadden, J. W., Coffey, R. C., Hadden, E. M., Lopez-Corrales, E., and Sunshine, G. H. 1975. Effects of levamisole and imidazole on lymphocyte proliferation and cyclic nucleotide levels. Cell. Immunol., 20:98–103.

Hayward, A. R., and Graham, L. 1976. Increased E-rosette formation by foetal liver and spleen cells incubated with theophylline. Clin. Exp. Immunol., 23:279–284.

Hill, H. R., and Quie, P. G. 1975. Defective neutrophil chemotaxis associated with hyperimmunoglobulinemia E. In Bellanti, J. A., and Dayton, D. H. (eds.): The Phagocytic Cell in Host Resistance. New York, Raven Press, pp. 249–266.

Huskisson, E. C., Dieppe, P. A., Scott, J., Trapnell, G., Balme, H. W., and Willoughby, C. A. 1976. Immunostimulant therapy with levamisole for rheumatoid arthritis. Lancet, 1:393–395.

Ippen, H., and Qadripur, S. A. 1975. Levamisol zur behandlung von hautkrankheiten. Dtsch. Med. Wochenschr., 100(34):1710–1711.

Jedrzejczak, W. W. 1976. Phytohaemagglutinin (PHA) skin test in predicting prognosis of cancer patients. Int. Arch. Allergy Appl. Immunol., 51:574–582.

Johnson, R. K., Houchens, D. P., Gaston, M. R., and Goldin, A. 1975. Effects of levamisole (NSC-177023) and tetramisole (NSC-102063) in experimental tumor systems. Cancer Chemother. Rep., 59:697–705.

Levo, Y., Rotter, V., and Ramot, B. 1975. Restoration of cellular immune response by levamisole in patients with Hodgkin's disease. Biomedicine, 23:198–200.

Liauw, H. L., and Stecher, V. J. 1977. Effect of levamisole on the chemotaxis of neutrophils and monocytes. In Chirigos, M. A. (ed.): Control of Neoplasia by Modulation of the Immune System. New York, Raven Press, vol. 2, pp. 51–56.

Lichtenfeld, J. L., Desuer, M. R., Wiernick, P. H., Moore, S., and Mardiney, M. R., Jr. 1977. Amplification by levamisole of human lymphocyte responsiveness to immunological stimuli *in vitro*. In Chirigos, M. A. (ed.): Modulation of Host Immune Resistance in the Prevention or Treatment of Induced Neoplasias. Fogarty International Center Proceedings, No. 28. pp. 17–21.

Lieberman, R., and Hsu, M. 1976. Levamisole mediated restoration of cellular immunity in peripheral blood lymphocytes of patients with immunodeficiency diseases. Clin. Immunol. Immunopathol., 5:142–146.

Lima, A. O., Javierre, M. Q., Silva, W. D., and Sette Camara, D. 1974. Immunological phagocytosis: Effect of drugs on phosphodiesterase activity. Experientia, 30(8):945–946.

Lods, J. C., Dujardin, P., and Halpern, G. M. 1976. Levamisole and bone-marrow restoration after chemotherapy. Lancet, 1:548.

Mantovani, A., and Spreafico, F. 1975. Allogeneic tumor enhancement by levamisole, a new immunostimulatory compound: Studies on cell-mediated immunity and humoral antibody response. Eur. J. Cancer, 11:537–544.

Merluzzi, V. J., Badger, A. M., Kaiser, C. W., and Cooperband, S. R. 1975. *In vitro* stimulation of murine lymphoid cell cultures by levamisole. J. Clin. Exp. Immunol., 22:486–492.

Olkowski, Z. L. 1978. Cyclic adenosine monophosphate levels in lymphocytes from patients with melanoma and squamous cell carcinoma treated with levamisole. In Chirigos, M. A. (ed.): Immune Modulation and Control of Neoplasia by Adjuvant Therapy. New York, Raven Press, vol. 7 (in press).

Perk, K., Chirigos, M. A., Fuhrman, F., and Pettigrew, H. 1975. Some aspects of host response to levamisole after chemotherapy in a murine leukemia. J. Natl. Cancer Inst., 54:253–256.

Persico, F. J., and Potter, W. A. 1978. The effect of levamisole on an *in vitro* model of cellular immunity. In Chirigos, M. A. (ed.): Immune Modulation and Control of Neoplasia by Adjuvant Therapy. New York, Raven Press, vol. 7 (in press).

Pike, M. C., and Snyderman, R. 1976. Augmentation of human monocyte chemotactic responsiveness by levamisole. Nature, 201:136–137.

Potter, C. W., Carr, I., Jennings, R., Rees, R. C., McGinty, F., and Richardson, V. M. 1974. Levamisole inactive in treatment of four animal tumours. Nature, 249:567–569.

Ramot, B., Biniaminov, M., Shoham, C., and Rosenthal, E. 1976. The unblocking effect of levamisole on E-rosette forming cells *in vivo* and *in vitro* in Hodgkin's disease patients. N. Engl. J. Med., 294:809–811.

Renoux, G., and Renoux, M. 1972. Levamisole inhibits and cures a solid malignant tumor and its pulmonary metastases in mice. Nature [New Biol.], 240:217–218.

Renoux, G., Renoux, M., and Aycardi, D. 1976. Levamisole promotes the killing of Listeria monocytogenes by macrophages (Abstract). Fed. Proc., 35(3):336.

Renoux, G., Renoux, M., and Palat, A. 1977. Influences of levamisole on T cell reactivity and on survival of intractable cancer patients. In Chirigos, M. A. (ed.): Modulation of Host Immune Resistance in the Prevention or Treatment of Induced Neoplasias. Fogarty International Center Proceedings, No. 28, pp. 77–79.

Sadowski, J. M., and Rapp, F. 1975. Inhibition by levamisole of metastases by cells transformed by herpes simplex virus type I (38776). Proc. Soc. Exp. Biol. Med., 149:219–222.

Sampson, D., Peters, T. G., Lewis, J. D., Metzig, J., and Kurtz, B. E. 1977. Dose independence of immunopotentiation and tumor regression induced by levamisole. Cancer Res., 37:3526–3529.

Schreiber, A. D., Parsons, J., and Cooper, R. A. 1975. Effect of levamisole on the human monocyte IgG receptor. Blood, 46(6):1018.

Schulze, H. J., and Raettig, R. J. 1973. Steigerung der activitaet von peritonealmakrophagen der maus durch levamisole. Verh. Dtsch. Ges. Inn. Med., 79:622–623.

Seftel, H. C., and Heinz, H. J. 1968. Comparison of piperazine and tetramisole in treatment of ascariasis. Br. Med. J., 4:93–98.

Shibata, H. R., Jerry, L. M., Lewis, M. G., Mansell, P. W., Capek, A., and Marquis, G. 1976. Immunotherapy of human malignant melanoma with irradiated tumor cells, oral BCG and levamisole. Ann. NY Acad. Sci., 277:355–357.

Spreafico, F., Vecchi, A., Mantovani, A., Poggi, A., Franchi, G., Anaelerio, A., and Garrotini, S. 1975. Characterization of the immunostimulants, levamisole and tetramisole. Eur. J. Cancer., 11:555–563.

Sunshine, G., Lopez-Corrales, E., Hadden, E. M., Coffey, R. G., Wanebo, H., and Hadden, J. W. 1977. Levamisole and imidazole: *In vitro* effects in mouse and man and their possible mediation by cyclic nucleotides. In Chirigos, M. A. (ed.): Modulation of Host Immune Resistance in the Prevention or Treatment of Induced Neoplasias. Fogarty International Center Proceedings, No. 28, pp. 31–37.

Thienpont, D., Brugmans, J., and Abadi, K. 1969. Tetramisole in the treatment of nematode infections in man. Am. J. Trop. Med. Hyg., 18:520–528.

Thienpont, D., Vanparijs. O.F., Raeymaekers, A. H. M., Vanderbeck, J., Demoen, P. J. A., Allewijn, F. T. N., Marsboom, R. P. H., Niemegeers, C. J. E., Schellekins, K. H. L., Janssen, P. A. J. 1966. Tetramisole (R8299), a new patent broad spectrum antihelminthic. Nature, 209:1084–1086.

Thornes, R. D. 1975. Adjuvant therapy of cancer via the cellular immune mechanism or fibrin by induced fibrinolysis and oral anticoagulants. Cancer, 35:91–97.

Van Ghinckel, R. F., and Haebeke, J. 1978. Effect of levamisole on spontaneous rosette-forming cells in murine spleen. Eur. J. Immunol. (in press).

Van Huele, R., De Cree, J., Adriaenssens, K., and De Hauwere, R. 1976. Levamisole therapy for cellular immunologic deficiency with high IGE values. Acta Paediatr. Belg., 29:41–46.

Verhaegen, H., De Cock, W., De Cree, J., Verbroggen, F., Verhaegen-De Clercq, M., and Brugmans, J. 1975. *In vitro* restoration by levamisole of the E-rosette forming cells after inhibition by azathioprene. Lancet, 1:978.

Versijp, G., van Zwet, T. L., and van Furth, R. 1975. Levamisole and functions of peritoneal macrophages. Lancet, 1:798.

Whitcomb, M. E., Merluzzi, V. J., and Cooperband, S. R. 1976. The effect of levamisole on human lymphocyte mediator production *in vitro*. Cell. Immunol., 218:272–277.

Woods, W. A., Fliegelman, M. J., and Chirigos, M. A. 1975. Effect of levamisole (NSC-177023) on DNA synthesis by lymphocytes from immunosuppressed C57Bl mice. Cancer Chemother. Rep., 59:531–536.

Immunotherapy of Human Cancer,
The University of Texas System Cancer Center
M. D. Anderson Hospital and Tumor Institute.
Raven Press, New York © 1978.

Transfer Factor and Immunotherapy for Cancer

H. Sherwood Lawrence, M.D.

Infectious Disease and Immunology Division, Department of Medicine, New York University School of Medicine, New York, New York

IMMUNOLOGIC CONCOMITANTS OF TUMOR INITIATION

I have presented elsewhere an interpretation of the immunologic plight of the tumor-bearing host and considered the detailed evidence that leads to this viewpoint (Lawrence, 1970, 1974). Briefly, this concept accepts the in vivo reality that mutant, neoplastic cells do arise in multicellular organisms at a greater or lesser rate from birth onwards. Current information would suggest that the oncogenic event may result from dedifferentiation, with resultant display of embryonal antigens; from chemical carcinogens intricately complexed to and altering self-antigens; or from oncogenic viral perturbations of cells, resulting in new, tumor-associated membrane antigens.

In each instance, the host, confronted with cells bearing either new or altered antigen mosaics that differ from his or her own histocompatibility antigens, mounts an immune response with various degrees of intensity. When such differences are markedly disparate, the potentially neoplastic cell or cells are recognized as overtly foreign and rejected as an allograft. When the antigenic differences between the potentially neoplastic cell and host histocompatibility antigens are less marked, the responses are feeble, and the mechanism of recognition and/or rejection may be evaded or dampened.

The evidence for this view is admittedly slender and largely circumstantial, drawing heavily on the immunologic response of normal persons to overtly foreign, dissociated cell or solid tissue allografts introduced by other men from without, rather than having arisen more subtly de novo within the host. Nevertheless, additional support for this view may be expected to accrue from exploitation of recent observations made in several laboratories that have detected cell-mediated immunity to the patient's tumor antigens in healthy domiciliary contacts who are tumor free. This includes in vitro demonstration of specific lymphocyte cytotoxicity versus tumor target cells or migration inhibitory factor (MIF) production upon exposure of the contact's blood lymphocytes to the patient's tumor antigen. Moreover, transfer factor prepared from the lymphocytes of such domiciliary contacts has been shown to confer on and/or augment in the anergic patient specific immunity to his own tumor antigens, which has been associated with lymphocytic infiltration and regression of metastases (LoBuglio *et al.,* 1973; Levin *et al.,* 1975; Byers *et al.,* 1975).

IMMUNOLOGIC CONSEQUENCES OF TUMOR GROWTH

Having evaded recognition and/or attempted disposal despite their foreign caste, such mutant neoplastic cells may multiply at varying generation times, shedding antigen in the process and triggering antibody production as well as formation of tumor antigen-antibody complexes (Hellström and Hellström, 1977). The latter may serve to blindfold reactive lymphocytes that ordinarily would seek out and initiate attempts to reject the tumor as an allograft, and camouflage tumor target cells.

The clinical consequences of this derangement may be seen in the lack of cell-mediated immune responses of the patient's lymphocytes (proliferation, cytotoxicity) upon exposure to his tumor antigens in vitro when suspended in autologous sera or plasma. This abrogation of cell-mediated immunity is restored when such potentially reactive, educated lymphocytes are washed and resuspended in normal plasma or tissue culture media.

Another phenomenon that is becoming recognized both experimentally and clinically is that whenever antibody production is in the ascendency, cell-mediated immune responses are depressed; conversely, elevation of cell-mediated immune responses suppresses antibody production presumably via stimulation of suppressor cell activity (Lawrence, 1976b). The clinical consequences of this aberration may be seen in the well-documented cutaneous anergy to common recall antigens (purified protein derivative, streptokinase-streptodornase, *Candida*) as well as the incapacity to be sensitized to new antigens (dinitrochlorobenzene) detected in patients with metastatic disease.

Thus, the tumor-bearing patient appears a captive of an exuberant but ineffective immune response that facilitates target-cell protection and is inappropriate for target-cell rejection. Such a patient appears chained to an immunologic treadmill committed to unrestrained antibody production with progressive and sustained depression of cell-mediated immune responses, upon which rejection of solid tissue allografts depends (Lawrence, 1974, 1977).

IMMUNOLOGIC INTERVENTION—STRATEGIES AND LIMITATIONS

Thus, viewed in this light, the tumor-bearing patient represents a unique example in nature of an individual tolerating an allograft without the external administration of immunosuppressive drugs, such as are required for renal transplant recipients. The reasons for this paradox appear to us to be that (1) the tumor is only masquerading as an allograft, comprising a mix of antigen mosaics recognized as "self" and punctuated with foreign antigens that express only weak or trivial histocompatibility differences and therefore evoke feeble cell-mediated immune responses; and (2) the immune response evoked is predominantly humoral antibody, which we have suggested elsewhere functions as nature's own immunosuppressive device that has evolved to dampen the explosive, delayed-type, inflammatory and cytotoxic consequences that would naturally result from uninhibited cell-mediated immune responses (Lawrence, 1976a).

How, then, are we to deflect the tumor-bearing individual from this ineffective immune response and convince the patient to recognize his tumor for the allograft it is and reject it forthwith? First, the limitation imposed by the patient is that of generalized depression or absence of cell mediated immune responses, an internally achieved immunosuppressed state. Second, the limitation imposed by a replicating antigen, resulting in antigenic overload and a state of high-zone tolerance, presents a persistent barrier to the initial development as well as prolonged maintainence of any transient augmentation of cell-mediated immunity that may be induced by immunotherapeutic measures. The approach to immunologic intervention should be preceded by appropriate measures to reduce the antigenic burden before attempts at immunotherapy are instituted. When undertaken, immunotherapy should be aimed at initially restoring the patient's capacity to develop cell-mediated immune responses in general and, concomitantly, specific immunity to the tumor antigens in particular.

TRANSFER FACTOR IN CANCER IMMUNOTHERAPY

Transfer factor is a dialyzable, low molecular weight (<10,000), nontoxic moiety that is prepared from mononuclear cells of immune donors and that selectively restores and/or augments both specific and nonspecific delayed-type hypersensitivity and cell-mediated immune responses in recipients without concomitant immunoglobulin production (Lawrence, 1955, 1969, 1974; Lawrence *et al.,* 1963). The availability of a potent preparation of proven capacity to initiate and/or boost both specific and nonspecific cell-mediated immune responses without toxic side effects fostered the application of transfer factor to immunotherapy for cancer. Graft versus host and other adverse reactions, such as may follow lymphocyte infusions into immunosuppressed patients, are avoided by the use of transfer factor. The fact that both specific immunity to the tumor and nonspecific augmentation of cell-mediated immune responses in general are achieved by transfer factor in the absence of the transfer of antibody production to tumor antigens could be viewed as an additional benefit.

As experience with the use of transfer factor in the immunotherapy for cancer is largely anecdotal at this stage, no firm conclusions can be drawn. However, some inferences can be drawn from the reported studies that are applicable to all types of immunotherapy.

Background Studies: Can Transfer Factor Restore Cell-Mediated Immunity to Anergic Cancer Patients?

Our laboratory conducted an early, prospective study on the incidence of anergy and its relation to metastatic disease preoperatively in 150 patients with a diversity of cancers compared with 80 control patients. Each group was evaluated for cutaneous delayed-type hypersensitivity reactivity to streptokinase-streptodornase (SK-SD), purified protein derivative (PPD), diphtheria toxoid, histoplasmin, coccidioidin, and mumps antigens (Solowey *et al.,* 1968). We found that 110 of 150 cancer patients were anergic to all skin test antigens used, whereas 66 of 80 control patients without cancer responded to at least one antigen. Additionally, 94 (85%) of 110 anergic cancer patients were found to have metastatic disease at subsequent operation, compared with 29 of 40 cancer patients who had responded to one antigen and were found free of metastatic disease.

To test whether such anergic individuals were able to respond to dialyzable transfer factor, 14 patients were given a single injection of SK-SD-positive transfer factor obtained from normal, immune donors. The technique of local transfer was used to assess the reaction to SK-SD challenge of a skin site prepared with transfer factor compared with SK-SD challenge of a remote, unprepared site. Of 14 anergic cancer patients, all responded with marked delayed-type hypersensitivity reactions to SK-SD at the prepared site. However, unlike those of normal persons, the reactions to SK-SD at remote sites (a measure of systemic transfer of delayed-type hypersensitivity) were feeble (approximately 10 mm of induration) and could not be elicited upon retest a week later.

With the miniscule dose of transfer factor used in the above group of patients, no clinical improvement was anticipated or observed. Nevertheless, these studies did demonstrate that anergic cancer patients with metastatic disease possess immunocompetent cell populations capable of response and that delayed-type hypersensitivity and cell-mediated immune responses can be augmented by administration of transfer factor prepared from normal persons. However, the initial responses observed were less intense, and the duration of augmented immunity was shorter than that observed in normal recipients of transfer factor.

Is Pooled, "Nonspecific" Transfer Factor Effective Immunotherapy for Breast Cancer?

With our colleagues at the Memorial Sloan-Kettering Cancer Center, we next turned to the larger question of whether pooled, "nonspecific" transfer factor would have any value as immunotherapy for patients with advanced, metastatic, inflammatory breast cancer (Oettgen *et al.,* 1974). The source of the pooled transfer factor preparations was 177 healthy female donors over 45 years of age. This choice was based on our assumption that some donors, via immunologic surveillance, would possess cell-mediated immunity to breast tumor antigens following successful encounters with mutant breast cells from puberty onward.

For this study, five patients were given 1 to 4 ml of dialyzable transfer factor subcutaneously daily or thrice weekly for periods as short as three weeks and as long as one year (310 days). The total dose of transfer factor administered to individual patients was equivalent to 20 to 257 ml packed white blood cells where 20 ml contained 17 billion cells. Either tuberculin (PPD) or SK-SD was used as a marker to detect the systemic transfer of cutaneous delayed-type hypersensitivity, which occurred in three of five patients. In only one of the five patients was a temporary regression of the metastatic lesions observed; this regression lasted for six months before relapse.

From this limited study, no conclusions were drawn concerning the potential usefulness of pooled, "nonspecific" transfer factor as immunotherapy for breast cancer. However, detailed ancillary studies for toxicity allowed the conclusion that transfer factor, used even in these massive amounts (257 ml = 217 billion cell equivalents) repeatedly (125 injections) for a long time (310 days), is a nontoxic material with no harmful hematologic, immunologic, enzymatic, biochemical, or clinical side effects. The dosage regimen used in this study also gives some clue to the margin of safety, as the transfer factor prepared from 10^9 lymphocyte equivalents represents the average dose used to treat patients with congenital immunodeficiency or infectious diseases.

Using breast-tumor-specific transfer factor, other investigators (Silva *et al.,* 1976) have noted more favorable clinical responses associated with flare of metastatic skin depots and longer periods (e.g., more than 16 months) of stabilization of disease.

Osteogenic Sarcoma—A Case for Tumor-Specific Transfer Factor?

Levin *et al.* (1975) have treated 13 patients with osteogenic sarcoma and compared the immunologic and clinical effects of tumor-specific versus nonspecific transfer factor. Of great interest was their finding that domiciliary contacts of patients with osteogenic sarcoma would have specific cell-mediated immunity, as evidenced by lymphocyte in vitro cytotoxicity to osteogenic sarcoma target cells (Byers *et al.,* 1975). Administration of tumor-specific transfer factor prepared from such donors to the 13 patients with osteogenic sarcoma resulted in augmentation of each patient's cell-mediated immunity to his tumor, as measured by (1) lymphocyte-mediated cytotoxicity to osteogenic sarcoma target cells; (2) lymphocytic infiltration and inflammatory responses induced in metastatic lesions of which biopsies had been done; and (3) general augmentation of cell-mediated immunity, as measured by increased numbers of E-rosettes. Of particular interest was the observation that when this augmentation of cell-mediated immunity following one dose of tumor-specific transfer factor was allowed to wane with time, the subsequent administration of an equivalent dose of nonspecific transfer factor had no detectable effect in the same patient. However, another subsequent injection of tumor-specific transfer factor into the same patient again resulted in augmentation of tumor-specific, cell-mediated immune responses. Based on regression of metastases and no new metastases during a period ranging from 3 to 20 months, the clinical response following administration of tumor-specific transfer factor was rated favorable in only 8 of 13 patients studied.

This investigative group has updated and expanded on the results of this study in more recent publications (Fudenberg *et al.,* 1974; Fudenberg, 1976; Byers *et al.,* 1976).

Neidhart and LoBuglio (1974) also report on clinical and immunologic improvement of another patient with osteogenic sarcoma following administration of tumor-specific transfer factor prepared from the patient's father, whose lymphocytes produced MIF in the presence of the patient's tumor antigens. Transfer factor was administered in doses of 15 units (1 unit $= 10^8$ lymphocyte equivalents) twice monthly and resulted in augmentation of the patient's cell-mediated immune responses to her own tumor antigens, as measured by the acquisition of MIF production. The patient remained free of disease as of 17 months following initiation of tumor-specific transfer factor therapy.

A summary by Meier and LoBuglio (in press) of later experience indicated that three of five osteosarcoma patients treated with transfer factor have done well for 7, 8, and 17 months after surgery whereas the remaining two patients relapsed at 4 and 12 months. An additional two patients with metastatic osteosarcoma in remission induced by combination chemotherapy remained free of disease with transfer factor therapy alone for 11 and 28 months, respectively. LoBuglio *et al.* (1973) also had treated a patient with alveolar sarcoma with tumor-specific transfer factor, prepared from the lymphocytes of the patient's identical twin, which resulted in cell-mediated immune response (acquisition of MIF production) by the patient to his own tumor antigens following two injections of 15 units each. The patient gained weight, became asymptomatic, and refused further therapy; the pulmonary lesions remained stable for a year but flared up at 14 months, and the patient died.

Transfer Factor Immunotherapy Compared with Combined Chemotherapy

Ivins *et al.* (1976) compared the results of transfer factor immunotherapy versus combined chemotherapy (methotrexate-Adriamycin-vincristine) in 26 randomized patients with clinically localized osteogenic sarcoma after surgery. In the group treated with transfer factor alone, delayed-type hypersensitivity reactions to skin test markers were converted, as evidence of transfer factor activity, in 8 of 14 patients. All of the patients receiving transfer factor had an increase in the proliferative responses of lymphocytes to phytohemagglutinin and concanavalin A; however, no clear-cut pattern could be established between augmented blastogenic responses and subsequent clinical course.

As of the most recent evaluation, all of the eight patients treated with transfer factor are alive, and four of these are free of disease. Among the 18 patients treated with combination chemotherapy, 14 are alive, 12 of whom are free of disease. The cumulative incidence of metastases in the group treated with transfer factor is 8.7 and in the group treated with chemotherapy, 5.1 per 100 patient-months.

Transfer Factor Immunotherapy Plus Combined Chemotherapy

Bearden *et al.* (1976) studied six patients with localized osteogenic sarcoma treated with combined tumor-specific transfer factor and chemotherapy after surgery. In the preliminary report, three patients remained free of recurrence for 7, 11, and 17 months, and the remaining three patients relapsed at 4, 14, and 16 months after amputation. For the patients who relapsed, therapy had been started after a lapse of two months rather than the recommended three weeks after amputation. The tumor-specific transfer factor used in this study was obtained from osteosarcoma patients' household contacts with high levels of lymphocyte target-cell cytotoxicity to tumor cells or disease-free osteosarcoma patients in complete remission for at least two years.

Repeated injections of tumor-specific transfer factor were followed in some of these patients by substantial increases in lymphocyte cytotoxicity to tumor target cells and stimulation of MIF production by tumor antigens. Minimal immunostimulation of direct cytotoxicity was observed in two patients who had early recurrences (Thor *et al.,* 1976).

Immunotherapy for Malignant Melanoma

In early attempts at immunotherapy for melanoma, Nadler and Moore (1965) obtained viable leukocytes from paired patients immunized with each other's tumor and transferred immune leukocytes back into the tumor donor. Five of 14 patients treated in this fashion improved, and one patient experienced complete remission of disease, with no recurrence one year later.

Krementz *et al.* (1974) confirmed this observation in 56 patients with melanoma immunized with each other's tumor extracts and cross-transfused with leukocytes in plasma. The incidence and severity of complications to the transfused cells, however, led the authors to prepare transfer factor from such cells and employ it as a safer form of immunotherapy.

It should be emphasized that in addition to the usual transfusion reactions reported here, immunotherapy with viable leukocytes or lymphocytes given to immunodeficient patients can result in graft versus host disease at worst or, at best, require the patient to reject the transferred cells and thereby prepare his own transfer factor in vivo. It would seem more reasonable to spare the patient's immunologic apparatus this additional burden and prepare transfer factor from such cells in vitro rather than require the patient to do so in vivo.

Brandes *et al.* (1971) used a similar cross-sensitization protocol for a patient with metastatic melanoma and used frozen and thawed leukocyte extracts obtained from the sensitized patient as a source of transfer factor. The leukocyte extract was infiltrated locally around metastatic nodules and given systemically as well, and resulted in vigorous inflammatory responses and rejection of metastatic tumor nodules in the skin, associated with a systemic febrile response and circulating lymphoblasts. The patient died subsequently of brain hemorrhage.

Spitler *et al.* (1973) treated nine melanoma patients with melanoma-specific, dialyzable transfer factor that had been prepared from cohabitants of the respective patients with demonstrable in vitro reactivity to the patients' melanoma antigens (lymphocyte transformation, MIF production). Only two of the nine patients so treated responded, immunologically with acquisition of lymphocyte transformation to their own melanoma antigens and clinically with regression of metastatic lesions. One patient remained in remission for 1½ years before new metastases developed, despite continued transfer factor therapy and coincident with loss of lymphocyte transformation and MIF production to melanoma antigens.

Spitler *et al.* (1976), in a subsequent study, compared the results of treating four patients with widely disseminated melanoma with transfer factor alone to the results of treating six patients with disseminated melanoma that was not widespread with transfer factor plus bacillus Calmette-Guérin (BCG) combined immunotherapy. There was no clinical or immunologic effect in any of the former group of four patients. Two of the six patients who received transfer factor plus BCG had complete regression of all tumor nodules coincident with combined immunotherapy; regression lasted for three years in one patient. The other patient who had responded had a recurrence with cerebral metastases and died. The two patients who responded favorably expressed lymphocyte stimulation to melanoma antigens. Smith *et al.* (1973) also report favorable responses of four of ten patients with melanoma who experienced reactions of tumor rejection and regression of metastatic lesions following administration of melanoma-specific transfer factor.

Silva *et al.* (1976) report stabilization of melanoma for more than six months in two of nine patients with metastatic disease treated with transfer factor. Vetto *et al.* (1976a) also have reported regression of metastatic tumor nodules in three of 11 patients with melanoma treated with transfer factor.

Bukowski *et al.* (1976) administered transfer factor to six patients with stage IV melanoma and observed no detectable effect on objective clinical responses despite increased lymphocyte cytotoxicity to melanoma cells detected in three patients. These investigators repeated the study with a group of stage III melanoma patients and compared the responses of five untreated patients with five patients who received transfer factor. Preliminary assessment of these patients reveals no apparent differences.

Jewell *et al.* (1976) compared the responses of 28 patients with stage II or III melanoma. The patients were randomly selected partners treated either with allogeneic tumor cell extracts followed by exchange of viable leukocytes between partners, or with irradiated whole tumor cells followed by exchange of transfer factor between partners. Objective clinical responses (greater than 50% regression of tumor mass) occurred in four of the 19 patients treated with transfer factor compared with none of nine patients in the leukocyte-treated group, eight of whom had progressive disease. Additionally, conversion of cutaneous delayed-type hypersensitivity reactions and MIF production occurred only in the group treated with transfer factor.

Other findings of interest related to the regression of tumor, which was observed in four of six patients who had received transfer factor prepared from partners immunized with autogenous tumor but in none of 16 patients who received transfer factor prepared from partners immunized with allogeneic tumor. From this limited experience, the authors call attention to the possibility that transfer factor may be superior to viable cell transfer and that the specificity of transfer factor for the host tumor may play a role in the effects achieved.

Transfer Factor Therapy for Miscellaneous Tumors

Nasopharyngeal Cancer

Goldenberg and Brandes (1972, 1976) report that nasopharyngeal carcinoma regressed in a patient treated with Epstein-Barr (E-B) virus-immune transfer factor obtained from donors who had recovered from infectious mononucleosis. In addition to clinical improvement, there was evidence from biopsy of intense lymphocytic infiltration of the tumor following the administration of transfer factor, which was associated with a fall in the antibody titer to E-B viral capsid antigen in addition to conversion of cutaneous delayed-type hypersensitivity reactions to PPD, *Candida, T. rubrum,* and mumps antigens. The patient was given transfer factor on a weekly basis with bleomycin therapy during an episode of relapse, and the disease remained stable for the following two years, until the patient relapsed and died. As an outgrowth of these studies, a double-blind randomized clinical trial is in progress in Hong Kong under the auspices of the Canadian Research Council. In this trial, half the patients are receiving conventional radiotherapy and half are receiving radiotherapy plus transfer factor obtained from normal donors with a history of infectious mononucleosis and/or detectable antibody to E-B viral capsid antigen. Depending on the results, a similar trial of transfer factor for Burkitt's lymphoma may be considered by this group.

Renal Cell Carcinoma

Fudenberg *et al.* (1974) have indicated that two of three patients with hypernephroma had marked improvement in their clinical status after receiving hypernephroma-specific transfer factor. Vetto *et al.* (1976b) also report on the arrest of pulmonary metastases of nine months' duration in one patient with renal cell carcinoma treated with transfer factor.

Montie *et al.* (1977) have reported on ten patients with disseminated renal carcinoma treated with tumor-specific transfer factor. The donors of transfer factor had greater than 50% cell inhibition of renal cell carcinoma lines in a microcytotoxicity assay and were family members when possible. No regression, but stabilization of metastases was observed in three patients for one, three, and six months, respectively, and in two other patients for four and five months, respectively, before rapid progression of disease despite continued transfer factor therapy. Two additional patients free of disease at the beginning of transfer factor therapy have remained so. No adverse local or systemic effects were noted following administration of transfer factor, and an increase in active E-rosettes appeared to correlate with stabilization of metastases.

Papillomatosis of the Larynx

Quick *et al.* (1975) report clinical and immunologic improvement in two children with laryngeal papillomatosis treated with transfer factor obtained from persons recovered from either condyloma acuminatum or papillomatosis. Following transfer factor therapy, both patients acquired the respective cutaneous delayed-type hypersensitivity and in vitro lymphocyte transformation responses (SK-SD, PPD) of the respective donors as well as an improved ability of their lymphocytes to kill the tumor cells in culture. Administration of the transfer factor prepared from the person who had recovered from papillomatosis resulted in a significant clinical response in both children, which was associated with a retardation of the growth of tumors and gross as well as histologic improvement in the appearance of the extirpated lesions coincident with marked infiltration of lymphocytes and plasma cells and necrosis of tumor cells. This histologic improvement was observed only following transfer factor administration, and after a four-month lapse of therapy, the original appearance with few cellular infiltrates recurred. Upon resumption of transfer factor therapy, there was a renewed influx of lymphocytes and plasma cells as described above; this was associated with clinical improvement.

Other Tumors

The number of individual case reports that comprise an assorted group of tumors appearing to manifest a favorable response to transfer factor therapy is growing: rhabdomyosarcoma, adenocarcinoma of colon (Vetto *et al.,* 1976a,b), vaginal carcinoma (Silva *et al.,* 1976), and mycosis fungoides (Zachariae *et al.,* 1975).

Transfer Factor Therapy for Infections in Hodgkin's Disease and Leukemia

The possible role of transfer factor as adjunctive immunotherapy for any malignancy or a select group of malignancies is difficult to predict from the anecdotal reports outlined above. Transfer factor possibly can be applied more immediately to treatment of the infectious complications that occur secondary to the immunosuppression produced by the tumor itself and compounded by the therapy employed. The rationale for this approach is based on the cumulative favorable experience with transfer factor in the immunotherapy for disseminated infectious diseases caused by viruses, fungi, and mycobacteria (Lawrence, 1974; Ascher *et al.,* 1976).

Drew *et al.* (1973) report on the use of transfer factor in a patient with Hodgkin's disease in whom disseminated herpes zoster developed during immunosuppressive therapy. Zoster-immune transfer factor was administered after therapy with arabinosyl adenine had failed to halt progression of the lesions. Upon administration of transfer factor, intense erythema developed around the vesicles and this was followed by crusting and healing of all the lesions. The culture positive for zoster virus became negative, and the patient's lymphocyte transformation test to zoster antigen became converted from a negative to a positive response. No new lesions of zoster appeared after the course of transfer factor.

Ng (1977) also has reported on transfer factor treatment of a patient with stage IV Hodgkin's disease in whom disseminated varicella developed after chemotherapy. Following administration of transfer factor plus hyperimmune globulin, the patient's lymphocyte transformation test and MIF production converted from negative to positive in the presence of varicella-zoster antigen. The patient became afebrile, the existing lesions became crusted, and no new lesions developed. This improvement was followed by a relapse and pseudomonas septicemia, with subsequent death of the patient. Kahn *et al.* (1976) have reported on similar clinical and immunologic improvement following transfer factor therapy for patients with rheumatoid arthritis and disseminated lupus in whom herpes zoster infections developed as a result of immunosuppressive therapy.

In 15 children with acute lymphoblastic leukemia in remission, Hayes and Mauer (1975) studied the effects of transfer factor on in vivo and in vitro responses of cell-mediated immunity. They found that transfer factor induced positive, cutaneous delayed-type hypersensitivity responses in all of seven children receiving two drugs and in two of eight children receiving four drugs.

Steele and Canales (1977) have studied varicella-immune transfer factor as a prophylactic immunization against varicella-zoster infections in children with acute lymphoblastic leukemia. Ten of 12 children in remission developed positive reactivity whereas none of three children in relapse responded. Three children who developed cell-mediated immunity to varicella-zoster antigen when exposed to chickenpox subsequently did not develop the disease. Follow-up studies at nine months revealed that all children still had positive responses to varicella-zoster antigen.

COMMENTARY AND CONCLUSIONS

I have attempted to give a tempered and circumspect assessment of the current state of the art for the immunotherapy of cancer with transfer factor. This is as it should be, in view of the anecdotal nature of the scattered clinical studies with small, heterogeneous groups of patients. This limitation will be alleviated only when the controlled, double-blind clinical trials in progress yield more extensive, factual data. These current trials are being done for nasopharyngeal cancer (Canadian National Research Council, Hong Kong), osteogenic sarcoma (Southwestern Cooperative Study Group, Mayo Clinic Study Group), and malignant melanoma (Harvard, New York University, University of California at San Francisco, and Temple Study Group).

The initial attempts at immunotherapy for cancer with transfer factor have given suggestive evidence of beneficial effects clinically (regression of metastases), histologically (lymphocytic infiltration of tumor), and immunologically (acquisition of cell-mediated immunity to tumor antigens, recall of delayed-type hypersensitivity responses, augmentation of lymphocyte proliferation and cytotoxicity responses, and conversion of MIF production).

The beneficial effects of immunotherapy with transfer factor that have accrued from patients with recalcitrant, disseminated intracellular infections caused by viruses, fungi, or mycobacteria are more readily apparent, and the clinical results more precisely documented. Unlike cancer, these infections are terminated after administration of transfer factor. Moreover, cultural evidence of eradication of the microbe or virus is readily demonstrated in association with augmentation of cell-mediated immunity and increased microbicidal activity of phagocytes. Additionally, the clinical signs of infection, such as fever, and laboratory signs of inflammation return to normal values as the patient recovers. These objective signs of eradication of an infection have been validated repeatedly in clinical trials that have established the effectiveness of antibiotic therapy.

An implicit and perhaps misleading assumption is that a particular cancer is a single disease entity—like coccidioidomycosis for example. Lack of the ability to fulfill Koch's postulates in relation to cancer leaves the etiology and pathogenesis unknown and the whole disease process a description of an aberration of cell growth. This ambiguity is compounded by the fact that our interpretation of the immunologic plight of the tumor-bearing patient is vastly oversimplified and requires extensive clarification before the dynamic and complex relationships between host and tumor are fully comprehended. Nevertheless, despite wide gaps in our knowledge, the model of the tumor as an allograft and the use of immunologic means to encourage the host to reject his tumor have conditioned most approaches to active or passive immunotherapy.

Finally, we come to a nagging doubt of whether any form of adjuvant cancer therapy, including immunotherapy, can be expected to rid the host of every last cancer cell or alter the as yet undefined aberration in the host that permitted the process to unfold de novo. Unhappily, there are no easy answers available and there is doubt, in some quarters, that even the proper questions are being posed.

It may be asking a great deal to expect any dramatic therapeutic benefit from administration of transfer factor to cancer patients, given the vagaries and variables of the patients selected, the type, duration, and stage of the particular cancer, and the source, potency, amount, and duration of transfer factor administered. Some of these variables may be reduced with the precise biochemical definition of transfer factor and its mechanism of action, as well as standardization of the unitage and dosage. Helpful clues to our understanding of the contribution of the host response in curbing tumor growth may be anticipated from the studies in progress. In any event, tempered by this spirit of restraint, we look forward to the results of the controlled clinical trials of transfer factor in cancer patients.

A recently discovered bovine transfer factor (Klesius *et al.,* 1975; Klesius and Fudenberg, 1977), which can protect cattle from coccidiosis and which is active when given to monkeys, could provide a potent, well-standardized, and virtually unlimited source of material. Because hormonal peptides of bovine origin have been administered to humans safely for several decades, it would only require immunizing cattle with human tumor types to obtain a transfer factor with appropriate specificity. Indeed, access to the large amounts of transfer factor provided by cattle could result in sequencing this low molecular weight peptide-nucleotide complex, which may not prove too difficult to synthesize.

ACKNOWLEDGMENTS

Work from the author's laboratory was supported by research grants 2 R01 AI-01254-22, 2 P01 CA-16247-04, and training grant 5 T01 AI-00005-18 from the U.S. Public Health Service; and research grant IM-134 from the American Cancer Society.

REFERENCES

Ascher, M. S., Gottlieb, A. A., and Kirkpatrick, C. H. (eds.) 1976. Transfer Factor. Basic Properties and Clinical Applications. New York, Academic Press, pp. 439–520.

Bearden, J. D., III, Thor, D. E., and Coltman, C. A. 1976. Adjunctive transfer factor in osteogenic sarcoma. I. Clinical implications of chemotherapy and immunotherapy. In Ascher, M. S., Gottlieb, A. A., and Kirkpatrick, C. H. (eds.): Transfer Factor. Basic Properties and Clinical Applications. New York, Academic Press, pp. 553–560.

Brandes, L. J., Galton, D. A. G., and Wiltshaw, E. 1971. New approach to immunotherapy of melanoma. Lancet, 2:293–295.

Bukowski, R. M., Deodhar, S., and Hewlett, J. S. 1976. Immunotherapy of human neoplasms with transfer factor. In Ascher, M. S., Gottlieb, A. A., and Kirkpatrick, C. H. (eds.): Transfer Factor. Basic Properties and Clinical Applications. New York, Academic Press, pp. 543–548.

Byers, V. S., Levin, A. S., Hackett, A. J., and Fudenberg, H. H. 1975. Tumor-specific cell-mediated immunity in household contacts of cancer patients. J. Clin. Invest., 55:500–513.

Byers, V. S., Levin, A. S., LeCam, L., Johnston, J. O., and Hackett, A. J. 1976. Discussion paper: Tumor-specific transfer factor therapy in osteogenic sarcoma: A two-year study. Ann. NY Acad. Sci., 277:621–627.

Drew, W. L., Blume, M. R., Miner, R., Silverberg, I., and Rosenbaum, E. H. 1973. Herpes zoster: Transfer factor therapy. Ann. Intern. Med., 79:747–748.

Fudenberg, H. H. 1976. Dialyzable transfer factor in the treatment of human osteosarcoma: An analytic review. Ann. NY Acad. Sci., 277:545–557.

Fudenberg, H. H., Levin, A. S., Spitler, L. E., Wybran, J., and Byers, V. 1974. The therapeutic uses of transfer factor. Hosp. Prac., 9:95–104.

Goldenberg, B. J., and Brandes, L. J. 1972. Immunotherapy of nasopharyngeal carcinoma with transfer factor from donors with previous infectious mononucleosis (Abstract). Clin. Res., 20:947.

Goldenberg, B. J., and Brandes, L. J. 1976. *In vivo* and *in vitro* studies of immunotherapy of nasopharyngeal carcinoma with transfer factor. Cancer Res., 36:720–723.

Hayes, L. B., and Mauer, A. M. 1975. Transfer factor activity in children receiving combination immunotherapy (Abstract). Proc. Am. Assoc. Cancer Res., 16:108.

Hellström, K. E., and Hellström, I. 1977. Immunologic enhancement of tumor growth. In Green, I., Cohen, S., and McCluskey, R. T. (eds.): Mechanisms of Tumor Immunity. New York, John Wiley and Sons, pp. 147–174.

Ivins, J. C., Ritts, R. E., Pritchard, D. J., Gilchrist, G. S., Miller, G. C., and Taylor, W. F. 1976. Transfer factor versus combination chemotherapy: A preliminary report of a randomized postsurgical adjuvant treatment study in osteogenic sarcoma. Ann. NY Acad. Sci., 277:558–574.

Jewell, W. R., Thomas, J. H., Morse, P., and Humphrey, L. J. 1976. Comparison of allogeneic tumor vaccine with leukocyte transfer and transfer factor treatment of human cancer. Ann. NY Acad. Sci., 277:516–521.

Kahn, A., Thaxton, S., Hill, J. M., Hill, N. O., Loeb, E., and MacLellan, A. 1976. Clinical trials with transfer factor. In Ascher, M. S., Gottlieb, A. A., and Kirkpatrick, C. H. (eds.): Transfer Factor. Basic Properties and Clinical Applications. New York, Academic Press, pp. 583–590.

Klesius, P. H., Kramer, T., Burger, D., and Malley, A. 1975. Passive transfer of coccidian oocyst antigen and diphtheria toxoid hypersensitivity in calves across species barriers. Transplant. Proc., 7:449–452.

Klesius, P. H., and Fudenberg, H. H. 1977. Bovine transfer factor: *In vivo* transfer of cell-mediated immunity to cattle with alcohol precipitates. Clin. Immunol. Immunopathol., 8:238–246.

Krementz, F. T., Mansell, P. W. A., Hornung, M. O., Samuels, M. S., Sutherland, C. A., and Benes, E. N. 1974. Immunotherapy of malignant disease: The use of viable sensitized lymphocytes or transfer factor prepared from sensitized lymphocytes. Cancer, 33:394–401.

Lawrence, H. S. 1955. The transfer in humans of delayed hypersensitivity to streptococcal M-substance and to tuberculin with disrupted leukocytes. J. Clin. Invest., 34:219–230.

Lawrence, H. S. 1969. Transfer factor. Adv. Immunol., 11:195–266.

Lawrence, H. S. 1970. Transfer factor and cellular immune deficiency disease. N. Engl. J. Med., 283:411–419.

Lawrence, H. S. 1974. Transfer factor in cellular immunity. Harvey Lect., 68:239–350.

Lawrence, H. S. 1976a. Infectious "self + X" mosaics: An invitation to autoimmunity with potential for restoration by transfer factor. In Dumonde, D. C. (ed.): Infection and Immunology in the Rheumatic Diseases. Oxford, Blackwell Scientific Publications, pp. 563–577.

Lawrence, H. S. 1976b. Summation of symposium. In Ascher, M. S., Gottlieb, A. A., and Kirkpatrick, C. H. (eds.): Transfer Factor. Basic Properties and Clinical Applications. New York, Academic Press, pp. 741–753.

Lawrence, H. S. 1977. Transfer factor in transplantation immunobiology. Transplant. Proc., 9:1319–1325.

Lawrence, H. S., Al-Askari, S., David, J. R., Franklin, E. C., and Zweiman, B. 1963. Transfer of immunological information in humans with dialysates of leukocyte extracts. Trans. Assoc. Am. Phys., 76:84–91.

Levin, A. S., Byers, V. S., Fudenberg, H. H., Wybran, J., Hackett, A. J., Johnston, J. O., and Spitler, L. E. 1975. Osteogenic sarcoma—Immunologic parameters before and during immunotherapy with tumor-specific transfer factor. J. Clin. Invest., 55:487–499.

LoBuglio, A. F., Neidhart, J. F., Hilberg, R. W., Metz, E. N., and Balcerzak, S. P. 1973. The effect of transfer factor therapy on tumor immunity in alveolar soft part sarcoma. Cell. Immunol., 7:159–165.

Meier, C. R., and LoBuglio, A. F. 1978. Transfer factor: A potential agent for immunotherapy of cancer. World J. Surg. (in press).

Montie, J. E., Bukowski, R. M., Deodhar, S. D., Hewlett, J. S., Stewart, B. H., and Straffon, R. A. 1977. Immunotherapy of disseminated renal carcinoma with transfer factor. J. Urol., 117:553–556.

Nadler, S. H., and Moore, G. E. 1965. Autotransplantation of human cancer. JAMA, 191:105–106.

Nadler, S. H., and Moore, G. E. 1966. Clinical immunologic study of malignant disease: Response to tumor transplants and transfer of leukocytes. Ann. Surg., 164:482.

Neidhart, J. A., and LoBuglio, A. F. 1974. Transfer factor therapy of malignancy. Semin. Oncol., 1:379–385.

Ng, R. P. 1977. Disseminated varicella infection: Treatment with transfer factor in a patient with Hodgkin's disease. Scand. J. Infect. Dis., 9:139–140.

Oettgen, H. F., Old, L. J., Farrow, J. H., Valentine, F. T., Lawrence, H. S., and Thomas, L. 1974. Effects of dialyzable transfer factor in patients with breast cancer. Proc. Natl. Acad. Sci. USA, 71:2319–2323.

Quick, C. A., Behrens, H. W., Brinton-Darnell, M., and Good, R. A. 1975. Treatment of papillomatosis of the larynx with transfer factor. Ann. Otol. Rhinol. Laryngol., 84:607–613.

Silva, J., Allen, J., Wheeler, R., Bull, F., Morley, G., and Plouffe, J. 1976. Transfer factor therapy of disseminated neoplasms. In Ascher, M. S., Gottlieb, A. A., and Kirkpatrick, C. H. (eds.): Transfer Factor. Basic Properties and Clinical Applications. New York, Academic Press, pp. 573–578.

Smith, G. V., Morse, P. A., Deraps, G. D., Raju, S., and Hardy, J. D. 1973. Immunotherapy of patients with cancer. Surgery, 74:59–65.

Solowey, A. C., Rapaport, F. T., and Lawrence, H. S. 1968. Cellular studies in neoplastic diseases. In Curtoni, E. S., Mattiuz, P. L., and Tosi, R. M. (eds.): Histocompatibility Testing. Baltimore, Williams & Wilkins, pp. 75–78.

Spitler, L. E., Levin, A. S., and Wybran, J. 1976. Combined immunotherapy in malignant melanoma. Regression of metastatic lesions in two patients concordant in timing with systemic administration of transfer factor and bacillus Calmette-Guerin. Cell. Immunol., 21:1–19.

Spitler, L. E., Wybran, J., Fudenberg, H. H., Levin, A. S., and Lewis, M. 1973. Transfer factor therapy of malignant melanoma (Abstract). Clin. Res., 21:221.

Steele, R. W., and Canales, L. 1977. Transfer factor in the prevention of varicella-zoster infections in childhood leukemia (Abstract). Pediatr. Res., 11:506.

Thor, D. E., Cottman, C. A., Bearden, J. D., III, Williams, T. E., and Flippen, J. H. 1976. Adjunctive transfer factor in osteogenic sarcoma. II. Methodology and results of immunological studies. In Ascher, M. S., Gottlieb, A. A., and Kirkpatrick, C. H. (eds.): Transfer Factor. Basic Properties and Clinical Applications. New York, Academic Press, pp. 563–569.

Vetto, R. M., Burger, D. R., Nolte, J. E., and Vandenbark, A. A. 1976a. Transfer factor immunotherapy in cancer. In Ascher, M. S., Gottlieb, A. A., and Kirkpatrick, C. H. (eds.): Transfer Factor. Basic Properties and Clinical Applications. New York, Academic Press, pp. 523–530.

Vetto, R. M., Burger, D. R., Nolte, J. E., and Vandenbark, A. A. 1976b. Transfer factor therapy in patients with cancer. Cancer, 37:90–97.

Zachariae, H., Grunnet, E., Ellegaard, J., and Thestrup-Pedersen, K. 1975. Transfer factor as an additional therapeutic agent in mycosis fungoides. Acta Allergol., 30:272–285.

Immunotherapy of Human Cancer,
The University of Texas System Cancer Center
M. D. Anderson Hospital and Tumor Institute.
Raven Press, New York © 1978.

Active-Specific Immunotherapy

Ariel C. Hollinshead, Ph.D.

Department of Medicine, The George Washington University Medical Center, Washington, D.C.

The design of an active-specific immunotherapy trial includes the careful selection of tumor-associated antigens (TAA) free of interfering, harmful, or inhibitory material and combined with the best adjuvant vehicle for slow delivery that the vaccinologist can find. An appropriately selected multimodality protocol, in which these antigens will be used, will permit active-specific excitation, both local and systemic, which results in an exclusive attack on the malignancy through primary immunologic programming. In this report, I will discuss each of these criteria, with pertinent examples. Other forms of active-specific therapy in the future may well be designed for secondary messages with the use of intermediate substances or may be engineered and programmed at the genetic level.

Tumor cell surfaces are enormously complex, and there is constant modulation, redistribution, loss or alteration of cell surface components, aggregation, localized nonspecific or specific coupling or agglutination with nonmembranous substances to prevent complement-mediated immune lysis, and constant fluctuation in microvillous structures for a chameleon-like quality, providing what Nicolson and Poste (1976) have termed "immunoevasive" properties. The TAA on tumor cells comprise only 1% to 3% of the total cell surface. More often than not, these substances are protected, and usually are not identified by conventional serologic means with patient sera because shed TAA and TAA antibody in the blood stream are in minute quantity. Highly sensitive assays, such as the enzyme-linked immunoabsorbent assay and radioimmunoassay, are necessary to detect them. Sometimes these "new" antigens turn out to be reprogrammed embryonic or fetal antigens. Others are identified as pieces of the structural components of a virus (virion) or nonstructural components induced by activated genetic or epigenetic viral mechanisms in the tumor cell. TAA can be portions of enzymes or endocrine-related products, or may be induced by carcinogens or an ancient, bacterial, genetic insertion activated during transformation. Probably, many of these substances are merely weak histocompatibility antigens that

---

Abbreviation used in this chapter: EDTA—ethylenediaminetetraacetic acid.

have undergone some structural change or modification. Exclusive chemical technique is required to ascertain whether these changes are merely quantitative, or are qualitative as well. However, it is this "exploitable difference" that must be studied, and appropriate tumor-associated materials must be selected to evaluate for use in active-specific immunotherapy trials.

Also important is an appreciation of the science of vaccinology and the selection of the best vehicle and mixture available based on reliable, classic studies of various forms of adjuvant and antigen. Prior to a phase II active-specific immunotherapy trial, reliable monitoring procedures are developed for use in pilot clinical studies to determine appropriate doses and timing of vaccine injection and interrelationships with conventional modes of therapy (surgery, radiotherapy, and chemotherapy). Thereby, a regimen with proper sequencing and with each component used for maximum activity, for interaction with other moieties without cross-interference, can be selected.

It is important to study the singular effect of this form of immunotherapy prior to or parallel with control studies combining it with chemotherapy or other forms of immunotherapy. Once the base lines have been established and the criteria fulfilled for phase I studies, including pilot clinical studies, as delineated by Hollinshead and Stewart (1977), then a phase II trial is undertaken and, if successful, is repeated (phase III trial) in multiple clinical centers prior to release as a general procedure available to qualified physicians.

IDENTIFICATION AND ISOLATION OF TAA

There are many time-honored methods for identifying and separating tumor-related components. However, TAA to be used in active-specific immunotherapy trials have special requirements. It is here that our talents in organic chemistry, biochemistry, and immunochemistry must be tempered by immunobiologic considerations. It is important to separate and identify those components that will remain immunoreactive and produce cell-mediated immune responses in the host. Moreover, once these components are selected, they must be studied for their ability to convert or boost the appropriate cell-mediated immune responses.

Although other means of measuring these reactivities are being developed, and in vitro tests may be useful for some forms of cancer, the ideal form of testing for such products at present is by delayed hypersensitivity reactions to skin tests conducted in an appropriate, controlled procedure. For example, Hollinshead *et al.* (unpublished data) used such procedures to isolate immunoreactive components from bladder cancer cell membranes, as illustrated in Figure 1. The procedures were similar to those developed for identifying TAA in various forms of cancer (Hollinshead *et al.,* 1972, 1974, 1976; Hollinshead and Herberman, 1973, 1975). The characteristics of these antigens are then studied, as shown in Table 1, and compared with the characteristics of other immunoreactive TAA identified with different forms of cancer, e.g., ovarian TAA, as delineated in the table. By careful use of uniform procedures for initial identification, it

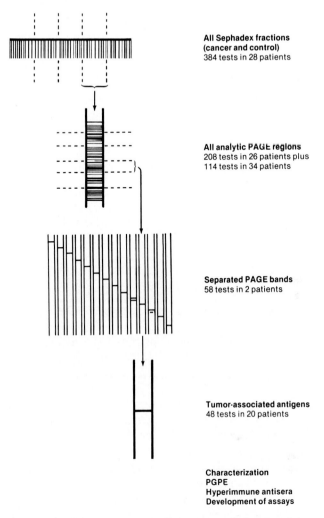

Figure 1. Separation and identification of soluble, bladder cancer cell membrane components that will remain immunoreactive and produce cell-mediated immune responses in the host. There were 812 skin tests with cancer, control, and recall antigens in 110 patients: 58 with bladder cancer and 52 with non-bladder cancers. Uniform analytical procedures are used for this form of initial identification to study tumor antigens associated with different forms of cancer for cross-reference and cross-controlled testing.

is possible to build an entire library of tumor antigens associated with different forms of cancer for cross-reference and cross-control testing. In this manner, the uniqueness or similarity of different forms and groups of cancers can be studied.

After these analytical procedures have accomplished their purpose and the characteristics of the antigen are known, preparative gel electrophoresis proce-

Table 1. *Characteristics of Cancer Cell Membrane Antigens That Induce Cell-Mediated Immune Responses**

Purified Antigen	Electrophoretic Mobility (cm)†	Presence	Chemical Composition‡
Bladder TAA	4.1	primary tumor, T-24 cells	protein
Bladder cancer tissue-associated antigen	7.1–7.2	primary tumor	protein
Ovarian TAA**	6.6–6.7	primary tumor	protein
Ovarian tissue-associated antigen††	8.35	primary tumor	glycoprotein

* Hollinshead *et al.,* unpublished data.

† Values indicate distance from tracking dye (bromphenol blue; 670 daltons) on gradient PAGE. PAGE stacked gels: 3.5%, 4.75%, 7%, and 10%. Calculations adjusted for relation of tracking dye to marker albumin in control PAGE.

‡ Staining individual gels with Coomassie brilliant blue, oil red O, and periodic acid—Schiff.

§ Tested by reseparation on sodium dodecyl sulfate PAGE for intact band, and by delayed hypersensitivity skin test and lymphocyte migration inhibition test of another aliquot for cell-mediated immune activity.

dures can be established for separating large quantities of the appropriate antigens for use in active-specific immunotherapy and for establishing monitoring procedures and assays, whereby appropriate hyperimmune antisera can be developed.

IDENTIFICATION OF INHIBITORY COMPONENTS

We described previously the existence of inhibitory antigens, or antigen-antibody complexes present on the cell surface that interfere with TAA-induced cell-mediated immune responses (Hollinshead *et al.,* 1973; Hollinshead, 1976). These inhibitory substances are composed of insoluble membrane components as well as glycoprotein-soluble membrane substances of fairly heavy molecular weight, which elute in the first peak of Sephadex G-200 separations and remain near the cathode in our analytical gradient polyacrylamide gel electrophoresis (PAGE) separations. These substances, in amounts that prevent the induction of cell-mediated immune responses to TAA, can be remixed with the TAA in a titration to determine the levels on each cell. It is necessary to free the TAA from these inhibitory cell-surface materials. As illustrated in Figure 2, the inhibitory factors have been shown to increase in each successive recurrent primary tumor, such as those described by Hitchcock *et al.* (1977). Hollinshead and Stewart (1977) have titrated the amounts of inhibitory antigens in the different forms of lung cancer and, as illustrated in Figure 2, found that the amounts differ among cancers of different histologic types in the same site. In addition, the level of inhibitory antigen is usually increased on metastatic cells but, as shown for melanoma (Fig. 2), quantities vary for metastases of different tissues.

Other inhibitory factors have been described, such as those that inhibit lymphoblastogenesis and are present on lymphoid cells (Smith *et al.,* 1970; Hersh *et al.,* 1974) and also in small amounts on cancer cells of some lines; recently, Han and Minowada (1977) showed that there is a large quantity of lymphoblasto-

Table 1, *continued*

Stability in Pure Form§			
Room Temp., 2 hr	4°C, 1 week	−70°C, 1 mo	Relation to Migration (cm) of Control Protein#
+	+	+	α_1-acid glycoprotein (40,000 d): 4.0
+	+	±	transferrin (76,500 d): 6.4–6.5 haptoglobin type 1 (100,000 d): 8.4
+	+	±	transferrin (76,500 d): 6.4–6.5
+	±	±	haptoglobin type 1 (100,000 d): 8.4

   # Estimation of precise migration of serum components of known molecular size on control gels. Specific components identified by reactions with monospecific antisera in gel double diffusion.
   ** Elicits a positive delayed hypersensitivity reaction to skin tests in patients with early ovarian cancer.
   †† Migrates just below ovarian carcinoembryonic antigen region. Occasionally elicits a positive delayed hypersensitivity reaction to skin tests in patients with advanced ovarian cancer as well as patients with other types of gynecologic cancer.

genesis inhibitory factor on lung cancer cells of certain lines. Chism *et al.* (1977) have pointed out the importance of taking into consideration the cell volume in inhibition assays.

Turk *et al.* (1976) have described control mechanisms in delayed-type hypersensitivity. They point out that there are two forms of delayed hypersensitivity. The stronger type of reaction, found in animals immunized with antigens and

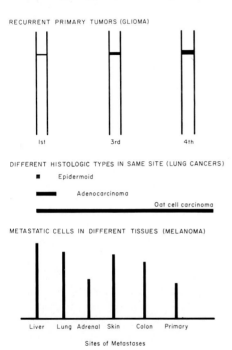

RECURRENT PRIMARY TUMORS (GLIOMA)

Ist   3rd   4th

DIFFERENT HISTOLOGIC TYPES IN SAME SITE (LUNG CANCERS)

■   Epidermoid

▬   Adenocarcinoma

▬▬   Oat cell carcinoma

METASTATIC CELLS IN DIFFERENT TISSUES (MELANOMA)

Liver Lung Adrenal Skin Colon Primary

Sites of Metastases

Figure 2. Major glycoproteins are present in greatly increased amounts on tumor cells. These materials prevent TAA-induced, cell-mediated immune responses and are probably one of several ways in which tumor cells escape immune surveillance in the cancer patient. These inhibitory antigens are seen to (1) increase with successive, recurrent primary malignancy, (2) be present in different amounts in different forms of cancer in the same organ site, and (3) in general, be present in greater amounts in metastatic tissue but to differ in concentrations on metastatic cells in different tissues.

Freund's complete adjuvant, has close similarities to the classic tuberculin reaction; the other form of skin reactivity develops into an Arthus or immediate-type skin reaction, frequently referred to as Jones-Mote hypersensitivity. The reactions are characterized by mononuclear cell infiltration consisting of varying proportions of lymphocytes and macrophages. Turk *et al.* point to work by others that shows that basophilic leukocytes are involved in the Jones-Mote reactions. In the induction of specific immunologic unresponsiveness, these workers have found that suppressor cells have a central as well as peripheral action, dependent on separate populations of cells. The relative proportion of suppressor cells is greater in the Jones-Mote form of delayed hypersensitivity than in the tuberculin-type reactions. Fudenberg and Smith (1977) have commented on antigen-specific suppressor cells detected in patients with pulmonary metastases. They state, "whether the inhibitory cells are cause or effect of metastases is unknown, and the mechanism of the observed inhibition also remains unknown. Nevertheless, it is tempting to speculate that the role of such immunologic suppression is at least as important in decreasing host resistance to metastases as that of the so-called 'blocking factors' (antigen-antibody complexes, free antigen) detected in the serum of patients with tumors."

PREPARATIVE METHODS OF TAA PRODUCTION

We first investigated the application of polyacrylamide gel preparative electrophoresis (PGPE) with the LKB 7900 Uniphor Electrophoresis system (Bromma, Sweden) to establish an alternate electrophoretic procedure for larger-scale purification of melanoma TAA. In the LKB Uniphor system, a single, large-diameter (2.0 to 2.5 cm) polyacrylamide gel is used as a support medium during electrophoresis. Recovery of separated sample is achieved through a uniquely designed elution chamber at the bottom end of the gel, which allows continuous collection of material separated during electrophoresis. Although the electrophoretic time is longer than that of the analytical, discontinuous-gradient PAGE system, the separated proteins are immediately available for concentration and storage at the end of the procedure. The composition of the polyacrylamide gel must be adjusted to allow complete migration of all sample proteins through the gel. Other experimental conditions, such as buffer composition and pH, are similar to those for the analytical system. The procedure with the LKB Uniphor has been satisfactory for some of the large-scale production of TAA.

As pointed out by Righetti and Secchi (1972), the effective maximal load limit per major protein component for any sample on the Uniphor system using preparative electrophoresis is approximately 10 mg. This factor may become critical in preparative electrophoresis of certain melanoma preparations if a large amount of a single, contaminating protein (e.g., albumin) with an electrophoretic mobility higher than that of TAA is present in the sample. Therefore, we are currently investigating the use of preparative isotachophoresis, using the Uniphor system as a potential alternative to preparative electrophoresis in cases when levels of contaminating protein are high. Mixing carrier-ampholines of various pH ranges with the sample allows initial stacking of the protein with interspaced carrier-ampholines. Their effect is maintained during the entire separation, and proteins are eluted from the system in sharp bands, thus avoiding the diffusion phenomena and cross-contamination that can occur during an electrophoretic separation. Isotachophoresis also allows the application of larger sample loads (100 to 300 mg) without affecting the efficiency of separation.

After preparation of TAA by the analytical, discontinuous-gradient PAGE technique, it is useful to prepare antisera to TAA to ascertain the reactivity of this antigen in common types of tests, such as double immunodiffusion and indirect immunofluorescence. An example of antisera prepared at this level of specificity is rabbit antiserum to ovarian TAA, the characteristics of which are delineated in Table 2. However, antiserum to TAA prepared at this fairly good level of purity is still not adequate for the development of the highly sensitive enzyme-linked immunoabsorbent assays or radioimmunossays.

The following is a detailed account of our experience in the preparation of hyperimmune, xenogeneic melanoma TAA antisera for the study of the biology of melanoma TAA and for further study in radioimmunoassay (Hollinshead *et al.,* unpublished data).

A semipurified preparation of melanoma TAA was used to prepare antiserum in rabbits. This antiserum was used to compare the properties of our TAA preparations with those of an antigen preparation used in the USSR (Gorodilova and Hollinshead, 1975; Gorodilova *et al.,* 1976). New Zealand white rabbits were injected with the glycolipoprotein (TAA), which was isolated by analytical PAGE, in a dose of 100 μg with Freund's complete adjuvant and a 100-μg

Table 2. *Characteristics of Xenogeneic Hyperimmune Antisera* to Ovarian Tumor-Associated Antigen†*

Double immunodiffusion tests
  Positive to purified O-TAA from:
    papillary serous cystadenocarcinoma, mucinous cystadenocarcinoma, undifferentiated adenocarcinoma, and serum albumin‡
  Negative to:
    AA-1 bladder cell line, J_{82} bladder cell line, T-24 bladder cell line, HCV_{29} bladder normal cell line, HSV-infected WI_{38} cells, WI_{38} cells, melanoma TAA, nevi, breast cancer TAA, normal ovarian tissue, adenocarcinoma lung TAA, colon cancer TAA, fetal black skin, fetal white skin, fetal bladder, fetal liver, fetal intestine, carcinoembryonic antigen, fibrosarcoma of the breast, meningioma cell line, acute lymphoid leukemia, gastric cancer, hemopexin, α_1-acid glycoprotein, and transferrin
Indirect immunofluorescence
  Preliminary tests with carefully washed ovarian cancer cells show a positive rim fluorescence not seen for control bladder cell line if albumin-absorbed antiserum is used.

---

  * Prepared in albino New Zealand rabbits inoculated monthly for five months with 15 μg O-TAA; fourth-month bleeding tested above.
  † Ovarian TAA is a fairly stable, single polypeptide, with molecular weight of approximately 78,000 daltons.
  ‡ This reaction disappeared after absorption of serum with 6 × crystallized serum albumin.

booster dose one month later. Two weeks after the last injection, the rabbits were bled. Precipitin patterns were analyzed in double diffusion agarose plate tests with the rabbit melanoma TAA antiserum when tested against melanoma TAA, neuroblastoma antigens, colon cancer antigens, fetal skin antigens, other less specific melanoma-associated antigens, and purified albumin. A specific precipitin band formed with the melanoma TAA, but not with the other antigens tested. A nonintersecting, different band formed with purified albumin. We used the antiserum to compare the USSR melanoma carbohydrate extract with our melanoma TAA by analysis of common precipitin patterns. The melanoma TAA present in the USSR extract (70 μg) was serologically identical to the US melanoma TAA (10 μg). A slightly skewed pattern developed because a stronger concentration of the USSR antigens was used. The additional band formed by the USSR antigen was similar to that for albumin. When the antiserum was absorbed against purified albumin, this band disappeared. This antiserum was used in several assay techniques (e.g., radioimmunoassay and indirect immunofluorescence) for preliminary work.

We soon realized that an antiserum of greater specificity would be necessary for more sensitive assay systems. For the production of this more specific antiserum, a Sephadex fraction from a metastatic melanoma was separated by PAGE, modified for preparative-sized samples (790 μg per gel). The purified TAA contained the glycolipoprotein plus a faint band, which was slightly more cathodic. Both the TAA band and the faint band close to it (Fig. 3) were used to immunize a 6- to 8-pound female New Zealand white rabbit. Antiserum produced by this animal has reacted in double diffusion tests with eight melanoma tumor preparations from both primary tumor and metastatic tissue. Multiple attempts with antigen derived from fetal skin, normal lung tissue from a melanoma patient, MCF_7 (a breast cancer cell line), and AB pooled sera (both whole and fractionated) to demonstrate cross-reactivity by this method have failed. When reacted with this antiserum and anti-whole human serum in adjacent wells, crude melanoma TAA produces two bands of precipitation, which cross and appear as a classic reaction of nonidentity. Cross-reactivity has been found with various other semipurified tumor extracts (breast, white blood cell, lung, colon). This reactivity appears to be identical in all samples in that the precipitin lines show identity reactions. However, partially purified melanoma extracts show several precipitin reactivities, only one of which shows an identity reaction with that found with other non-melanoma tumor extracts. Immuno-PAGE, with a stacked gel imbedded in 0.85% agarose after electrophoresis, has demonstrated this reactivity to be directed against a component located in the same region of the gel containing the glycolipoprotein described earlier (Fig. 4, center). Furthermore, this antiserum, unabsorbed, reacted in adjacent wells with melanoma TAA, and the previously described, absorbed antiserum produced the classic reaction of identity (Fig. 4, left).

In initial studies, Sephadex fractions containing TAA were iodinated by the method of Hunter (1973), which is essentially the chloramine-T method of

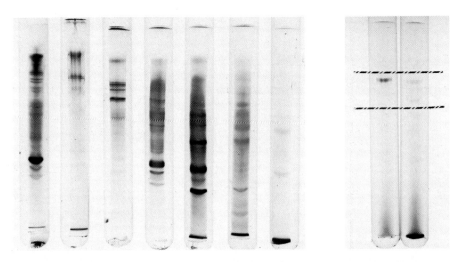

Figure 3. After identification and analysis by analytical procedures, techniques are modified for preparative procedures for vaccine production and for further purification of TAA for production of hyperimmune xenogeneic antisera. Left, Sephadex fraction from metastatic melanoma, selected for containing TAA, is separated by PAGE modified for preparative-sized samples (790 μg per gel) for vaccine production, as shown on right. This further purified TAA, which contains glycolipoprotein antigen plus slightly more cathodic faint band, was used to immunize a group of 6- to 8-pound New Zealand white rabbits, one of which produced good hyperimmune xenogeneic antiserum for further study.

Greenwood *et al.* (1963): Thirty to 60 μg of TAA fraction in 10 to 20 μl is oxidized by the addition of 50 μg of chloramine-T in 10 μl of 0.05 M phosphate buffer, pH 7.5, to the reaction mixture, which contains high-activity ^{125}I (supplied as NaI, New England Nuclear NEZ033H, greater than 350 mCi/ml) in a sodium hydroxide solution that is neutralized with hydrochloric acid and then adjusted to pH 7.5 with 0.5 M phosphate buffer. After 50 seconds, this reaction is stopped by the addition of 250 μg of sodium metabisulfite in 10 μl of buffer. Fifty microliters of buffer is added to the reaction mixture, and this combined volume is then transferred to a 0.9 (internal diameter) × 30 cm Sephadex G-75 column to separate bound from unreacted ^{125}I. Twenty-five 0.5-ml fractions are collected by an LKB RediRac fraction collector; from each fraction, a 10-μl sample is removed for counting in a Packard or Nuclear Chicago gamma spectrometer. These samples are counted for 1 or 1.2 seconds, depending on which gamma counter is used, and the elution profile and an estimate of degree of activity associated with protein are determined. Ten thousand counts per minute per nanogram is considered the minimum acceptable activity. Then, the protein peak of this separation is pooled and concentrated to a volume of less than 0.3 ml in an Amicon Model 10-PA Ultrafiltration cell fitted with either a UM10 or a YM10 membrane. This volume is loaded on a stacked-gradient polyacrylamide gel and electrophoresed at 4 milliamperes until the

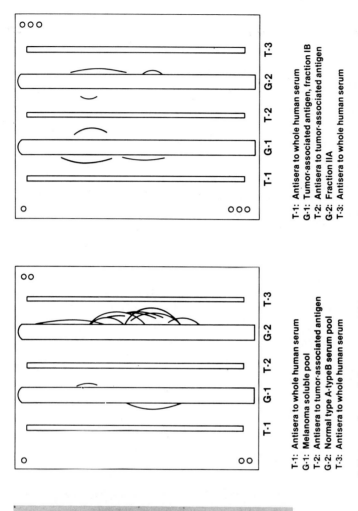

T-1: Antisera to whole human serum
G-1: Melanoma soluble pool
T-2: Antisera to tumor-associated antigen
G-2: Normal type A-typeB serum pool
T-3: Antisera to whole human serum

T-1: Antisera to whole human serum
G-1: Tumor-associated antigen, fraction IB
T-2: Antisera to tumor-associated antigen
G-2: Fraction IIA
T-3: Antisera to whole human serum

Figure 4. Antisera to TAA is first studied for reactivity to crude, partially separated TAA using double diffusion and immunoelectrophoresis. These tests are not sensitive enough but permit selection of the best antisera to be used in development of the more sensitive enzyme-linked immuncab-sorbent assay and radioimmunoassay tests. Left, In double diffusion tests, crude melanoma soluble pool (center well) reacts with (1) anti-TAA, unabsorbed and (2) anti-semipurified TAA, absorbed, but not with (3–6) antisera to other tumor antigens. Reaction produces two bands of precipitation, which join and produce classic reaction of identity. Center, Immunoelectrophoresis demonstrates reactivity to be directed against component located in same region of gel containing glycolipoprotein TAA. Right, Sephadex fraction IB contains most of melanoma TAA; neighboring fraction, IIA, contains smaller quantity. Antisera can be further processed through affinity chromatography or used with radioimmunoassay to identify peak TAA activity in finer separation for production of antisera.

bromphenol blue tracking dye, which is added to the upper chamber buffer at the beginning of the run, is just eluting from the anodic end of the gel. The gel is then removed from its glass tube and sliced with a scalpel into regions. The region(s) for measurement of TAA is then used in a double-antibody radio-immunoassay (Egan *et al.*, 1972).

To Beckman Microfuge tubes (400 μl) is added 0.05 M phosphate buffer containing 1 mg/ml Knox gelatin, 43 mM EDTA, and 0.01% sodium azide. Twenty microliters of patient serum is added to appropriate tubes containing 1 ng (approximately 10,000 cpm) of labeled TAA. Then, 10 μl of a 1:150 dilution of antiserum is added to each tube, and the volume brought up to 350 μl. The tubes are mixed in a Vortex and incubated for one hour at 37°C and then overnight at 4°C. After addition of 10 μl of a 1:20 dilution of an IgG fraction of burro anti-rabbit IgG to each tube, the tubes again are mixed in a Vortex, incubated for one hour at 37°C and then for three minutes at 0°C, and centrifuged for 20 minutes in a Beckman Model B Microfuge. Supernatants are aspirated; the pellets are washed once in buffer and centrifuged for another 10 minutes, and the wash is removed. Tubes are then counted for one minute each, and the percent bound in each test is determined. All tests are run in duplicate.

Patient sera whose TAA level falls outside of the effective range of the standard curve are either diluted or supplemented with more serum and retested. Quantities of TAA per milliliter are determined by calculating the value of the standard curve function at the percent bound of the patient serum. This function is obtained by applying a regression analysis, similar to that of Rodbard and Lewald (1970), to the points of the standard curve determination, which seem linear when the log of antigen is plotted versus the percent bound. Calculations of standard curve functions are made in duplicate for each assay. Sephadex fraction containing TAA was used as the inhibitory antigen for this determination, and a correction factor based on the relative amount of TAA in the sample was used to estimate actual quantities in serum.

Antiserum to TAA purified by PGPE was the primary antibody in a double-antibody radioimmunoassay. The second antibody was an IgG fraction of burro anti-rabbit IgG. We measured the binding of the 46 individual PAGE regions to the primary antibody. PAGE regions were individually reacted with antibody in the presence of pooled normal sera and soluble materials derived from normal adult and fetal tissues. The regions constituting the area not inhibited by these normal materials were used to obtain the standard curve, shown in Figure 5, by competition with cold Sephadex TAA dilutions. These same regions were then used in the radioimmunoassay to determine the amounts of TAA present in the sera of patients undergoing immunotherapy in our trials.

An example of the types of measurements that may be made with the melanoma radioimmunoassay is shown in Table 3. In preliminary pilot studies with different approaches to treatment, it was possible to study serum TAA levels. As shown in the table, patients with recurrent melanoma all have levels above

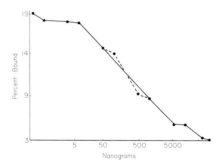

Figure 5. Radioimmunoassay (RIA) standard curve for melanoma TAA. Antisera to TAA (preparative purification) was primary antibody in double-antibody RIA. Second antibody was IgG fraction of burro anti-rabbit IgG. Crude, labeled, TAA-containing material was separated by PAGE and individually reacted with antibody in presence of pooled normal sera and soluble materials derived from normal adult and fetal tissues. Regions comprising area not inhibited by these normal materials were used to obtain standard curve by competition with cold Sephadex TAA dilutions. Thus, use of large batches of crude antigen as standard sources is possible and, at present, would be more economical for monitoring stages II and III immunotherapy trials.

normal. At present, any interpretation of the levels is anecdotal, but it is interesting to study these levels relative to the time since reductive surgery and to status of treatment. For example, patients 5 and 22 are alive, and patients 6 and 17 are dead. These figures are raw data without correction factors for precipitins. The use of specific TAA antisera and crudely separated antigens was possible. Further studies of more purified TAA would depend on sufficient material; however, large batches of crude, standard sources are currently used and may be more economic and dependable.

DEVELOPMENT AND SELECTION OF IMMUNOLOGIC TESTS AND THEIR USE IN MONITORING ACTIVE-SPECIFIC IMMUNOTHERAPY TRIALS

The selection of appropriate tests for immune monitoring is difficult because not all tests are suitable, and many tests are being improved and changed while others are in the developmental stage. There are four kinds of reactions for immune monitoring, namely, nonspecific and specific cellular and humoral immune reactions. Tests for nonspecific cellular immune reactions include skin tests with recall antigens, complete blood cell counts, lymphocyte counts, determination of red blood cell sedimentation rates, percentage and total B and T cells, and the lymphocyte migration inhibition test to determine levels of inhibitory or other tissue antigens. Nonspecific changes in humoral indicators might be measured by the enzyme-linked immunoabsorbent assay currently being developed to assess the prealbumin and α_1-acid glycoprotein components in cancer patient sera, which have been shown by Hollinshead *et al.* (1977) to have an interrelationship and to reflect, in general, relative amounts of tumor present.

Table 3. *Radioimmunoassay Determinations of TAA Levels in Patients with Recurrent Malignant Melanoma: Random Serum Samples**

Patient Code No.	Time Since Reductive Surgery and Treatment Status	Serum TAA (ng/ml)
More than one serum sample		
5	2 wk PO	461
	3 wk PO, 1 wk after 5 × 200 mg/m² DTIC	291
	3 mo PO, after 2 courses TAA	62
6	10 days PO, 6 days after 4 × 200 mg/m² DTIC	3,251
	1 mo PO, 3 days before death	9,143
13	3 mo before surgery	1,151
	2 mo before surgery, day of 1st course TAA	2,238
	2 days after 1st course TAA	149
	4 days PO, 2 mo after 2nd course TAA	3,251
	7 days PO	664
	2½ mo PO, 5 × 200 mg/m² DTIC	1,255
	(4 mo PO, patient died)	
11	3½ mo PO, day of 3rd course TAA	1,914
	4 mo PO; 20-mm nodule in right side of neck at 2 mo PO no longer palpable	552
	6½ mo PO; 30-mm nodule in left side of neck	1,934
	7½ mo PO; 30-mm nodule had enlarged, softened, decreased in size, and disappeared	733
15	Day of 3rd course TAA	468
	3 wk after 3rd course TAA	160
17	1 wk PO	484
	2 wk PO, 5 × 200 mg/m² DTIC	176
	2 mo PO, 1 mo after 1st course TAA	279
	1½ mo after 1st course TAA	29
	3 mo PO, 1 wk before death	3,722
22	5 mo PO; 2 courses TAA at 1 and 5 mo PO	17
	10 mo PO, 3rd course TAA	98
23	2 wk PO, 1st course TAA	259
	1½ mo PO, 2nd course TAA	144
26	1 mo PO, 5 × 200 mg/m² DTIC	3,069
	2 mo PO, 1 mo after 1st course TAA	143
	6 mo PO, after 3 courses DTIC and 1 course TAA	1,367
One serum sample		
12	10 mo PO, 7 mo after 3 courses TAA	630
	(Spot on lung 9 mo PO; chest X-ray film showed normal appearance 12 mo PO)	
16	5 mo PO; skin tests only	773
24	2 wk PO	91
28	2 mo PO, 1 wk after 1st course TAA	39
Normal controls	. . .	0 to 7

Abbreviations: mo, month(s); PO, after reductive surgery; wk, week(s).
* Hollinshead *et al.,* unpublished data.

In addition, radioimmunoassays for inhibitory antigens and complexes are being developed and may provide useful measurements. Hunter *et al.* (1977) have suggested that spleen lymphocytes and T-lymphocytes show increased rosette formation if there is histologic involvement. This raises the question of just how early during the development of cancer one can detect immune change, and just how sensitive are the different tests used for immune monitoring.

Specific cellular immune reactivities may be assessed with high, medium, and low doses of TAA in serial tests to determine if a patient is capable of producing an immune response, if anergic patients may be converted, and if immune response may be increased. In addition, the levels of inhibitory antigen can be titered. Complement fixation immunodiffusion tests are often useful when TAA have an association with virion components and can be measured for their immunologic properties in the presence of complement. Migration indices after incubation of TAA with peripheral blood leukocytes (Hollinshead *et al.*, 1976) may reflect completely or only partially the in vivo cell-mediated immune events. Specific humoral immune reactivities may be measured with such assays as the enzyme-linked immunoabsorbent assay for TAA alone or in the presence of interfering serum components or the radioimmunoassay for TAA or TAA complexes.

Arlen and Hollinshead (1977) have conducted phase I studies for melanoma TAA. Phase I studies with leukemia-associated antigens are discussed by Hersh *et al.* (1978) in this volume (see pages 83 to 97). Such pilot studies are necessary to establish various parameters, such as dose and timing, in different forms of immunotherapy (Piessens *et al.*, 1977; Serrou and Dubois, 1977).

PHASE II IMMUNOTHERAPY TRIALS

Vaccinology

Our phase II lung cancer immunotherapy trials followed a study of appropriate adjuvants and drugs in addition to the preparations already discussed.

An excellent review of Freund's adjuvant is found in "Pages From an Allergist's Notebook: Freund's Adjuvants" (1969). It summarizes the discovery by Rabinovitz, working in the laboratory of Koch in 1897, that *Mycobacterium butyricum* plus butter produced cellular reactions identical to those to pathologic tubercle bacilli. Grassberger, in 1899, found that emulsion of tubercle bacilli with paraffin oil is more effective and that the bacilli may be alive or killed and mixed with other bacteria. In 1935, Couland found that sensitization to tubercle bacilli could be induced by incorporating the bacilli in a paraffin of a high melting point (50°C), and in 1937, Saenz and colleagues repeated these studies. It is interesting to note that studies with skin tests for delayed hypersensitivity reactions are more than 40 years old.

The review goes on to describe the work by Freund in the 1940s, in which he found that (1) the addition of various foreign materials after injection of killed tubercle bacilli in mineral oil produced no effect; (2) killed tubercle bacilli in mineral oil emulsified or suspended with foreign material enhanced antibody production; (3) with many substances, tubercle bacilli were not necessary, and serum antibody production could be sustained for a long period with an incomplete adjuvant of mineral oil plus emulsifier only; and (4) the complete Freund's adjuvant produced a two-phase antibody formation; i.e., the emulsion was incomplete, and there was an immediate release of an aqueous portion of the emulsion, followed by a booster from the emulsified portion. The work by Freund and others shows that the antigen incorporated in the adjuvant remains at the site of injection for several months, but that it is also adjuvant-transported to the subpleural parts of the lungs and regional lymph nodes. Freund thought that the granulomata formed as a result of the complete adjuvant accounted for a large part of the antibody production. However, the review continues, in 1955, White and associates showed by means of fluorescent antibodies that antibody is present not only in draining lymph nodes of the injection site but also in lymph cells of the remote areas of the body. Other workers believed that granuloma formation was not necessary for antibody production. In 1948, Freund had shown that the presence of oil in the tissues attracted antigen cells, which took part in antibody formation; where there were no granulomata, large mononuclear cells, lymphocytes, and plasma cells gathered and occasionally phagocytosed the mineral oil droplets. The adjuvant consisted of 1.5 parts Arlacel A emulsifier to 8.5 parts of Bayol F or Klearol mineral oil (v/v) given as a 0.1-ml-deep subcutaneous injection. Freund found that this immunization could be repeated at two- or three-week intervals, and that, as a rule, a second or third injection with incomplete adjuvant was satisfactory.

The reviewer points out that today's oil adjuvants are tested for absence of carcinogens in one part in 1 billion or 10 billion. Arlacel A (Mannide monooleate), the emulsifying agent, is of a highly purified grade and is tested for deterioration products. Seventy-five thousand civilian and military personnel received emulsified influenza vaccine and experienced no immediate ill effects (Walter Reed Hospital, 1951 to 1953). Salk and Salk (1977) described the results of 10- and 18-year follow-up studies of 18,000 persons who received an adjuvant vaccine, 4,000 who received aqueous vaccine and 22,000 who received a saline placebo as a control. The death certificates, autopsy results, and terminal hospital records show no incidence of neoplasms, allergic diseases, or collagen diseases. The adjuvants have been used also in trachoma vaccines, for slow iodine release in patients with endemic hypothyroidism as well as for use in hundreds of allergy patients. Salk and Salk have emphasized that increases in antibody levels are more striking after inoculation of antigen with emulsified (adjuvant) vaccine than after inoculation with aqueous (saline) vaccine. They show that the antibody response is related directly to the quantity of antigen in both aqueous and adjuvant vaccine, and state that "Emulsification reduces the tendency toward febrile reactions, in part because of the smaller amounts of antigen required with the adjuvant, and in part because of the slower release of antigen." For virus vaccines, they suggest that the use of purified viral subunits or soluble viral products, or different adjuvant substances will eliminate the few local reactions that have been associated with the use of emulsified vaccines. In aqueous preparations, a large quantity of antigenic material is needed to stimulate immunity. Water-in-oil emulsified vaccines more effectively evoke and maintain higher antibody titers. Salk and Salk point out that the use of a potent immunologic adjuvant permits a more rapid and economical production of large quantities of vaccine because of the relatively small amounts of antigen needed. Newer forms of oil-in-water adjuvants are of great promise and are reviewed by Ribi *et al.* (1978) in this volume (see pages 131 to 154).

Shaw *et al.* (1964) again point out the fact that Freund's adjuvants generally direct the body to produce not only high-titer circulating antibody but also delayed-type hypersensitivity to the incorporated antigen. If an organ antigen is incorporated in complete adjuvant, an organ-specific disease is produced. These scientists showed that experimental "allergic" encephalomyelitis (EAE) was induced in guinea pigs by a single, intercutaneous injection of neural tissue antigens and Freund's complete adjuvant. Neither the Freund's adjuvant nor the neural tissue antigens alone were capable of inducing EAE in the guinea pigs; there was no evidence that either agent alone was responsible for the induction of EAE in thousands of guinea pigs tested. Other workers have pointed out the importance of combining antigen and adjuvant for desired effects. Brown *et al.* (1967) showed the necessity of complete adjuvant if testicular antigens were to induce characteristic orchitis. If the animals developed orchitis, they also developed delayed hypersensitivity, and antibody was not detected in the testes of any animal that had no delayed hypersensitivity.

The findings in all of these studies point to the great importance of using tumor antigens that are completely freed from normal tissue components to avoid damaging the normal tissue of the organ that contains the tumor. They also indicate the great importance of the appropriate balance of antigen and adjuvant, and the necessity of using a complete adjuvant in proper emulsion with the tumor-associated antigen.

Interrelationship with Chemotherapy

The selection of appropriate agents that are systemically effective is emphasized often (Schultz *et al.*, 1977) and must be considered when designing controlled trials. High-dose methotrexate with citrovorum factor is useful in osteogenic sarcoma treatment (Jaffe *et al.*, 1977) and, to some extent, in combination therapy for oat cell carcinoma of the lung (Israël *et al.*, 1977). The results of treatment with methotrexate in combination are not significantly better than those obtained with methotrexate as a single agent in the treatment of other forms of lung cancer (Schaerer *et al.*, 1977); there is some question as to whether methotrexate is at all effective. However, it is not the way methotrexate works as a chemotherapeutic agent that eventually proved its use worthwhile. Stewart *et al.* (1976)

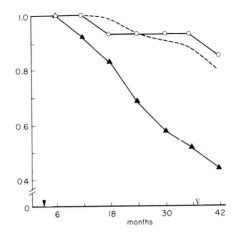

Figure 6. Active-specific immunotherapy trial life table analysis for 52 stage I lung cancer patients (as of September 1977). 0——0, active-specific immunotherapy group; -----, lower 95% confidence limit; ▲——▲, no immunotherapy. At end of three months postsurgery (▼), after three monthly courses of therapy, patients were given no further treatment and were followed to end of trial (▽), 36 months, and beyond. Differences between the two groups are significant ($p < .0001$).

have shown that methotrexate acts immunologically to cause a rebound over-shoot. This property of the drug was incorporated in a phase II active immuno-therapy trial in which a control group was compared with a group receiving methotrexate alone, a group receiving the vaccine alone, and a fourth group in which methotrexate was used to induce a rebound overshoot and the vaccine was administered, with proper timing, at the height of the overshoot. There was no difference between the survival rates for patients receiving the drug alone and in the control group, nor were there differences between the two groups receiving immunization. As shown in Figure 6, the effect of the vaccine in this phase II active-specific immunotherapy trial is highly significant. As described in detail elsewhere (Stewart *et al.,* 1977; Hollinshead and Stewart, 1977), the vaccine's systemic effects are reflected also in delayed hypersensitivity reactions, examples of which are shown in Figure 7. The results of this trial suggest that a phase III trial is appropriate.

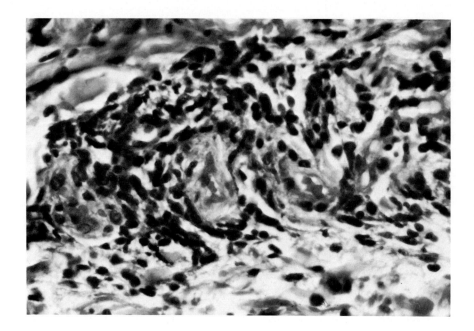

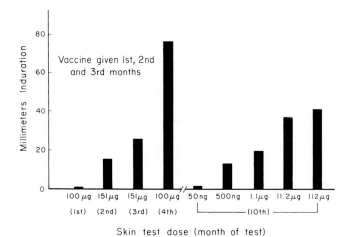

Figure 7. Above, Classic dual effect of appropriate vaccine involves systemic effects (see Fig. 6), which are reflected also in delayed hypersensitivity reactions, with 100% mononuclear cell infiltration. Below, In this example, patient with stage I epidermoid carcinoma of left lung mounts specific immune response to successive vaccination, and immunologic memory and appropriate form of specific response are retained, even at nanogram level, for a long time.

Thus, after identifying and isolating appropriate antigens, measuring inhibitors, developing appropriate monitors, and selecting appropriate adjuvants and drugs, phase II active-specific immunotherapy trials are possible.

ACKNOWLEDGMENTS

We are grateful to Drs. T. Stewart, J. Harris, M. Arlen, R. Yonemoto, H. Takita, H. Miller, W. Jaffurs, M. Hitchcock, R. Herberman, and many other colleagues, appropriately referenced in the text of this overview. The excellent research assistance of W. Queen, O. Lee, K. Tanner, and P. Jones and technical assistance of C. Bryck, R. Huff, and J. Woodard as well as the past assistance by Drs. R. Hansing and B. Das are gratefully acknowledged. We thank K. Kennard for administrative assistance and for professional manuscript preparation.

This work was supported in part by subcontract N01-CB-64007 with Roswell Park Memorial Institute; NCI-CB-64022 from the National Cancer Institute; IR26 CA17444-03 from the National Bladder Cancer Project, National Cancer Institute; and the Eugene T. Cole Cancer and Immunology Research Fund.

REFERENCES

Arlen, M., and Hollinshead, A. 1977. Tumor specific immune stimulation in patients with recurrent malignant melanoma (Abstract). 30th Annual Meeting of the Society of Surgical Oncology, Inc. (James Ewing).

Brown, P. C., Glynn, L. E., and Holborow, E. J. 1967. The dual necessity for delayed hypersensitivity and circulating antibody in the pathogenesis of experimental allergic orchitis in guinea-pigs. Immunology, 13:307–314.

Chism, S. E., Burton, R. C., Grail, D. L., Bell, P. M., and Warner, N. L. 1977. In vitro induction of tumor-specific immunity. VI. Analysis of specificity of immune response by cellular competitive inhibition: Limitations and advantages of the technique. J. Immunol. Methods, 16:245–262.

Egan, M. L., Lautenschleger, J. T., Coligan, J. E., and Todd, C. W. 1972. Radioimmunoassay of carcinoembryonic antigen. Immunochemistry, 9:289–299.

Fudenberg, H. H., and Smith, C. L. 1977. Human lymphocyte subpopulations and metastatic neoplasia. N. Engl. J. Med., 297:162–163.

Gorodilova, V. V., and Hollinshead, A. 1975. Melanoma antigens that produce cell-mediated immune responses in melanoma patients: Joint US-USSR study. Science, 190:391–392.

Gorodilova, V. V., Hollinshead, A., and Babakova, S. V. 1976. Cell immunity reaction in patients with melanoma. Vopr. Onkol., 12:1–5.

Greenwood, F. C., Hunter, W. M., and Glover, J. S. 1963. The preparation of ^{131}I-labeled human growth hormone of high specific activity. J. Biol. Chem., 89:114–123.

Han, T., and Minowada, J. 1977. Lymphoblastogenesis inhibitory factor produced by human lung cancer cell lines. J. Surg. Oncol., 9:243–248.

Hersh, E. M., Gutterman, J. U., Mavligit, G. M., Granatek, C. H., Rossen, R. D., Rios, A., Goldstein, A. L., Patt, Y., Rivera, E., Richman, S. P., Bottino, J., Farquhar, D., Morris, D., and Ezaki, K. 1978. Clinical rationale for immunotherapy and its role in cancer treatment. In: Immunotherapy of Human Cancer (The University of Texas System Cancer Center M. D. Anderson Hospital and Tumor Institute 22nd Annual Clinical Conference). New York, Raven Press, pp. 83–97.

Hersh, E. M., McCredie, K. B., and Freireich, E. J. 1974. Inhibition of in vitro lymphocyte blastogenesis by inhibitor produced by cultured human lymphoblasts. Clin. Exp. Immunol., 17:463.

Hitchcock, M. A., Hollinshead, A. C., Chretien, P., and Rizzoli, H. V. 1977. Soluble membrane antigens of brain tumors. I. Controlled testing for cell-mediated immune responses in a long surviving glioblastoma multiforme patient. Cancer, 40:660–666.

Hollinshead, A. C. 1976. Cell membrane antigens associated with human adult acute leukemia. Blood Cells, 2:257–265.

Hollinshead, A. C., Chretien, P. B., Lee, O., Tarpley, J. L., Kerney, S. E., Silverman, N. A., and Alexander, J. C. 1976. In vivo and in vitro measurements of the relationship of human squamous carcinomas to herpes simplex virus tumor-associated antigens. Cancer Res., 36:821–828.

Hollinshead, A. C., Chuang, C., Cooper, E. H., and Catalona, W. J. 1977. Interrelationship of prealbumin and α_1-acid glycoprotein in cancer patient sera. Cancer, 40:2993–2998.

Hollinshead, A. C., and Herberman, R. B. 1973. Separation of the major histocompatibility antigens from other antigens present on human leukemic and white blood cell membranes. In Dutcher, R. M., and Chieco-Bianchi, L. (eds.): Unifying Concepts of Leukemia (Bibl. Haematol., no. 39). Basel, S. Karger, pp. 828–837.

Hollinshead, A. C., and Herberman, R. B. 1975. Identification and characterization: Cell membrane antigens associated with the blast phase of human adult leukemia. In Ito, Y., and Dutcher, R. M. (eds.): Comparative Leukemia Research 1973, Leukemogenesis. Tokyo, University of Tokyo Press, pp. 339–348.

Hollinshead, A. C., Herberman, R. B., Jaffurs, W. J., Alpert, L. K., Minton, J. P., and Harris, J. E. 1974. Soluble membrane antigens of human malignant melanoma cells. Cancer, 34:1235–1243.

Hollinshead, A., Jaffurs, W., Alpert, L., and Herberman, R. 1973. Specific soluble membrane antigen of malignant and normal breast cells: Delayed hypersensitive skin reactions in cancer patients. In Maltoni, C. (ed.): Cancer Detection and Prevention (Proceedings of the Second International Symposium on Detection and Prevention of Cancer). Amsterdam, International Congress, Series no. 322, pp. 647–654.

Hollinshead, A., McCammon, J. R., and Yohn, D. S. 1972. Immunogenicity of a soluble transplantation antigen from adenovirus 12-induced tumor cells demonstrated in inbred hamsters (PD-4). Can. J. Microbiol., 18:1365–1369.

Hollinshead, A. C., and Stewart, T. H. M. 1977. Lung tumor antigens: Specific active immunotherapy trials. In: Detection Specific Sites (Proceedings of the Third International Symposium on Detection and Prevention of Cancer). New York, Marcel Dekker, vol. IV, part 2, p. 52.

Hunter, C. P., Pinkus, G., Woodward, L., Moloney, W. C., and Churchill, W. H. 1977. Increased T lymphocytes and IgMEA-receptor lymphocytes in Hodgkin's disease spleens. Cell. Immunol., 31:193–198.

Hunter, W. M. 1973. Radioimmunoassay. In Wier, D. M. (ed.): Handbook of Experimental Immunology, 2nd edition. Oxford, Blackwell Scientific Publications, ch. 17.

Israël, L., Depierre, A., Choffel, C., Milleron, B., and Edelstein, R. 1977. Immunochemotherapy in 34 cases of oat cell carcinoma of the lung with 19 complete responses. Cancer Treat. Rep., 61:343–347.

Jaffe, N., Frei, E., III, Traggis, D., Cassady, J. R., Watts, H., and Filler, R. M. 1977. High-dose methotrexate with citrovorum factor in osteogenic sarcoma—Progress report II. Cancer Treat. Rep., 61:675–679.

Pages from an Allergist's Notebook (EAB). 1969. Freund's adjuvants. Rev. Allergy, 23:389–400.

Piessens, W. F., Campbell, M., and Churchill, W. H. 1977. Inhibition or enhancement of rat mammary tumors dependent on dose of BCG. J. Natl. Cancer Inst., 59:207–211.

Nicolson, G. L., and Poste, G. 1976. The cancer cell: Dynamic aspects and modifications in cell-surface organization. N. Engl. J. Med., 295:253–258.

Ribi, E. R., McLaughlin, C. A., Cantrell, J. L., Brehmer, W., Azuma, I., Yamamura, Y., Strain, S. M., Hwang, K. M., and Toubiana, R. 1978. Immunotherapy for tumors with microbial constituents or their synthetic analogues. A review. In: Immunotherapy of Human Cancer (Proceedings of The University of Texas System Cancer Center M. D. Anderson Hospital and Tumor Institute 22nd Annual Clinical Conference). New York, Raven Press, pp. 131–154.

Righetti, P., and Secchi, C. 1972. Preparative polyacrylamide gel electrophoresis. J. Chromatogr., 72:165–175.

Rodbard, D., and Lewald, J. E. 1970. Computer analysis of radioligand assay and radioimmunoassay data. In: Steroid Assay by Protein Binding (Proceedings of Karolinska Second Symposium on Research Methods in Endocrinology). Stockholm, Karolinska Institute, pp. 79–103.

Salk, J., and Salk, D. 1977. Control of influenza and poliomyelitis with killed virus vaccines. Science, 195:834–847.

Schaerer, R., Sotto, J. J., Wiget, U., Perdrix, A., Bensa, J. C., and Ribaud, P. 1977. Chemotherapy of bronchogenic carcinomas by a combination of cyclophosphamide, methotrexate, vincristine and bleomycin. Eur. J. Cancer, 13:425–428.

Schultz, R. M., Papamatheakis, J. D., Luetzeler, J., and Chirigos, M. A. 1977. Association of macrophage activation with antitumor activity by synthetic and biological agents. Cancer Res., 37:3338–3343.

Serrou, B., and Dubois, J. B. 1977. Combination of radiotherapy and immunotherapy in the treatment of Lewis's tumour. Eur. J. Cancer, 13:489–491.

Shaw, C., Alvord, E. C., Jr., Fahlberg, W. J., and Kies, M. W. 1964. Substitutes for the mycobacteria in Freund's adjuvants in the production of experimental "allergic" encephalomyelitis in the guinea pig. J. Immunol., 92:28–40.

Smith, R. T., Bausher, J. A., and Adler, W. H. 1970. Studies of an inhibitor of DNA synthesis and a non-specific mitogen elaborated by human lymphoblasts. Am. J. Pathol., 60:495.

Stewart, T. H. M., Hollinshead, A., and Harris, J. E. 1976. Immunotherapy of lung cancer. Ann. NY Acad. Sci., 277:436–466.

Stewart, T. H. M., Hollinshead, A., Harris, J., Raman, S., Belanger, R., Crepeau, A., Crook, A., Hirte, W., Hooper, D., Klaasen, D., Rapp, E., and Sachs, H. 1977. A survival study of specific active immunotherapy in lung cancer. In Crispen, R. G. (ed.): Neoplasm Immunity: Solid Tumor Therapy (Proceedings of a Chicago Symposium, 1977). Philadelphia, Franklin Institute Press, pp. 37–48.

Turk, J. L., Polak, L., and Parker, D. 1976. Control mechanisms in delayed-type hypersensitivity. Br. Med. Bull., 32:165–170.

CLINICAL IMMUNOTHERAPY

Immunotherapy of Human Cancer,
The University of Texas System Cancer Center
M. D. Anderson Hospital and Tumor Institute.
Raven Press, New York © 1978.

Chemoimmunotherapy for Acute Myelocytic Leukemia

James F. Holland, M.D., J. George Bekesi, Ph.D., and Janet Cuttner, M.D.

Department of Neoplastic Diseases, Mount Sinai School of Medicine, New York, New York

We have explored the technique of immunization with tumor cells, and as the keystone of that effort, we have studied the removal of sialic acid from leukemic cell surfaces by incubation with *Vibrio cholerae* neuraminidase (Bekesi *et al.,* 1971, 1972). Other neuraminidases do not work, apparently because they have not nearly as much activity for the 2–6 linkage as does the *V. cholerae* neuraminidase. By incubating the cells, one eliminates their leukemogenicity but enhances their immunogenicity. Significant protection by these cells can be demonstrated in immunoprophylaxis experiments.

With chemoimmunotherapy, however, we have demonstrated a great augmentation of cure rate for mice bearing L1210 leukemia (Bekesi and Holland, 1974). With a nitrosourea alone, 20% of the animals in our study were cured. With immunization with the specific tumor (10^7 neuraminidase-treated L1210 leukemic cells) on day 3, 6, 9, 11, or 15 after the transplantation, as many as 90% of animals survived for 60 days or more (Fig. 1). If the tumor burden is allowed to become larger, i.e., if chemotherapy is delayed, the chemotherapy as well as the chemoimmunotherapy is less effective. Cure of the L1210 leukemia in animals with a nitrosourea alone allowed 90% to withstand only a 1,000-cell challenge. All of those cured by chemotherapy plus immunotherapy withstood a challenge of 10^4, and 90% withstood 10^5 to 10^6 cells (Fig. 2) (Bekesi *et al.,* 1974).

L1210 leukemia, a lymphocytic leukemia, is the first model system we used, as we did not have an appropriate myeloid leukemia model in our laboratories. L1210 leukemia is a transplanted tumor, and the possibility of genetic drift between tumor and host, allowing for changes that would propitiate immunotherapy, prompted us to study autochthonous AKR leukemia. Immunization, either intraperitoneal or subcutaneous, of newly diagnosed AKR leukemic mice with

---

Abbreviations used in this chapter: CCNU—1-(2-chloroethyl)-3-cyclohexyl-1-nitrosourea; DMSO—dimethyl sulfoxide; EDTA—ethylenediaminetetraacetic acid.

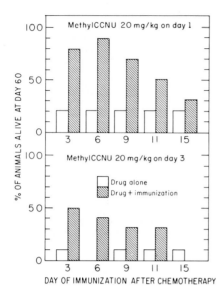

Figure 1. Effect of chemotherapy (methyl CCNU) and chemotherapy plus immuno-therapy (10^7 neuraminidase-treated L1210 leukemic cells) on survival of DBA/2 mice with L1210 leukemia.

neuraminidase-treated leukemic thymocytes from other AKR mice did not aug-ment survival time (Fig. 3). Reducing the leukemic body burden by chemother-apy and then giving immunotherapy, however, substantially extended survival (Fig. 4). Based on these observations in an autochthonous tumor (Bekesi and Holland, 1974; Bekesi *et al.*, 1976), we initiated a study of human acute myelo-cytic leukemia (AML).

Leukemic blasts from untreated patients with acute myelocytic leukemia who have leukocytosis are harvested with either a Haemonetics or an Aminco centri-

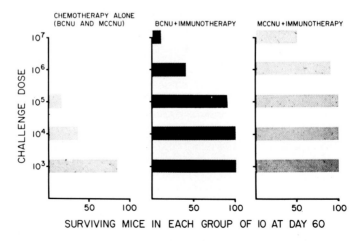

Figure 2. Refractoriness of DBA/2 mice to challenge with untreated L1210 tumor cells following chemotherapy or chemoimmunotherapy.

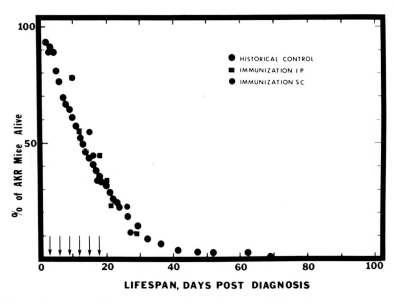

Figure 3. Effect of immunization with neuraminidase-treated leukemic thymocytes on survival of AKR leukemic mice.

fuge. If granulocytes represent more than 5% of harvested cells, they are removed by glass or nylon adherence. Thereafter, myeloblasts and other nonadherent cells are frozen in a programmed manner in 10% DMSO. They are thawed immediately prior to use, separated from nonviable cells by centrifugation on a human serum albumin cushion, and then incubated with *V. cholerae* neuraminidase. This enzyme, which requires calcium to attach to the cell surface, is removed by multiple washes in EDTA so that neuraminidase itself is not given to the patient, only the cells minus their sialic acid. Each batch of cells is reserved for a particular patient for at least six months. Each batch is analyzed for its sialic acid content and is tested to see if it is, in fact, immunogenic in mixed cell cultures. Those apparently not immunogenic are not used. Pooled cells are not used. Immediately after incubation with neuraminidase and washing, cells are injected into patients with AML in remission induced by chemotherapy. Some 50 intradermal sites are chosen in areas that we think will give stimulus to multiple lymph node areas. Multiple, intradermal areas of injection are a significant feature that differentiates this from other types of cellular immunotherapy (Holland and Bekesi, 1976). For some patients, we also have given injections of methanol extraction residue of bacillus Calmette-Guérin (MER). Microscopically, the cutaneous lesions manifesting delayed hypersensitivity reactions to cell injection show inflammatory mononuclear cells and immunoblasts. The leukemic cells disappear; we have given thousands of inoculations and there has never been an instance of leukemic cellular growth or tumefaction.

The results of a clinical trial with patients with AML randomly allocated

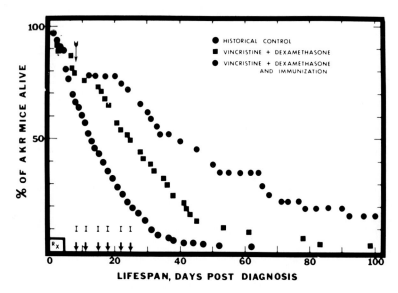

Figure 4. Effect of chemotherapy and chemotherapy plus immunization with neuraminidase-treated leukemic spleen cells on survival of AKR leukemic mice.

to receive chemotherapy only or chemotherapy plus neuraminidase-treated cells show important differences. Cytosine arabinoside and daunorubicin were used for remission induction, after which monthly courses of cytosine arabinoside in combination with a rotating cycle of thioguanine, cyclophosphamide, and CCNU were administered. Because remission in our control group appeared short, a group of patients in the Cancer and Leukemia Group B (CALGB) study #7421 was selected as a second control because they had been treated with a chemotherapeutic regimen identical to that for patients in our study. Since one way to get a specious treatment effect is to have a poor control, this CALGB control group represents the universe of patients treated with the same drugs. The difference in remission duration between the group receiving neuraminidase-treated cells and both control subsets is substantial (Fig. 5): Seven of 19 patients treated with cells exited complete remission at a median of 23 months, compared with five months for three of four of our control subjects and 10 months for 15 of 20 CALGB controls. Patients were disqualified if they were over 60 years of age, had received slightly altered chemotherapy, or had missed a marrow examination at the times set by the rigid protocol, or because of similar infractions. The disqualified patients were not those who were doing poorly and eliminated so that only patients responding well would remain. Eight of 12 disqualified patients treated with neuraminidase-treated cells were in remission for a median of 14 months, compared with six months for nine of 13 disqualified control subjects (Fig. 6). The effects of treatment on remission duration for the combined set of patients are shown in Figure 7.

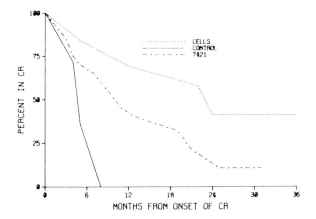

Figure 5. Effect of chemotherapy plus neuraminidase-treated cells versus chemotherapy only on remission duration for patients with acute myelocytic leukemia. Remission was induced by cytosine arabinoside and daunorubicin. CR, complete remission.

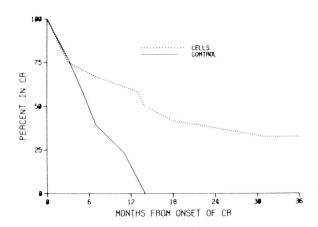

Figure 6. Effect of same treatment as in Figure 5 on remission duration for patients disqualified from the study because of infractions of protocol.

Five patients treated with tumor cells are alive and well beyond five years. The differences between patients treated with tumor cells and control subjects, both contemporaneous controls and the "universe" controls of CALGB patients who received the same chemotherapy, are significant ($p < .01$).

Furthermore, a group of patients was treated with MER in addition to the neuraminidase-treated cells (Fig. 7). This additional treatment compromises the immunizing effect and returns the patients to status, as if they were receiving chemotherapy alone.

We have been able to recognize in vitro correlates of this alteration in remission duration. Patients immunized with cells alone have progressively increasing

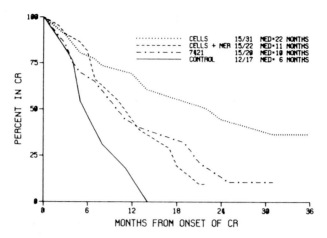

Figure 7. Effect of chemotherapy and chemoimmunotherapy on remission duration for AML patients, both qualified and disqualified. CR, complete remission.

response to phytohemagglutinin and pokeweed mitogen and an increasing number of T cells (Bekesi *et al.,* 1977). Patients who receive cells plus MER have a similarly increased number of T cells, but a progressive diminution in the responses to phytohemagglutin and pokeweed mitogen. We interpret this to be the appearance of a population of suppressor cells, evoked by MER, which alters the response of T and B cells to the mitogens. On cessation of MER administration to a few patients whose in vitro data suggested this phenomenon, the in vitro parameters have been restored and remission has continued. Even though they are part of the cells-plus-MER treatment subset, such patients appear to have longer remissions than those continued on a full dose of MER with the cells and who relapse prematurely. Thus, excess immunologic stimulation with the biologic equivalent of tumor enhancement appears possible.

We have demonstrated that MER can be given in lower doses by serial log dilutions, from 100 μg down to .001 μg. The graded responses titer the dermal reaction that is tolerable for each patient (Perloff *et al.,* 1977).

An investigation that has 733 patients entered is now in progress under the study chairmanship of Dr. Janet Cuttner in the Cancer and Leukemia Group B. It is an attempt to demonstrate the value of MER used alone as an immunotherapeutic agent. The design of the study calls for a standard chemotherapeutic regimen for remission induction: cytosine arabinoside and daunorubicin. A random segment of patients received MER on the first day of induction and monthly during maintenance. Another subset received MER during remission maintenance only. The third, control group received only chemotherapy (Cuttner *et al.,* 1977). At the most recent evaluation, which included 509 patients, there was an increase in remission frequency, 58%, associated with MER treatment in induction, versus 52% for those who did not receive MER among patients under 60 years of age. Adding the 180 patients over the age of 60 and adjusting the two groups for equal age distribution, 48% in the MER-treated group and 46% in the group who did not receive MER reached M1 marrow. Thus, MER makes no important difference to the total population of patients who are immunized on the first day of remission induction. However, among patients who had negative results of skin tests to a battery of recall antigens, MER administration on day 1 led to 57% remission, compared with 44% for those who received chemotherapy alone. Indeed, all the changes in this entire group reasonably can be ascribed to conversion of those patients anergic to recall antigens to reactor status by MER. Among such patients, remission frequency was increased to the same as for patients who had positive reactions to recall antigens.

There is a relationship between the diameter of the induration manifesting MER response and remission induction frequency: Of patients who were unresponsive to all the recall antigen tests, 73% reached complete remission if their MER inflammatory response was an induration greater than 2 cm in diameter versus 50% if less than 2 cm.

Another important effect of MER given on the first day of remission induction relates to infection. There was an equivalent amount of hemorrhage and infection during the first course of chemotherapy irrespective of whether MER was administered: two thirds of the patients acquired serious or life-threatening infections and one third experienced serious or life-threatening bleeding. In the MER-treated group who had a second course of chemotherapy, however, half as much infection and only 10% as much bleeding occurred, whereas these complications in the group that was not immunized persisted at the same, earlier high rate.

Preliminary data on remission duration are available for two different chemotherapeutic regimens of maintenance. One subset of patients received cytosine arabinoside and thioguanine in repeated courses. For patients who received this chemotherapy and no MER, the median remission duration is 12 months; for those who received MER in maintenance only, 17 months; and, for uncertain reasons, for those who received MER in both phases, induction and remission, only 12 months. The other maintenance chemotherapy subset received half as much thioguanine; with their monthly courses of cytosine arabinoside, they received vincristine and dexamethasone on alternate months. In this second subset, the median remission duration for patients who received only chemotherapy is 11 months; for those who received MER in maintenance only, 11 months; and for those who received MER in both phases, induction and remission, 19 months. The MER effects seem to be influenced by the chemotherapy, but because we are dealing with small sample sizes, representing only 200 patients in remission, the differences are not yet statistically significant. Other data suggest that specific doses of a particular immunostimulatory agent influence its effect (Perloff *et al.,* 1977). In addition, specific components of chemotherapeutic regimens may influence the effects of immunotherapy, just as may the timing of and relationship between the chemotherapy and immunotherapy.

Neuraminidase-treated cells appear to have specificity and to be a highly effective immunotherapeutic adjuvant, albeit expensive and complex. MER is relatively inexpensive, transportable, stable, safe, and noninfectious, and is subject to further refinement. In preliminary assessment of a large series of patients, it demonstrates some efficacy in acute myelocytic leukemia.

ACKNOWLEDGMENTS

This work was supported in part by contract CB-43879 and grants CA-15936 and CA-16118 from the National Cancer Institute, and by the T. J. Martell Memorial Foundation for Leukemia Research.

REFERENCES

Bekesi, J. G., and Holland, J. F. 1974. Combined chemotherapy and immunotherapy of transplantable and spontaneous murine leukemia in DBA/2 and AKR mice. Recent Results Cancer Res., 47:357.

Bekesi, J. G., Holland, J. F., and Roboz, J. P. 1977. Specific immunotherapy with neuraminidase-modified leukemic cells. Med. Clin. North Am., 61:1083.

Bekesi, J. G., Roboz, J. P., Walter, L., and Holland, J. F. 1974. Stimulation of specific immunity against cancer by neuraminidase treated tumor cells. Behring Inst. Mitt., 55:309.

Bekesi, J. G., Roboz, J. P., Zimmerman, E., and Holland, J. F. 1976. Treatment of spontaneous leukemia in AKR mice with chemotherapy, immunotherapy, interferon and virazole. Cancer Res., 36:631.

Bekesi, J. G., St. Arneault, G., and Holland, J. F. 1971. Increase of leukemia L1210 immunogenicity by Vibrio cholerae neuraminidase treatment. Cancer Res., 31:2130.

Bekesi, J. G., St. Arneault, G., Walter, L., and Holland, J. F. 1972. Immunogenicity of leukemia L1210 cells after neuraminidase treatment. J. Natl. Cancer Inst., 49:107.

Cuttner, J., Glidewell, O., and Holland, J. F. 1977. Advances in the treatment of acute leukemia. In Tagnon, H. J., and Staquet, M. J. (eds.): Recent Advances in Cancer Treatment. New York, Raven Press, pp. 13–18.

Holland, J. F., and Bekesi, J. G. 1976. Immunotherapy of human leukemia with neuraminidase modified cells. Med. Clin. North Am., 60:539.

Perloff, M., Holland, J. F., Lumb, G. J., and Bekesi, J. G. 1977. Effects of methanol extraction residue of bacillus Calmette-Guerin (MER) in man. Cancer Res., 37:1191.

Immunotherapy of Human Cancer,
The University of Texas System Cancer Center
M. D. Anderson Hospital and Tumor Institute.
Raven Press, New York © 1978.

Preliminary Results of Three Chemotherapy-Immunotherapy Protocols for Treatment of Acute Lymphoid Leukemia in Children

Georges Mathé, M.D., Francoise de Vassal, M.D., Léon Schwarzenberg, M.D., Miguel Delgado, M.D., Roy Weiner, M.D.,* Marianne Gil, M.D., Juan Pena-Angulo, M.D., Dominique Belpomme, M.D., Pierre Pouillart, M.D., David Machover, M.D., Jean-Louis Misset, M.D., José-Luis Pico, M.D., Claude Jasmin, M.D., Maurice Hayat, M.D., Maurice Schneider, M.D., Albert Cattan, M.D., Jean-Louis Amiel, M.D., Marina Musset, M.D., Claude Rosenfeld, M.D., and Patricia Ribaud, M.D.

Institut de Cancérologie et d'Immunogénétique (INSERM), Hôpital Paul-Brousse, and Dèpartement d'Hématologie, Institut Gustave-Roussy, 94800 Villejuif, France

Based on our experimental studies (Mathé, 1976), we conducted in 1962 the first comparative trial with active immunotherapy for acute lymphoid leukemia (ALL) (Mathé *et al.,* 1969). We compared the length of remission and survival of patients submitted to active immunotherapy, consisting initially of the application of bacillus Calmette-Guérin (BCG) as a nonspecific immunity adjuvant and/or irradiated leukemic cells as the specific stimulus, and patients not submitted to immunotherapy. After the introduction of 30 patients into the trial, we noted a significant difference in favor of immunotherapy, and therefore stopped introducing more patients into the trial, which we were not authorized to prolong or repeat for ethical reasons. Then, all the patients who had received immunotherapy were treated with both BCG and irradiated cells. Fifteen years later, seven of the 20 patients in the immunotherapy group are still in remission and one more is alive, whereas none of ten control patients not submitted to immunotherapy after maintenance chemotherapy is alive (Mathé, 1977; Mathé *et al.,* 1977).

Since this trial, we have conducted several successive trials with different protocols, adapting the pre-immunotherapy chemotherapy to the progress made by different groups in the world and by ourselves (Clarysse *et al.,* 1976; Simone,

---

Abbreviations used in this chapter: EORTC—European Organization for Research on Treatment of Cancer; V forms—voluminous forms; WHO—World Health Organization.
* Present address: Division of Medical Oncology, University of Florida, Gainesville, Florida.

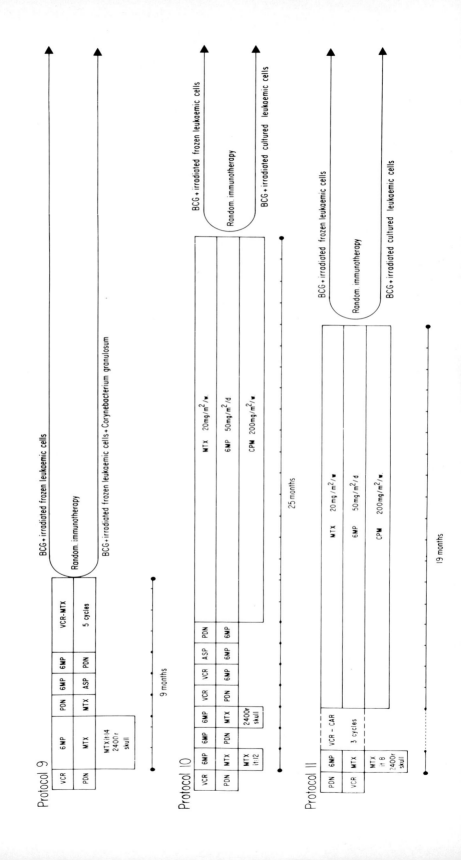

Protocol 9

VCR	Vincristine	$1.5\,mg/m^2/w$ (iv)
PDN	Prednisone	$40\,mg/m^2/d$ (po)
6MP	6-mercaptopurine	$50\,mg/m^2/d$ (po)
MTX	Methotrexate	$5\,to\,15\,mg/m^2 \times 2/w$ (im)
ASP	L-Asparaginase	$15000\,u/m^2/d$ (iv or im)
cycles	{ VCR $0.75\,mg/m^2$ days 1 and 2 (iv)	
	{ MTX $7.5\,mg/m^2$ every 6h for 48h (days 3 and 4) (im)	

Protocol 10

VCR	Vincristine	$1.5\,mg/m^2/w$ (iv)
PDN	Prednisone	$40\,mg/m^2/d$ (po)
6MP	6-mercaptopurine	$50\,mg/m^2/d$ (po)
MTX	Methotrexate	$5\,to\,15\,mg/m^2$ twice a w (im)
ASP	L-Asparaginase	$15000\,u/m^2/d$ (iv or im)
CPM	Cyclophosphamide	

Protocol 11

VCR	Vincristine	$1.5\,mg/m^2/w$ (iv)
PDN	Prednisone	$40\,mg/m^2/d$ (po)
6MP	6-mercaptopurine	$50\,mg/m^2/d$ (po)
MTX	Methotrexate	$5\,to\,15\,mg/m^2 \times 2/w$ (im)
cycles	{ VCR $1\,mg/m^2$ day 1 (iv)	
	{ ARC* $240\,mg/m^2/d \times 4d$ continous perf d2,3,4,5	
	{ PDN $40\,mg/m^2/d$ day 14 to 20 (po)	

* Arabinosylcytosine

Figure 1. Schematic representation of protocols 9, 10, and 11. (Reproduced from Mathé et al., 1978, with permission of Alan R. Liss, Inc.)

1976; Holland, 1978), and comparing different immunotherapeutic modalities in patients randomized after remission induction by cell-reducing, complementary chemotherapy. We report in this paper the preliminary results of treatment of ALL by three different protocols (Fig. 1).

MATERIAL AND METHODS

The modes of remission induction (by prednisone and vincristine) (Clarysse et al., 1976) were identical, and the cerebromeningeal preventive treatments (Aur et al., 1972; Pouillart et al., 1972; Mathé et al., 1975a) were not significantly different in the three protocols.

In the first (protocol 9), chemotherapy after remission induction comprised successive administration of binary combinations of drugs that were the most possibly efficient in the treatment of ALL (Clarysse et al., 1976). This treatment was short—nine months—and the patients then were randomized to either receive or not receive *Corynebacterium granulosum* (Schwarzenberg and Mathé, 1975) as a complement to BCG and irradiated cells.

After a certain application period, we learned that long-term chemotherapy for patients in remission was essential for obtaining a favorable result (Clarysse et al., 1976; Simone, 1976; Holland, 1978), and we started a new protocol, number 10, by which the pre-immunotherapy chemotherapy was much longer than that by protocol 9. The fundamental difference was the adjunction of 18 months' treatment with the combination of methotrexate, 6-mercaptopurine, and cyclophosphamide to seven months' post-remission chemotherapy of the same kind used in protocol 9.

We then set up protocol number 11. The total duration of post-remission chemotherapy was intermediate of those of protocols 9 and 10; it consisted essentially of 18 months' administration of the same combination of methotrexate, 6-mercaptopurine, and cyclophosphamide as in protocol 10. With protocols 10 and 11, we were comparing, in patients randomized after the end of chemotherapy, two modalities of immunotherapy: BCG and frozen, irradiated leukemic cells (Mathé, 1976) versus BCG and culture-produced, irradiated leukemic cells (Rosenfeld et al., 1977).

As no significant differences have yet appeared among the immunotherapy branches in these three different trials, it appears to us to be of interest to compare the respective results; although the trials do not use three randomized branches of the same protocol, but three different protocols, they are validly comparable because the distribution of the children is homogenous in regard to age, sex, and cytologic types of ALL according to the WHO Reference Center (Mathé and Rappaport, 1976) (Table 1).

The distribution is also homogenous in regard to our prognostic predictions, which were based on two factors. One factor takes into account the WHO Reference Center cytologic types of ALL (Mathé et al., 1971; Mathé and Rappaport, 1976): We have shown previously that the prognosis of the microlympho-

Table 1. *Distribution of Patients Treated by ICIG-ALL Protocols 9, 10, and 11**

Parameter	No. (%) of Patients per Protocol		
	9 (n = 31)†	10 (n = 14)‡	11 (n = 14)§
Sex			
Male	22 (71)	9 (64)	8 (57)
Female	9 (29)	5 (36)	6 (43)
Cytologic types #			
PLb	7 (23)	3 (21)	4 (29)
PLc	13 (42)	3 (21)	3 (21)
MLb	4 (13)	5 (36)	4 (29)
mLb	2 (6)	1 (7)	2 (14)
Unclassified	5 (16)	2 (14)	1 (7)
Prognostic factors			
mLb, V⁻ MLb, PLc	10 (32)	4 (29)	4 (29)
PLb, V⁺ MLb, PLc	16 (52)	7 (50)	7 (50)
Unclassified	5 (16)	3 (21)	3 (21)

* Reproduced from Mathé *et al.,* 1978, with permission of Alan R. Liss, Inc.
† Patients aged 2 to 13 years: < 5 yr., 12 (39%); 5 to 10 yr., 14 (45%); >10 yr., 5 (16%).
‡ Patients aged 1 to 13 years: < 5 yr., 8 (57%); 5 to 10 yr., 4 (29%); >10 yr., 2 (14%).
§ Patients aged 3 to 14 years: < 5 yr., 7 (50%); 5 to 10 yr., 4 (29%); >10 yr., 3 (21%).
\# PLb, prolymphoblastic; PLc, prolymphocytic; MLb, macrolymphoblastic; mLb, micro-lymphoblastic.

blastic type is most often good, that the prognosis of the prolymphoblastic type is most often unfavorable, and that the prognosis of the macrolymphoblastic and prolymphocytic types is intermediate (Mathé *et al.,* 1971). The second factor takes into account the volume of the neoplasm: We have observed previously that the so-called V⁺ forms (characterized in this report by leukemic cells $\geq 10^4/$ cu mm and by large splenomegaly and adenomegalies) have a poorer prognosis than the V⁻ forms [leukemic cells $< 10^4/$cu mm; no large splenomegaly or adenomegalies (Mathé *et al.,* 1975b)]. Hence, the population of patients was stratified into two groups to be compared for prognosis: (1) those with microlymphoblastic and V⁻ macrolymphoblastic and prolymphocytic disease types, and (2) those with prolymphoblastic and V⁺ macrolymphoblastic and prolymphocytic types.

RESULTS AND DISCUSSION

The remission rates were 29 of 31 (94%) with protocol 9, 14 of 14 (100%) with protocol 10, and 13 of 14 (93%) with protocol 11 (Mathé *et al.,* 1978). Figure 2, which shows the curves of duration of the first remission, as established by the "direct" method, shows that these curves break to form a tendency toward a plateau at about the 24th month. This plateau concerns about 50% of the children treated by protocol 9 (only one relapse between the 24th and 54th months), 43% of those treated by protocol 10, and 54% of those treated by protocol 11. The differences among the three percentages are not significant.

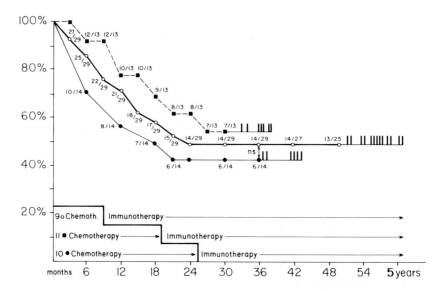

Figure 2. Cumulative curves of duration of first remission (established by "direct" method) for children treated by protocols 9, 10, and 11. (Reproduced from Mathé *et al.,* 1978, with permission of Alan R. Liss, Inc.)

No correlation, then, is found between remission duration and the length of the pre-immunotherapy chemotherapy, and one can conclude that the long-term first remission rate is on the order of 50% with these three protocols.

We cannot exclude the possibility that a nine-month chemotherapy regimen provides the maximum that maintenance chemotherapy can do on the remission curves. This is not the generally accepted concept, however, at least for exclusive maintenance chemotherapy (Jacquillat *et al.,* 1973; Clarysse *et al.,* 1976; Simone, 1976; Holland, 1978). Thus, the fact that the curve for protocol 9 is identical to the curve for protocol 11 between the ninth and 25th months (immunotherapy versus chemotherapy) indicates that the actions of immunotherapy and maintenance chemotherapy during this period are similar. The results of an EORTC Hemopathies Working Party (personal communication 1977, 1978) randomized trial comparing, after one year of chemotherapy, active immunotherapy comprising administration of BCG and irradiated cells with further maintenance chemotherapy support this conclusion.

We know that two controlled studies (Medical Research Council, 1971; Heyn *et al.,* 1978) have failed to confirm the efficacy of active immunotherapy in children. Their conclusions should be restricted to the preparations and modalities of application of BCG used in their trials. Hence, these interesting trials do not disprove the action of active immunotherapy of other modalities, such as those used in our trials [application of a preparation of living Pasteur strain BCG that was active in our experimental screening (Mathé *et al.,* 1973) and that induces a bacteremia, shown experimentally as a condition necessary for action of the BCG (Khalil *et al.,* 1975) and considered present in man only if followed by a slight increase in the patient's temperature (about 38°C for at least one day)]. Negative results have been registered also in immunotherapy trials for other diseases, especially acute myeloid leukemia, melanoma, and bronchus cancer, for which the results of other trials have shown the efficacy of this therapeutic weapon (Pouillart *et al.,* 1976; McKneally *et al.,* 1977; see also Terry and Windhorst, 1978).

Comparing the results of these three trials (protocols 9, 10, and 11) to the most recent results obtained with long-term maintenance chemotherapy by other groups, we find that they are better than most, and at least as good as the best ones. Our long-term first remission rate, of the order of 50%, is equal to, or higher than, that obtained by the Memphis Group in the so-called total therapy VII 1970–1971 trial, which was performed at about the same time: Treatment with the most efficient branch of this protocol resulted in a plateau for 43% of the subjects, and with the other branches, plateaux for 32%, 23%, and 18% of the subjects (Simone, personal communication). Other results of only prolonged maintenance chemotherapy (Bernard *et al.,* 1975b; Clarkson *et al.,* 1975; Fernbach *et al.,* 1975; Lonsdale *et al.,* 1975) did not show, at the time of publication, a plateau of first remission curves; late relapses after maintenance chemotherapy may reach up to 35% (Bernard *et al.,* 1975a), whereas we have observed no relapses between five and 14 years in patients receiving active immunotherapy (Mathé *et al.,* 1976).

Figure 3 shows the cumulative survival curves for patients in our trial. One

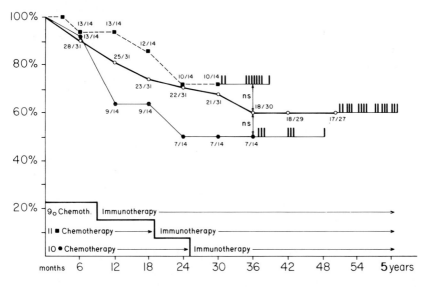

Figure 3. Cumulative curves of duration of survival (established by "direct" method) for children treated by protocols 9, 10, and 11 (Reproduced from Mathé *et al.,* 1978, with permission of Alan R. Liss, Inc.)

sees that they form plateaux for 60%, 50%, and 71% of the patients treated with protocols 9, 10, and 11, respectively. These percentages are also higher than, or as high as, those with the best branches of the protocols for maintenance chemotherapy trials described in the literature (Bernard *et al.,* 1975b; Clarkson *et al.,* 1975; Fernbach *et al.,* 1975; Lonsdale *et al.,* 1975; Lee *et al.,* 1976; Holland, 1978).

Tolerance

There were no deaths during the cumulative 863 months of immunotherapy with these three protocols, as opposed to six (five pneumopathies and one digestive tract hemorrhage) during the same number of months of chemotherapy.

Currently, none of more than 300 patients receiving immunotherapy have died (Schwarzenberg *et al.,* 1976), whereas in the literature, one finds between 4% (Lampert *et al.,* 1975) and 24% (Jacquillat *et al.,* 1975) mortality (Gee *et al.,* 1974; Aur *et al.,* 1975; Mandelli *et al.,* 1975; Simone, 1975; Smyth *et al.,* 1975) among patients in remission under maintenance chemotherapy. The EORTC Hemopathies Working Party (personal communication 1977, 1978) confirmed this important fact, noting four deaths among the 29 randomized patients under maintenance chemotherapy, and none among the 29 patients submitted to immunotherapy.

No long-term aftereffects have been observed in the patients submitted to five-year immunotherapy (Schwarzenberg *et al.,* 1976). The scarified areas leave no unsightly blemishes after immunotherapy has been stopped. Presently, we are comparing the long-term side effects on spermatogenesis and lymphocyte chromosomes in patients who received short-term and those who received long-term maintenance chemotherapy.

Prediction of Prognosis and Adaptation of Treatment

Our earlier studies (Mathé *et al.,* 1971, 1975b) led us to consider patients with the microlymphoblastic type and the V$^-$ macrolymphoblastic and prolymphoblastic types of disease to have good prognoses, and those with the prolymphoblastic type and the V$^+$ macrolymphoblastic and prolymphocytic types to have poor prognoses. When we began protocols 9, 10, and 11, the study of immunologic markers of leukemic cells, which also enables us to predict the prognosis (Belpomme *et al.,* 1974, 1977), was not yet operational for all patients.

The important differences observed between the patients treated by protocol 9 and those treated by the three protocols 9, 10, and 11, inclusively, and for whom, at the onset of their disease, we had predicted prognosis based on the cytologic typing of the WHO Reference Center (Mathé *et al.,* 1971; Mathé and Rappaport, 1976) and the volume of the neoplasm (Mathé *et al.,* 1975b) confirm our previously published conclusions (Fig. 4 and 5). One sees in Figure 4 that the long-term first remission rate for patients with a predicted good

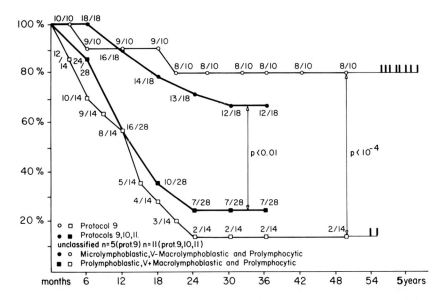

Figure 4. Cumulative curves of duration of first remission (established by "direct" method) according to prognostic factors for children treated by protocol 9, and children treated by protocols 9, 10, and 11, inclusively. (Reproduced from Mathé *et al.*, 1978, with permission of Alan R. Liss, Inc.)

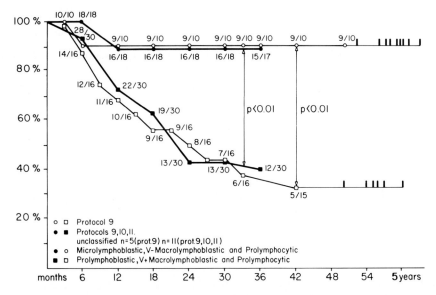

Figure 5. Cumulative curves of duration of survival (established by "direct" method) according to prognostic factors for children treated by protocol 9, and children treated by protocols 9, 10, and 11, inclusively. (Reproduced from Mathé *et al.*, 1978, with permission of Alan R. Liss, Inc.)

prognosis is of the order of 80% for protocol 9, and 66% for the three protocols overall. On the other hand, the long-term first remission rate for the patients with a predicted poor prognosis is of the order of 14% with protocol 9, and 25% with the three protocols overall. Differences of the same order are shown by survival curves (Fig. 5).

This observation may explain why, when treating all ALL patients identically with any of the successive protocols, we have made no progress as far as the long-term first remission rate is concerned; it seems that all these protocols provide almost the maximum action for the patients with good prognoses, whereas they are poorly effective, whatever the modality, for the patients with predicted poor prognoses. Hence, we were led to adapt later protocols to the predicted prognoses of the patients with two different approaches: By our protocol 12, we give more intensive chemotherapy to the patients with predicted poor prognoses and we submit patients with good prognoses to the same type of treatment as that by the protocols described in this paper; whereas by protocol 16, we submit patients with poor prognoses to a different immunotherapeutic approach, based on the interspersion of chemotherapy and immunotherapy. According to the preliminary result of Ekert *et al.* (1975, 1978), treatment of ALL in children with such a procedure is far superior to that of their historical controls.

REFERENCES

Aur, R. J. A., Simone, J. V., Hustu, H. O., and Verzosa, M. 1972. A comparative study of central nervous system irradiation and intensive chemotherapy early in remission of childhood acute lymphocytic leukemia. Cancer, 29:381–391.

Aur, R. J. A., Verzosa, M., Hustu, O., Simone, J., and Barker, L. 1975. Leucoencephalopathy (LEP) during initial complete remission (CR) in children with acute lymphocytic leukemia (ALL) receiving methotrexate (MTX) (Abstract). Proc. Am Assoc. Cancer Res., 16:92.

Belpomme, D., Dantchev, D., Du Rusquec, E., Grandjon, E., Huchet, R., Pouillart, P., Schwarzenberg, L., Amiel, J. L., and Mathé, G. 1974. T and B lymphocyte markers on the neoplastic cell of 20 patients with acute and 10 patients with chronic lymphoid leukemia. Biomedicine, 20:109–118.

Belpomme, D., Mathé, G., and Davies, A. J. S. 1977. Clinical significance and prognostic value of the T-B immunological classification of human primary acute lymphoid leukemias. Lancet, 2:555–558.

Bernard, J., Weil, M., and Jacquillat, C. 1975a. Prognostic factors in human acute leukemias. In Fliedner, T. M., and Perry, S. (eds.): Workshop on Prognostic Factors in Human Acute Leukemia. Oxford, Pergamon Press, pp. 97–121.

Bernard, J., Weil, M., and Jacquillat, C. 1975b. Treatment of acute lymphoblastic leukemia. Wadley Med. Bull., 5:1–11.

Clarkson, B. D., Dowling, M. D., Gee, T. S., Cunningham, I. B., and Burchenal, J. H. 1975. Treatment of acute leukemia in adults. Cancer, 36:775–795.

Clarysse, A., Kenis, Y., and Mathé, G. 1976. Cancer Chemotherapy: Its Role in the Treatment Strategy of Hematologic Malignancies and Solid Tumors. New York, Springer-Verlag, 566 pp.

Ekert, H., and Jose, D. G. 1975. Chemotherapy and BCG in acute lymphocytic leukaemia. Lancet, 2:713–714.

Ekert, H., Jose, D. G., Waters, K. D., Smith, P. J., and Mathews, R. N. 1978. Intermittent chemotherapy and BCG in continuation therapy of children with acute lymphocytic leukemia. In Terry, W. D., and Windhorst, D. (eds.): Immunotherapy of Cancer: Present Status of Trials in Man. New York, Raven Press, pp. 483–492.

Fernbach, D. J., George, S. L., Sutow, W. W., Ragab, A. H., Lane, D. M., Haggard, M. E., and Lonsdale, D. 1975. Long-term results of reinforcement therapy in children with acute leukemia. Cancer, 36:1552–1559.

Gee, T. S., Haghbin, M., Tan, C., Murphy, M. L., Dowling, M. D., and Clarkson, B. D. 1974. Differences in response in adults (15 years) and children with acute lymphoblastic leukemia (ALL) on a single therapeutic regimen (Abstract 720). Proc. Am. Assoc. Cancer Res., 15:164.

Hemopathies Working Party of the EORTC. 1978. Immunotherapy versus chemotherapy as maintenance treatment of acute lymphoblastic leukemia. In Terry, W. D., and Windhorst, D. (eds.): Immunotherapy of Cancer: Present Status of Trials in Man. New York, Raven Press, pp. 471–481.

Heyn, R., Joo, P., Karon, M., Nesbit, M., Shore, N., Breslow, N., Weiner, R., Reed, A., Sather, H., and Hammond, D. 1978. BCG in the treatment of acute lymphocytic leukemia. In Terry, W. D., and Windhorst, D. (eds.): Immunotherapy of Cancer: Present Status of Trials in Man. New York, Raven Press, pp. 503–512.

Holland, J. 1978. Acute lymphocytic leukemia and lymphomas: Status of chemotherapy. In Terry, W. D., and Windhorst, D. (eds.): Immunotherapy of Cancer: Present Status of Trials in Man. New York, Raven Press, pp. 441–450.

Jacquillat, C., Weil, M., Gemon, M. F., Auclerc, G., Loisel, J. P., Delobel, J., Flandrin, G., Schaison, G., Izrael, V., Bussel, A., Dresch, C., Weisgerber, C., Rain, D., Tanzer, J., Najean, Y., Seligmann, M., Boiron, M., and Bernard, J. 1973. Combination therapy in 130 patients with acute lymphoblastic leukemia (Protocol 06 LA 66-Paris). Cancer Res., 33:3278–3284.

Jacquillat, C., Weil, M., Gemon, M. F., Boiron, M., and Bernard, J. 1975. Acute lymphoblastic leukemia in adults. In Mandelli, F., Amadori, S., and Mariani, G. (eds.): Therapy of Acute Leukemias. Rome, Minerva Medica, pp. 113–126.

Khalil, A., Rappaport, H., Bourut, C., Halle-Pannenko, O., and Mathé, G. 1975. Histologic reactions of the thymus, spleen, liver and lymph nodes to i.v. and s.c. BCG injections. Biomedicine, 22:112–121.

Lampert, F., Heinze, G., Wundlisch, G. F., Olischlager, A., Klose, K., Usener, M., and Neidhardt, M. 1975. Cranial irradiation and combination chemotherapy of childhood acute lymphoblastic leukaemia. In Mandelli, F., Amadori, S., and Mariani, G. (eds.): Therapy of Acute Leukemias. Rome, Minerva Medica, pp. 595–599.

Lee, S. L., Kopel, S., and Glidewell, O. 1976. Cytomorphological determinants of prognosis in acute lymphoblastic leukemia of children. Semin. Oncol., 3:209–217.

Lonsdale, D., Gehan, E. A., Fernbach, D. J., Sullivan, M. P., Lane, D. M., and Ragab, A. H. 1975. Interrupted vs continued maintenance therapy in childhood acute leukemia. Cancer, 36:341–352.

Mandelli, F., Amadori, S., Anselmo, M. P., Del Principe, D., Deriu, L., Digilio, G., Isacchi, G., and Multari, G. 1975. Total therapy in acute lymphoid leukemias. In Mandelli, F., Amadori, S., and Mariani, G. (eds.): Therapy of Acute Leukemias. Rome, Minerva Medica, pp. 609–615.

Mathé, G. 1976. Cancer Active Immunotherapy, Immunoprophylaxis and Immunorestoration: An Introduction. New York, Springer-Verlag, 405 pp.

Mathé, G. 1977. Human models for cancer active immunotherapy. Biomedicine, 26:1–5.

Mathé, G., Amiel, J. L., Schwarzenberg, L., Schneider, M., Cattan, A., Schlumberger, J. R., Hayat, M., and De Vassal, F. 1969. Active immunotherapy for acute lymphoblastic leukaemia. Lancet, 2:697–699.

Mathé, G., Amiel, J. L., Schwarzenberg, L., Schneider, M., Cattan, A., Schlumberger, J. R., Hayat, M., and De Vassal, F. 1977. Follow-up of the first (1962) pilot trial on active immunotherapy of acute lymphoid leukaemia. A critical discussion. Biomedicine, 26:29–35.

Mathé, G., De Vassal, F., Delgado, M., Pouillart, P., Belpomme, D., Joseph, R., Schwarzenberg, L., Amiel, J. L., Schneider, M., Cattan, A., Musset, M., Misset, J. L., and Jasmin, C. 1976. 1975 current results of the first 100 cytologically typed acute lymphoid leukaemia submitted to BCG active immunotherapy. Cancer Immunol. Immunother., 1:77–86.

Mathé, G., De Vassal, F., Schwarzenberg, L., Delgado, M., Weiner, R., Gil, M. A., Pena-Angulo, J., Belpomme, D., Pouillart, P., Machover, D., Misset, J. L., Pico, J. L., Jasmin, C., Hayat, M., Schneider, M., Cattan, A., Amiel, J. L., Musset, M., Rosenfeld, C., and Ribaud, P. 1978. Preliminary results of three protocols for the treatment of acute lymphoid leukaemia of children: Distinction of two groups of patients according to predictable prognosis. Med. Pediatr. Oncol., 4:17–27.

Mathé, G., Halle-Pannenko, O., and Bourut, C. 1973. BCG in cancer immunotherapy. II. Results obtained with various BCG preparations in a screening study for systemic adjuvants applicable to cancer immunoprophylaxis or immunotherapy. Natl. Cancer Inst. Monogr., 39:107–112.

Mathé, G., Pouillart, P., and Schwarzenberg, L. 1975a. Meningeal localisation of acute leukemias. Acta Neuropathol. (Berl.), 6:235–239.

Mathé, G., Pouillart, P., Schwarzenberg, L., Hayat, M., De Vassal, F., and Lafleur, M. 1975b. Prognostic factors in acute leukemias. In Fliedner, T. M., and Perry, S. (eds.): Workshop on Prognostic Factors in Human Acute Leukemia. Oxford, Pergamon Press, pp. 145–162.

Mathé, G., Pouillart, P., Sterescu, M., Amiel, J. L., Schwarzenberg, L., Schneider, M., Hayat, M., De Vassal, F., Jasmin, C., and Lafleur, M. 1971. Subdivision of classical varieties of acute leukemias. Correlation with prognosis and cure expectancy. Eur. J. Clin. Biol. Res., 16:554–560.

Mathé, G., and Rappaport, H. 1976. Histological and Cytological Typing of Neoplastic Diseases of Haematopoietic and Lymphoid Tissues. Geneva, World Health Organization, 45 pp.

McKneally, M. F., Maver, C. M., and Kausel, H. W. 1977. Intrapleural BCG immunostimulation in lung cancer. Lancet, 1:1003.

Medical Research Council. 1971. Treatment of acute lymphoblastic leukemia. Comparison of immunotherapy (BCG), intermittent methotrexate, and no therapy after a five month intensive cytotoxic regimen (Concord trial). Br. Med. J., 4:189–194.

Pouillart, P., Mathé, G., Palangié, T., Schwarzenberg, L., Huguenin, P., Morin, P., Gautier, M., and Parrot, R. 1976. Trial of BCG immunotherapy in the treatment of resectable squamous cell carcinoma of the bronchus (stages I and II). Cancer Immunol. Immunother., 1:271–273.

Pouillart, P., Schwarzenberg, L., Schneider, M., and Amiel, J. L. 1972. Les méningites lymphoblastiques. Fréquence, prévention et traitement. Nouv. Presse Med., 1:387–390.

Rosenfeld, C., Goutner, A., Venuat, A. M., Choquet, C., Pico, J. L., Doré, J. F., Liabeuf, A., Durandy, A., Desgrange, C., and De Thé, G. 1977. An effective human leukaemic cell line: Reh. Eur. J. Cancer, 13:377–379.

Schwarzenberg, L., and Mathé, G. 1975. Results obtained with active immunotherapy using corynebacteria (C. parvum or C. granulosum) in the treatment of acute lymphoid leukemia. In Halpern, B. (ed.): *Corynebacterium parvum:* Application in Experimental and Clinical Oncology. New York, Pergamon Press, pp. 372–375.

Schwarzenberg, L., Simmler, M. C., and Pico, J. L. 1976. Human toxicity of BCG applied in cancer immunotherapy. Cancer Immunol. Immunother., 1:69–76.

Simone, J. V. 1975. Treatment of childhood acute lymphocytic leukemia. In Mandelli, F., Amadori, S., and Mariani, G. (eds.): Therapy of Acute Leukemias. Rome, Minerva Medica, pp. 73–95.

Simone, J. V. 1976. Factors that influence haematological remission duration in acute lymphocytic leukaemia. Br. J. Haematol., 32:465–472.

Smyth, A. C., Wiernik, P. H., and Serpick, A. A. 1975. Therapy of adult acute lymphocytic leukemias (ALL) with thioguanine, oncovin, daraprin and dexamethasone (TODD) (Abstract). Proc. Am. Assoc. Cancer Res., 15:236.

Terry, W. D., and Windhorst, D. (eds.) 1978. Immunotherapy of Cancer: Present Status of Trials in Man. New York, Raven Press, 696 pp.

Immunotherapy of Human Cancer,
The University of Texas System Cancer Center
M. D. Anderson Hospital and Tumor Institute.
Raven Press, New York © 1978.

Immunotherapy for Malignant Melanoma

Jordan U. Gutterman, M.D., Giora M. Mavligit, M.D.,
Stephen P. Richman, M.D., Robert S. Benjamin, M.D., Anne
Kennedy, B.A.,* Charles M. McBride, M.D.,† Michael A.
Burgess, M.B.B.S., Shelley L. Bartold, Ph.D.,* Edmund A.
Gehan, Ph.D.,* and Evan M. Hersh, M.D.

*Departments of Developmental Therapeutics, *Biomathematics, and †Surgery, The University of Texas System Cancer Center M. D. Anderson Hospital and Tumor Institute, Houston, Texas*

In this report, we summarize updated results of adjuvant immunotherapy with bacillus Calmette-Guérin (BCG) for patients with recurrent malignant melanoma. In addition, we describe preliminary results of a new, three-drug chemoimmunotherapy regimen for patients with disseminated disease. The rationale and background of the use of BCG immunotherapy have been described elsewhere (Gutterman *et al.,* 1973, 1974).

MATERIALS AND METHODS

Between November 1971 and March 1976, 105 patients with regional lymph node metastases were entered in the study of BCG adjuvant immunotherapy. All patients had recurrent melanoma and were eligible for the study after surgical removal of all clinical evidence of disease.

Forty patients were entered into the first trial, which was conducted between November 1971 and October 1974. Nineteen patients received high-dose Tice strain BCG and 21 patients received low-dose Tice BCG, as described earlier (Gutterman *et al.,* 1973). In the second trial, October 1974 to March 1976, 40 patients with < 5 involved nodes received fresh frozen Pasteur strain BCG. Twenty-five patients with ≥ 5 involved nodes were included in another trial conducted October 1974 to March 1976; they received chemotherapy with DTIC, 250 mg/m² daily for five days, every 21 days and fresh frozen Pasteur strain BCG, 6 × 10⁸ viable units on days 7, 12, and 17.

The surgical control group consisted of 260 patients with stage IIIB melanoma who had been treated with surgery alone at M. D. Anderson Hospital between

---

Abbreviations used in this chapter: DTIC—dimethyl triazeno imidazole carboxamide; WHO—World Health Organization.

I. PRECHEMOTHERAPY IMMUNOTHERAPY

   INTRAVENOUS *Corynebacterium parvum*

   <u><60 YEARS</u>   <u>≥60 YEARS</u>

   0.25 mg/m² DAYS 1,2   0.2 mg/m² × 14 DAYS

   0.5 mg/m² DAY 3

   1.0 mg/m² DAY 4

   2.0 mg m² DAYS 5–14

II. CHEMOTHERAPY

                           DTIC 250 mg/m² DAYS 15–19

   RANDOMIZATION

                           DTIC 250 mg/m² DAYS 15–19
                           + ACTINOMYCIN D 1.5 mg/m² DAY 15 ONLY

III. IMMUNOTHERAPY

   SUBCUTANEOUS *Corynebacterium parvum*

   2 mg/m²   DAYS 21, 26, 31

   REPEAT CHEMOTHERAPY EVERY 3 WEEKS

IV. IMMUNOTHERAPY REINTENSIFICATION WITH INTRAVENOUS
   Corynebacterium parvum × 14 DAYS GIVEN AFTER EVERY
   3 COMPLETE CYCLES OF CHEMOTHERAPY AND SUBCUTANEOUS
   Corynebacterium parvum

Figure 1. Regimen of chemoimmunotherapy for disseminated malignant melanoma.

January 1965 and October 1971. Variables of these patients were examined in a fashion comparable to that for the patients in our study. The natural histories of these surgical control patients will be examined in detail in another report.

In September 1975, we initiated a study for patients with disseminated melanoma. All patients received immunotherapy with *Corynebacterium parvum* administered intravenously, as indicated in Figure 1. Patients then were randomized to receive DTIC alone or DTIC plus actinomycin D (Gutterman *et al.*, 1977).

The statistical methods used included a generalized Wilcoxon test and a one-tailed analysis for testing differences between remission or survival curves (Gehan, 1965) and the methods of Kaplan and Meier (1958) for calculating and plotting remission and survival curves.

RESULTS

Immunotherapy

Results of clinical follow-up studies have been described previously (Gutterman *et al.*, 1973). The postoperative disease-free intervals for the surgically treated control and the BCG-treated groups of stage IIIB patients with less than five involved nodes are shown in Figure 2. There has been a statistically

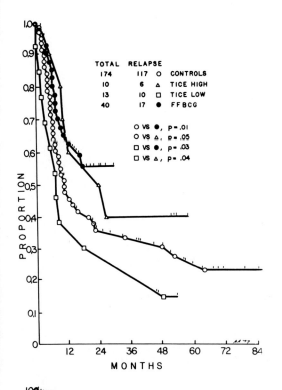

Figure 2. Disease-free intervals for stage III melanoma patients with less than five involved nodes receiving adjuvant BCG therapy.

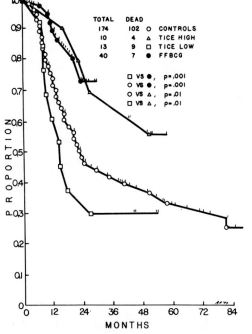

Figure 3. Survival rates for stage III melanoma patients with less than five involved nodes receiving adjuvant BCG therapy.

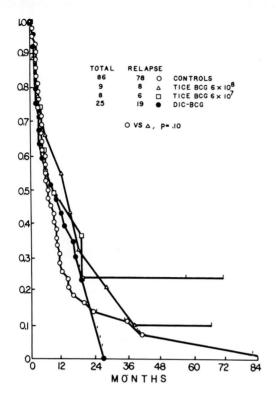

Figure 4. Disease-free intervals for stage III melanoma patients with five or more involved nodes receiving adjuvant BCG therapy.

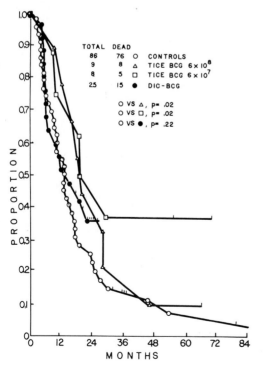

Figure 5. Survival rates for stage III melanoma patients with five or more involved nodes receiving adjuvant BCG therapy.

Table 1. *Response Rates for Patients with Disseminated Malignant Melanoma Receiving Chemoimmunotherapy*

	No. (%) Responding to Therapy		
Response	C. parvum + DTIC ± Act-D (1975*)	DTIC + BCG (1972*)	DTIC (1967*)
Remission	26/81 (32)	24/89 (27)	17/111 (15)
Stabilization	27/81 (34)	28/89 (32)	33/111 (30)
Progression	28/81 (34)	37/89 (41)	61/111 (55)

* Initial year of study.

significant prolongation of the postoperative disease-free interval for patients treated with either high-dose Tice or fresh frozen Pasteur strain BCG compared with the control group. No benefit was derived for those patients treated with low-dose Tice BCG. The survival for the group of patients with less than five involved nodes is shown in Figure 3. Patients treated with the high doses of BCG (Tice or fresh frozen) have had a highly significant prolongation of survival. Only 4 of 10 patients treated with high-dose Tice and 7 of 40 treated with fresh frozen BCG have died.

In contrast to these encouraging results, little benefit has been derived for patients with five or more involved nodes. There has been no statistical improvement in the postoperative disease-free interval for patients treated with BCG alone or DTIC plus BCG (Fig. 4), and there has been little improvement in the postoperative survival time (Fig. 5).

Chemoimmunotherapy

The overall response rates for patients with disseminated malignant melanoma receiving chemoimmunotherapy are presented in Table 1. Thirty-two percent (26) of 81 patients achieved remission; 34% (27), stabilization; and 34% (28), disease progression. All patients treated with *C. parvum* and DTIC plus actinomycin D, as well as patients under the age of 60 treated with DTIC and the

Table 2. *Response Rates for Patients with Disseminated Malignant Melanoma Receiving Chemoimmunotherapy, According to Patient Age*

	No. (%) Responding to Therapy			
	< 60 yr		≥ 60 yr	
Response	C. parvum + DTIC + Act-D	C. parvum + DTIC	C. parvum + DTIC + Act-D	C. parvum + DTIC
Remission	11/31 (36)	8/20 (40)	5/15 (33)	2/15 (14)
Complete	4/31 (13)	2/20 (10)	3/15 (20)	1/15 (7)
Partial	7/31 (23)	6/20 (30)	2/15 (13)	1/15 (7)
Stabilization	10/31 (32)	6/20 (30)	6/15 (40)	5/15 (33)
Progression	10/31 (32)	6/20 (30)	4/15 (27)	8/15 (54)

Table 3. *Correlation of Remission Rate with Fever Induced by 14-Day Course of* C. parvum, *2 mg/m²*

| | No. of Patients Responding/Total Patients* | | | |
| | Days 5–9 | | Days 10–14 | |
Therapy	98.6°–102.9°F	≥ 103°F	98.6°–102.9°F	≥ 103°F
C. parvum +DTIC + Act-D	4/14	7/15	3/18	7/11
C. parvum + DTIC	4/11	4/6	5/12	3/5
Total	8/25 (31%)	11/21 (50%)	8/30 (27.5%)	10/16 (62.5%)†

* < 60 years old.
† Difference in remission at days 10–14, < 103°F vs. ≥ 103°F, $p = .04$.

high dose of *C. parvum* had remission rates ranging from 33% to 40% (Table 2). Only those patients over the age of 60 who were treated with *C. parvum* and DTIC without actinomycin D had a low response rate (14%).

Table 3 shows that the response rate correlates with the degree of fever induced by the 14-day course of *C. parvum* prior to chemotherapy. Patients who had a daily temperature of at least 103°F for the entire 14 days had a high response rate compared with patients who did not have high temperature. Thus, 10 (63%) of 16 patients who maintained a fever of 103°F or greater for the entire 14 days achieved a partial or complete remission. In comparison, 8 (27.5%) of 30 patients who had temperatures of 98.6° to 102.9°F responded.

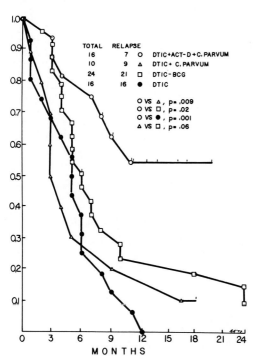

TOTAL	RELAPSE		
16	7	○	DTIC+ACT-D+C. PARVUM
10	9	△	DTIC+ C. PARVUM
24	21	□	DTIC-BCG
16	16	●	DTIC

○ VS △ , p= .009
○ VS □ , p= .02
○ VS ● , p= .001
△ VS □ , p= .06

Figure 6. Durations of remission for patients with disseminated malignant melanoma receiving chemo-immunotherapy.

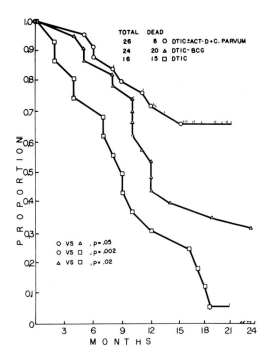

Figure 7. Survival rates for patients with disseminated malignant melanoma responding to chemoimmunotherapy.

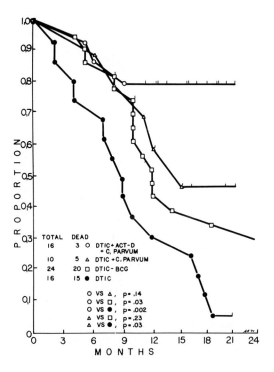

Figure 8. Survival rates for patients with disseminated malignant melanoma responding to different regimens of chemoimmunotherapy.

The durations of remission for patients treated in this study are significantly longer than those for patients treated with DTIC alone but are not significantly longer compared with remissions of patients treated with DTIC plus BCG (Fig. 6). Patients treated with *C. parvum* and DTIC plus actinomycin D have had the longest remissions. Their remissions are significantly longer than those of patients treated with *C. parvum* and DTIC only (Fig. 6).

Figure 7 shows survival rates for the patients treated by the *C. parvum*-DTIC protocol. Only 8 of the 26 responders overall have died. The survival of the responding patients is significantly longer than that of responding patients treated with other, previous regimens. Figure 8 shows survival rates for the responders according to the therapy regimen. Only 3 of the 16 patients receiving *C. parvum* and DTIC plus actinomycin D have died. At the most recent evaluation, however, the survival of responding patients in this group was not statistically longer than that of responding patients treated with *C. parvum* and DTIC without actinomycin D (Fig. 8).

DISCUSSION

These early results suggest that, when given in adequate numbers of viable units, BCG is capable of prolonging the postoperative disease-free interval and survival, particularly among patients with tumor metastatic to < 5 lymph nodes. Similar data have been reported by Morton and co-workers (1977) as well as those conducting the WHO melanoma trial (Beretta *et al.,* 1978). However, it seems that BCG has maximal benefit in the treatment of primary melanoma.

The preliminary results of chemoimmunotherapy with intravenous *C. parvum* and DTIC plus actinomycin D are encouraging. A more extensive report of this trial will be reported elsewhere.

ACKNOWLEDGMENT

This work was supported by contract 33888 and grant 05831 from the National Cancer Institute.

REFERENCES

Beretta, G., Adamus, J., Aubert, C., Bonadonna, G., Cochran, A., DeMarsillac, J., Durand, J., Ikonopisov, R. L., Kiss, B., Kulakowski, A., Lejeune, F., Mechl, Z., Milton, G. W., Peter, H. H., Priario, J., Rumke, P., Tomin, R., and Veronesi, U. 1978. Controlled study for prolonged chemotherapy, immunotherapy, and chemotherapy plus immunotherapy as an adjuvant to surgery in stage I-II malignant melanoma: Preliminary report, International Group for the Study of Melanoma. In Terry, W. D., and Windhorst, D. (eds.): Immunotherapy of Cancer: Present Status of Trials in Man. New York, Raven Press, pp. 65–71.
Gehan, E. A. 1965. A generalized Wilcoxon text for comparing arbitrarily singly censored samples. Biometrika, 52:203–223.
Gutterman, J. U., Mavligit, G., Benjamin, R., Burgess, M. A., and Hersh, E. M. 1977. An effective

new chemoimmunotherapy regimen for disseminated malignant melanoma (DMM). Proc. Am. Soc. Clin. Oncol., 18–300 #C-135.

Gutterman, J. U., Mavligit, G., Gottlieb, J. A., Burgess, M. A., McBride, C. M., Einhorn, L., Freireich, E. J, and Hersh, E. M. 1974. Chemoimmunotherapy of disseminated malignant melanoma with dimethyl triazeno carboxamide and bacillus Calmette-Guerin. N. Engl. J. Med., 291:592.

Gutterman, J. U., Mavligit, G., McBride, C., Frei, E., III, Freireich, E. J, and Hersh, E. M. 1973. Active immunotherapy with BCG for recurrent malignant melanoma. Lancet, 1:1208.

Kaplan, E. L., and Meier, P. 1958. Nonparametric estimation from incomplete observations. J. Am. Statist. Assoc., 53:457–481.

Morton, D. L., Eilber, F. R., Holmes, E. C., Townsend, C. M., Jr., Mirra, J., and Weisenburger, T. H. 1977. Adjuvant therapy in melanoma and sarcomas. In Salmon, S. E., and Jones, S. E. (eds.): Adjuvant Therapy of Cancer. Amsterdam, Elsevier/North-Holland Biomedical Press, pp. 191–198.

Immunotherapy of Human Cancer,
The University of Texas System Cancer Center
M. D. Anderson Hospital and Tumor Institute.
Raven Press, New York © 1978.

Immunology and Immunotherapy of Human Sarcomas

Joseph G. Sinkovics, M.D., Carl Plager, M.D., Nicholas
Papadopoulos, M.D., Marion J. McMurtrey, M.D.,* Jimmy J.
Romero, B.S., Ruth Waldinger, R.N.,† and Marvin M.
Romsdahl, M.D., Ph.D.*

*Department of Medicine, Section of Clinical Tumor Virology and Immunology and Solid Tumor Clinics (Service), and Departments of *Surgery and †Nursing, The University of Texas System Cancer Center M. D. Anderson Hospital and Tumor Institute, Houston, Texas*

HISTORICAL CONTRIBUTION OF DR. W. B. COLEY

In the last decade of the past century, the astute surgeon Dr. William B. Coley read about a patient whose recurrent and finally inoperable "round cell sarcoma" of the neck completely regressed after a natural erysipelas infection. Setting himself characteristically after the truth, he traced this patient and found him in good health without evidence of tumor. Difficult years followed for Dr. Coley: He tried to cure cancer by inducing erysipelas around large tumors. Erysipelas in itself was an infection of high mortality those days. The cultural characteristics of streptococci that caused erysipelas were not well known either. Yet, Dr. Coley recorded success; for example, in 1892, he cured a patient of an inoperable "spindle cell sarcoma." To make his treatment safer and better standardized, Dr. Coley began to use "toxins" of streptococci. Prodigiosus bacteria were then known to increase the virulence of certain other bacteria with which they were cocultivated. Dr. Coley therefore decided to grow erysipelas-causing streptococci in prodigiosus cultures. Coley's toxin preparations were derived from these mixed cultures. This procedural innovation had introduced a new element in this treatment modality: endotoxin. These gram-negative rods, now known as *Serratia marcescens,* produce endotoxin. Thus, Dr. Coley, without knowing that he was working with one of the most powerful biologic agents (for the most profound and diverse effects of endotoxin in man, see Fig. 1), opened an era of human tumor immunotherapy.

Coley's toxin preparations were produced by Parke-Davis laboratories, and the preparation was available to practicing physicians. Many patients thus were treated and their case histories have been presented in detail in an anecdotal

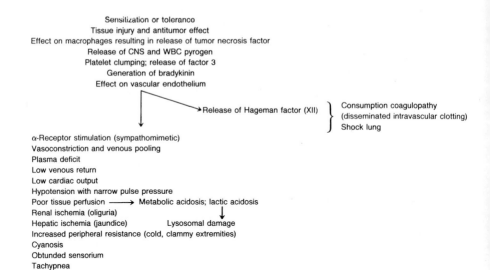

Figure 1. Effects of endotoxin in man. CNS, central nervous system; WBC, white blood cells.

fashion. Even though this mode of presentation does not measure up to modern requirements for proof of effectiveness of a treatment regimen, the overwhelming impression one gathers from reading these case histories is that treatment of patients with a variety of advanced neoplasms was effective in producing partial and probably complete remissions. Sarcomas of soft tissues and bone were prominent among the responsive tumors (Coley, 1893, 1898, 1908; Nauts, 1974, 1975a,b, 1976). The possible mechanisms of this treatment regimen were not understood.

It is in this present era of tumor immunology when Dr. Coley's pioneering contribution assumes its full importance, although it has not received adequate recognition. We know now that activated macrophages distinguish between cell populations growing in an orderly, contact-inhibited fashion and in a disorderly, contact-uninhibited fashion. Macrophages attack disorderly parenchymal cells. We have learned that in the wake of a delayed hypersensitivity reaction, in which lymphocytes and macrophages cooperate, cells expressing the antigen that elicited the reactions and also bystander cells within the radius of the reaction are destroyed. Malignant tumors of the skin have been destroyed by delayed hypersensitivity reactions induced around them (Klein *et al.,* 1975). We have just begun to understand the complex interaction of molecular mediators released from reactive lymphocytes and macrophages. Prominent among these mediators are cytotoxins, macrophage activating and macrophage migration inhibitory factors, mediators of helper and suppressor lymphocytes, skin reaction factor, interferon, factors inhibitory to nucleic acid synthesis, and tumor necrosis factor. In the context of Dr. Coley's discovery, tumor necrosis factor of macrophage origin may be the most important. Endotoxin in itself is not overtly toxic to cultured tumor cells. Primed and activated macrophages, however, release a molecular mediator that can destroy tumor cells. Macrophages can be primed with mycobacteria, but it is exposure of macrophages to endotoxin that best elicits the release of tumor necrosis factor (Carswell *et al.,* 1975). It is still not known if it was this powerful system that Dr. Coley's toxin treatment activated in all those patients whose anecdotal case histories documented successful treatment of inoperable malignant neoplasms. However, Dr. Coley provided the lead to which some good rationale has been added recently.

IMMUNE ASSESSMENT OF PATIENTS WITH SARCOMA

General Immunity

Patients with sarcomas tested against recall antigens seldom display defective immunity unless the tumors are far advanced, and skin test reactivity to recall antigens has no prognostic value (Pinsky *et al.,* 1974; Kotz *et al.,* 1976; Pritchard *et al.,* 1976). Immune competence of patients with sarcomas is rapidly restored after surgical removal of the tumor (Golub *et al.,* 1974). Newly acquired immunity, as assayed with dinitrochlorobenzene (DNCB) skin tests, has no prognostic value for patients with sarcomas (Kotz *et al.,* 1976), but DNCB reactivity has been found to correlate with the extent of the disease: 11 of 13 patients with stage I, 5 of 8 patients with stage II, and 7 of 19 patients with stage III sarcomas were reactive in the DNCB primary skin sensitization test (Eilber *et al.,* 1975a).

The blastogenic response of lymphocytes to phytohemagglutinin (PHA) has provided little, if any, prognostic information for patients with sarcomas (Kotz *et al.,* 1976), but blastogenic response to concanavalin A seems to decrease significantly in patients with advancing sarcomas (Pritchard *et al.,* 1976). There have been contradictory findings in patients with osteogenic sarcoma. In one study, these patients were immunocompetent when tested for PHA reactivity but failed to distinguish by in vitro lymphocyte-mediated reactions normal autologous fibroblasts from autologous tumor cells (McMaster *et al.,* 1973, 1974). In another study, the lymphocytes of patients with osteosarcoma failed to respond to PHA; curiously, the lymphocytes of patients with soft tissue sarcomas were reactive to PHA (Twomey and Chretien, 1975). Patients with Kaposi's sarcoma also were found to display various immune defects (Master *et al.,* 1970; Taylor *et al.,* 1971; Dobozy *et al.,* 1973; Taylor and Ziegler, 1974). The dependence of this tumor on immunosuppression of the host is well documented in those cases that occurred in organ transplant recipients; in some of these cases, the tumors regressed after discontinuation of immunosuppressive treatment (Myers *et al.,* 1974; Hardy *et al.,* 1976).

Sarcoma-Directed Immunity

Extensive literature concerning antibody- and lymphocyte-mediated immune reactions of patients with sarcomas tested against autologous tumor cells or allogeneic sarcoma cells has been reviewed recently (Sinkovics *et al.,* 1977b). In the latter assay, adequate selectivity, i.e., reactions to sarcoma cells without reactions to carcinoma, melanoma, or other unrelated tumor cells, was sought. There is no doubt that patients with sarcomas display both antibody- and lymphocyte-mediated immune reactivity to autologous sarcoma cells (Morton *et al.,* 1969; Sinkovics *et al.,* 1974). Immune reactivities of patients with sarcomas directed to allogeneic sarcoma cells are stronger and more frequent than reactivities directed to carcinoma and other unrelated tumor cells (Kay *et al.,* 1976; Sinkovics *et al.,* 1976b). However, the possession of immune faculties reactive to sarcoma cells is not confined to patients with sarcomas and to their closest relatives or intimate contacts (Byers *et al.,* 1975a) inasmuch as strong reactors are readily found in the healthy human population (Bukowski *et al.,* 1976; Kay *et al.,* 1976). Thus, it is not known if the sarcoma-directed immune reactivity detected in patients with sarcomas does truly develop in response to growing tumors. Possibly, such immune reactions are widely spread in the healthy human population but undergo quantitative or qualitative depreciation before or during tumor growth and are reconstituted coincidentally with successful removal of the tumor.

In selected patients, results of serial quantitative testing of humoral or cell-mediated, sarcoma-directed immunity appear to change according to clinical status. For example, complement-fixing cytolytic antibodies seemingly specific for sarcoma cells decline with large tumor burden but rise after surgical removal of tumor (Wood and Morton, 1971). Lymphocytes cytotoxic to sarcoma cells and serum factors blocking or potentiating this effect also correlate with therapy-induced regression or therapy-resistant growth of tumors (Sinkovics *et al.,* 1975b). However, contradictions between the in vitro assays and the patients' clinical status also have been found (Table 1). For example, tumor growth has been observed in immunocompetent patients who also displayed sarcoma-directed immune reactions (lymphocytes cytotoxic to sarcoma cells; serum factors potentiating this effect but without demonstrable blocking factors) (Sinkovics *et al.,* 1972b, 1975a).

It has been suggested that sarcoma cells may express antigens that serve as targets for immune reactions of the host; in these cases, good immunologic control of the tumor and prolonged tumor-free survival may occur in immuno-reactive patients (Sinkovics *et al.,* 1976a). It has also been postulated that sarcomas can grow in an immunocompetent human host without the expression of antigens that may serve as targets for the immune reactions of the host; thus, patients displaying sarcoma-directed immune reactions (even without blocking serum factors) may succumb to the disease (Sinkovics *et al.,* 1976a). In a series of lymphocyte-mediated cytotoxicity assays, cross-reactions between soft tissue

Table 1. Discrepancy Between Clinical Course and In Vitro Cytotoxicity Assays of Nonselective and Selective Lymphocytes to Established, Allogeneic, Human Tumor Cell Lines

| | | | Percent Growth Reduction of Tumor Cell Lines* | | | | | | | | | | |
| | | | 2043 | | 2118 | | 2089 | | 2322 | | 2454 | | 3123 | |
Patient	Lymphocytes†	Day	2	4	2	4	2	4	2	4	2	4	2	4
1‡	Ly		−42	40	...	...	...	...	−14	8	35	19	...	...
	Se Ly		−10	−50	...	...	...	...	−5	23	27	7	...	...
2§	Ly		15	21	35	42	−69	41	−17	64	...	...	47	61
	Se Ly		68	24	39	75	34	50	0	69	...	...	71	28

* Minus sign indicates growth stimulation. Cytotoxicity assay done in duplicates in LabTek chamber/slides (Sinkovics et al., 1975a). See Sinkovics et al., 1977b for descriptions of cell lines.

† Ly, purified peripheral blood lymphocytes; Se, heat-inactivated blood serum.

‡ Young man with osteosarcoma metastatic to lungs, surviving longer than four years. Patient's lymphocytes stimulate growth of squamous carcinoma cells (line 2043) and are only weakly cytotoxic to chondrosarcoma cell lines 2322 and 2454.

§ Young man with osteosarcoma metastatic to lungs, rapidly succumbing. Patient's lymphocytes display nonselective cytotoxicity, potentiated by patient's serum, to squamous carcinoma (2043) and kidney carcinoma (2118) cell lines. Rhabdomyosarcoma cell line 2089 is first stimulated, then inhibited by lymphocytes, and is inhibited by serum and lymphocytes. Lymphocytes as well as serum and lymphocytes strongly inhibit chondrosarcoma cell line 2322 by day 4 (but not by day 2), and also inhibit neurofibrosarcoma cell line 3123.

and bone sarcoma cells were found; patients with sarcomas had circulating lymphocytes that were cytotoxic not only to cultured sarcoma cells but also to cultured melanoma and carcinoma cells (Sinkovics et al., 1977d; Sinkovics and Plager, 1977). The attacker cell population was not subfractionated; thus, natural killer cells, tumor-specific cytotoxic lymphocytes, and the recently recognized suppressor cells (Yu et al., 1977) acted together in these relatively crude assays. However, two major points still emerged: (1) Patients with sarcomas are not overtly immunoincompetent; i.e., they possess a relatively large supply of cytotoxic lymphocytes; and (2) Ewing's sarcoma differs from other sarcomas; e.g., the lymphocytes of patients with this tumor reacted strongly to one allogeneic Ewing's sarcoma cell line (Sinkovics et al., 1977b) but displayed only weak or mediocre reaction to bone and soft tissue sarcoma cells or to carcinoma and melanoma cells (Sinkovics and Plager, 1977; Sinkovics et al., 1977d).

Osteoclasts are thought to form the benign giant cell tumors of the bone. These tumors may be transformed into osteogenic sarcomas or fibrosarcomas (malignant fibrous histiocytomas) of the bone, especially after irradiation. According to one report, the large, multinucleated cells of this tumor are not osteoclasts but defensive macrophages. The elongated cells, formerly thought to be stromal cells, represent highly antigenic tumor (osteosarcoma) cells that are contained by host immune mechanisms; in athymic mice, not the large, multinucleated cells but the small, elongated cells grew out as malignant tumor (Byers et al., 1975b).

Three types of resistance of human sarcoma cells to cytotoxic lymphocytes have been observed: (1) Soluble substances released from sarcoma cells render cytotoxic lymphocytes noncytotoxic (Sinkovics et al., 1972a). These soluble substances may represent the sialomucin coat of sarcoma cells, sarcoma antigens, or molecular mediators capable of inactivating cytotoxic lymphocytes. (2) Nonexpression of target antigens by sarcoma cells has been demonstrated by the fact that sarcomas growing in fully immunocompetent patients (in whose immune reaction pattern, blocking serum factors could not be detected) have been recognized (Sinkovics et al., 1976a). (3) In advanced passages of certain human sarcoma cell lines, human lymphocytes are often cytotoxic, but frequently, resistant colonies of sarcoma cells emerge. In some cultures, the resistant cells appear and behave as fibroblasts reverted from neoplastic to normal growth pattern (Fig. 2 and 3). It is possible that certain clones of lymphocytes can elicit cell differentiation; this phenomenon would represent a hitherto unrecognized function of lymphocytes (Sinkovics, 1976a).

The unreliability of presently available in vitro assays for the monitoring of sarcoma-directed immunity is reflected by fluctuations of such reactivity in serially tested, healthy persons (Kay et al., 1976). Thus, serial assays should be done with cryopreserved attacker cells against target sarcoma cells of the same batch so that variations inherent in the antigenic expression of the target cells and in assays set individually in time sequence be eliminated.

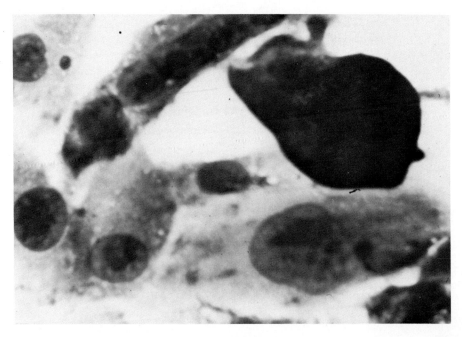

Figure 2. Malignant-appearing cells from passage 33 of human chondrosarcoma cell line 1459 (Sinkovics *et al.,* 1971a,b, 1972a). One cell is in mitosis.

ACTIVE IMMUNIZATIONS

Sarcoma-Specific Antigens

When immune reactivity of patients with sarcoma cells was first discovered, the antigens evoking this reactivity were believed to be those of an oncornavirus (Morton *et al.,* 1969; Sinkovics *et al.,* 1970b,c, 1971b; Giraldo *et al.,* 1971). This possibility was supported by the cross-reactivity of these antigens among various histologic subtypes of sarcomas; the transfer of antigen-synthesizing capability from sarcoma cells to normal human embryonic fibroblasts with filtrates of sarcoma cells (the phenomenon of antigenic conversion); the transfer of haphazard, contact-uninhibited growth pattern from sarcoma cell cultures to normal human embryonic fibroblasts with filtrates of sarcoma cells (the phenomenon of "focus formation"); the occasional appearance of type C virus particles or of filamentous structures resembling unenveloped viral nucleocapsids in cultured sarcoma cells; and the display of sarcoma-directed immune reactions by intimate contacts of patients with sarcomas (for reviews, see Sinkovics and Harris, 1976; Sinkovics *et al.,* 1977b). Further, oncornaviral fragments were demonstrated in human sarcoma cells (Kufe *et al.,* 1972). Finally, osteosarcomas

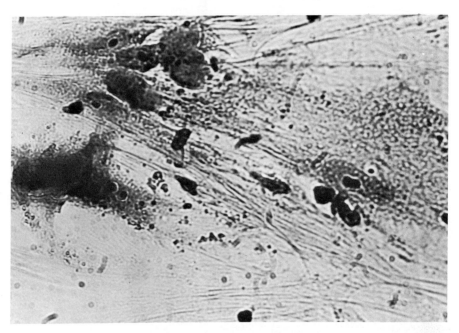

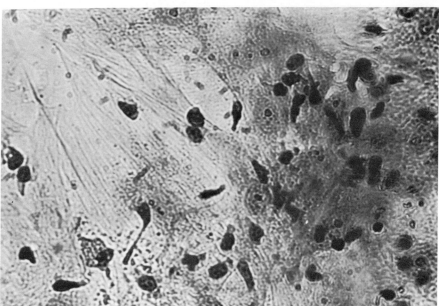

Figure 3. Top, When added to cell line 1459, purified lymphocytes of a healthy donor were cytotoxic. Many lymphocytes entered elongated cells (emperipolesis). Bottom, Remaining cells of line 1459 became fibroblast-like in appearance and growth pattern. One of several possible interpretations is that differentiation of malignant mesenchymal (sarcoma) cells can be effected by a unique lymphocyte population (Sinkovics, 1976a).

induced in hamsters after the inoculation of human osteosarcoma filtrates expressed antigens that reacted with the sera of osteosarcoma patients (Pritchard *et al.,* 1974).

More recent studies have failed to confirm that the antigens expressed in human sarcoma cells are of oncornaviral origin. The diffuse cytoplasmic antigen (S2) is probably an oncofetal antigen, whereas the granular cytoplasmic antigen (S1) resembles most of the Forssman antigens (Mukherji and Hirshaut, 1973; Hirshaut *et al.,* 1974; Sethi and Hirshaut, 1976). The complement fixing S3 antigen differs from both of these antigens because S1 antibody is highly prevalent in patients having all types of solid tumors, including malignant lymphomas, whereas S3 antibody occurs in low titers and only occasionally in patients with malignant lymphomas. Antibody to S2 antigen occurs even less frequently than antibody to S3 in patients with lymphomas. Only S3 antibodies increase after removal of sarcomatous tumors (suggesting binding of S3 antibody to tumor cells in vivo). Even though no oncornaviral glycoprotein antigens or structural oncornaviral proteins, including reverse transcriptase, can be demonstrated in human sarcoma cells, the antigenic changes displayed by these cells can result from the effects of an oncornaviral genome present in these cells. Human sarcoma cells are clearly "nonproducers" of virions but may harbor strongly suppressed and well-integrated oncornaviral genomes.

Cultures of Kaposi sarcoma cells often contain a herpes-type virus (Wang *et al.,* 1975) resembling cytomegalovirus (Giraldo *et al.,* 1972). The relationship of this virus to the tumor is entirely unknown. It is possible that the virus is carried into the tumor by B-lineage reactive lymphocytes, but it is also possible that the viral genome exists in the tumor cells, codes for neoantigens, and contributes to the initiation of these tumors.

The osteoclasts of Paget's osteitis deformans have been considered transformed and neoplastic for some time. These osteoclasts can be suppressed by mithramycin or actinomycin D. Patients with Paget's disease of the bone have an increased incidence of osteogenic sarcomas. Subviral structures have been detected in the osteoclasts of Paget's disease (Rebel *et al.,* 1975; Mills and Singer, 1976); thus, this entity may represent a slow virus disease.

Recently, solubilized antigen was prepared from human osteosarcoma cells; lymphocytes of osteosarcoma patients undergo blastogenic response upon exposure to this antigen (Gainor *et al.,* 1976). Erythrocytes may be coated with this antigen and agglutinated with sera of patients (Gamblin *et al.,* 1977). Xenogeneic immune sera against this antigen also were produced (Marsh *et al.,* 1972). In a study by Singh *et al.* (1977), rabbits immunized with cultured human osteosarcoma cells yielded an immune RNA of lymphoid tissue origin that could render normal human peripheral blood lymphocytes cytotoxic to two human osteosarcoma cell lines; cytotoxicity to other human tumor cell lines (adenocarcinoma of the stomach and, curiously, rhabdomyosarcoma and mesenchymoma) did not increase.

Extracts (3M potassium chloride) of Ewing's sarcomas or cells cultured from this tumor stimulated migration factor release from leukocytes of patients with Ewing's sarcoma; the leukocytes of normal donors or patients with tumors other than Ewing's sarcoma (breast and lung carcinoma) responded weakly. The leukocytes of a few patients with Ewing's sarcoma responded to lung and breast carcinoma extracts. Unfortunately, cross-reactions between soft tissue, bone, and Ewing's sarcoma cells were not studied (McCoy et al., 1977).

Sarcoma-Specific Immunization

Attempts at immunotherapy with sarcoma cells or cell lysates for patients with sarcomas are not extensive. The osteosarcoma immunotherapy trial of Memorial Sloan-Kettering Cancer Center has not been analyzed recently. In this trial, the control group was not followed as closely as the immunized groups; for example, chest X rays were done less frequently in the control group than in the immunized groups. Thus, the time from surgery to appearance of metastases appears longer in the control group (Marcove et al., 1973). However, disease-free interval was significantly longer for those patients who received lysed vaccine than for those who received whole cell vaccine; thus, there is suggestive evidence that the clinical course of human osteosarcoma can be altered by immunologic manipulations.

In another study, patients with sarcomas received active immunization with allogeneic or autologous X-irradiated sarcoma cells, neuraminidase-treated sarcoma cells, or sarcoma cell lysates, such as viral oncolysates (Rosato et al., 1974; Green et al., 1976; for review, see Sinkovics et al., 1977b). Laboratory monitoring of these patients indicated improvement in one or more of the following parameters: lymphocyte-mediated cytotoxicity, serum factors potentiating lymphocyte-mediated cytotoxicity (Sinkovics et al., 1977b), and decrease in serum factors blocking lymphocyte-mediated cytotoxicity (Currie, 1973). However, no clinical benefits from these vaccinations were well documented.

Immunostimulation Combined with Sarcoma-Specific Immunization

Corynebacterium parvum added to conventional treatment of patients with metastatic sarcomas has been claimed to increase survival rate (Israël and Edelstein, 1975): In a conventionally treated group, survival rates at 6, 12, and 24 months were 65%, 43%, and 0%, respectively; whereas in a group receiving conventional treatment plus immunotherapy, survival rates at 6, 12, and 30 months were 84%, 84%, and 39%, respectively.

In other trials, nonspecific immunostimulation with BCG was combined with presumably sarcoma-specific active immunization with allogeneic sarcoma cells or cell lysates. In the California trial, patients with stages I and II soft tissue sarcomas received postoperative adjuvant immunotherapy with bacille Calmette-Guérin (BCG) and allogeneic sarcoma cells. No evidence of disease was found in 11 of 18 postoperatively immunized patients and in 5 of 15 patients treated surgically only. Tumors recurred or metastases appeared in the immunized patients in 4 to 25 months (mean, 15 months, and median, 12 months) versus 1 to 24 months (mean, 7.3 months, and median, 6 months) in the surgically treated patients. Three of 17 patients who received adjuvant immunotherapy after removal of tumors remained alive and free of tumors, whereas none of eight stage III patients treated with surgery alone survived. Similar attempts at immunotherapy for osteogenic sarcoma failed to significantly alter the course of the disease (Eilber *et al.,* 1975b; Townsend *et al,* 1976).

Viral oncolysates were used in the chemoimmunotherapy for patients with malignant melanoma (McMurtrey *et al.,* 1977; Sinkovics *et al.,* 1977a) and metastatic sarcomas. Based on evaluations of all patients in October 1976 and February 1977, the progression of disease was significantly delayed in patients for whom tumor-directed immunization was added to conventional treatment and nonspecific immunostimulation. Among those with metastatic sarcomas, 66% and 72% of 49 conventionally treated patients had progressive disease at the first and second evaluations, respectively. These patients had received chemotherapy with vincristine, cyclophosphamide, doxorubicin, actinomycin D, and dimethyl triazeno imidazole carboxamide in addition to radiotherapy and surgery. Of 19 patients receiving the conventional treatment plus nonspecific immunostimulation by scarification with Chicago BCG, 40% and 53% had progressive disease when analyzed in October 1976 and February 1977, respectively. The third group of patients with metastatic sarcomas received conventional treatment as outlined above, BCG, and active immunization with allogeneic sarcoma viral oncolysates. Of these 19 patients, 14% and 32% had progressive disease at the first and second evaluations, respectively. These patients are being submitted to a computer-assisted analysis, which will include a balance of prognostic factors and will express survival based on life table analysis.

In the preliminary assessment, disease progression appears to be controlled best in the group receiving viral oncolysates (Sinkovics, 1977; Sinkovics *et al.,* 1977c). For this group, chemotherapy was administered on days 1 through 5 and immunotherapy on days 17 and 24. It is evident that with longer observation and treatment, the incidence of progressive disease increases most in those groups to which immunotherapy was administered. At the first analysis (October 1976), only patients receiving treatment for six months or more were included. It is possible that by the end of the second year, most patients who received immunotherapy will have succumbed to progressive disease. Thus, the next logical step should be to administer more intensive immunotherapy (days 9, 13, 17, and 24 within each 28-day course). However, no major granting agency has extended its support to this proposal.

LYMPHOCYTE TRANSFER

Adoptive immunization with transfer of immune lymphocytes is an attractive modality of immunotherapy. It works in syngeneic animals and between donors and recipients rendered mutually tolerant to noncompatible transplantation antigens (Sinkovics, 1976b). When donors and recipients are not histocompatible, the donor cells may be rejected or may immunologically attack the recipient. A low-grade, chronic, homologous disease in the tumor-bearing recipient may exert antitumor effects; thus, mouse leukemias and sarcomas can be treated by adoptive immunization (Sinkovics, 1976c).

In man, cross-transfusion of lymphocytes and plasma from donors who rejected the recipients' allotransplanted tumors only occasionally brings about well-documented tumor responses (Neff and Enneking, 1975), although some in vitro measurable parameters (migration inhibitory factor, cytotoxic lymphocytes) improve in the recipients (Sinkovics et al., 1973; Neidhart and LoBuglio, 1974). Lymphocyte transfusions with or without documented antitumor immunity of the donor could transfer various immune faculties (skin test reactivity, cytotoxic lymphocytes, serum factors potentiating this effect) to the recipients, but without significant antitumor effects (Krementz et al., 1974; Roth et al., 1975; Sutherland et al., 1976; Yonemoto, 1976).

In a study of patients with osteosarcoma who received postoperatively the cross-transplant, cross-transfusion type of treatment, 33% of 32 patients were clinically tumor free at two years. This was not significantly better than the 22% clinically tumor-free patients of the 145 historical control patients in the series at Memorial Sloan-Kettering Cancer Center (Neff and Enneking, 1975).

LYMPHOCYTE PRODUCTS

Interferon

Interferon is recognized not only as an inhibitor of virus synthesis but as a regulator of cell growth. The growth of osteosarcoma cells can be inhibited in vitro by human interferon preparations (Strander and Einhorn, 1977). In Sweden, interferon has been used as adjuvant therapy for osteogenic sarcoma. Twenty-eight patients with osteogenic sarcoma received treatment with human interferon, 3×10^6 units intramuscularly daily for one month before and during surgery, and the same dose thereafter three times weekly for more than 17 months. Sixty-four percent of these patients were clinically tumor free and 73% were alive at 2½ years, whereas 30% of the 23 patients treated concurrently by conventional means (amputation) experienced no evidence of disease and 35% were alive at 2½ years. Only 15% of historical control patients had no evidence of disease at 2½ years (Strander, written personal communication, 1977).

Transfer Factor

Recent reports indicate controversy concerning the immunologic specificity of transfer factor when used for the treatment of human tumors: One group claims specificity for osteogenic sarcoma when transfer factor is prepared from donors with immune reactivity to this tumor (Byers *et al.,* 1976; Fudenberg, 1976), whereas another group could not document such specificity (Ivins *et al.,* 1976). At the Mayo Clinic, a change in the natural history of osteogenic sarcoma has been observed in that populations of patients treated conventionally (by amputation) have shown gradually prolonged survival in the past decade. In a recent clinical trial, 18 postamputation patients were randomized to receive adjuvant chemotherapy with methotrexate, doxorubicin (Adriamycin), and vincristine (Oncovin) (MAO), and 17 postamputation patients were randomized to receive adjuvant treatment with transfer factor. The transfer factor donors were long tumor-free survivors of osteogenic sarcoma (Ivins *et al.,* 1976). To this group of transfer factor recipients, 13 more nonrandomized patients were added. In both treatment groups (chemotherapy and transfer factor) approximately 50% had no evidence of disease at two years. With an unexpected improvement in the group treated concurrently by conventional means (surgery only), patients receiving either modality of adjuvant therapy did not do significantly better than this control group. However, more than 70% of the group of 15 patients receiving transfer factor with skin test conversion from nonreactivity to reactivity (as tested with recall antigens to which the transfer factor donor was reactive and the recipient was nonreactive) remained clinically tumor free at 30 months, whereas only 20% of the 15 recipients of transfer factor who did not demonstrate skin test conversion were clinically tumor free at this time (Pritchard, written personal communication, 1977).

HUMAN TUMOR IMMUNOLOGY AND IMMUNOTHERAPY

The contribution of most immunotherapeutic regimens to the treatment of human tumors so far has been so marginal that one cannot be certain of the true value of this new modality. Locoregional applications of immunotherapy carry the highest promise: Inoculation of BCG into melanoma nodules or into the pleural cavity after resection of bronchogenic carcinoma and induction of delayed hypersensitivity reactions in the vicinity of skin cancers are the most successful, whereas systemic application of immunotherapy seldom, if ever, produces convincing and highly significant benefits. Successful claims of systemic immunotherapy frequently succumb to the following criticisms: (1) Prognostic factors are not evenly distributed between control (conventionally treated) and treated (by conventional means plus immunotherapy) groups of patients; (2) the results of immunotherapy are significantly better only if the control group is historical, no matter how "carefully matched" for prognostic factors; and (3) an early delay of disease progression among the patients receiving immunotherapy is frequently lost upon prolonged follow-up of treated and control groups of patients. Thus, determination of the efficacy of systemic immunotherapy for human tumors remains an unresolved, investigational clinical problem.

Another major unresolved problem is the possible contribution of tumor-specific immunity to nonspecific immunostimulation in the treatment of human tumors. As extensively reviewed recently (Sinkovics, 1976), tumor-specific immunity plays an important role in the immunotherapy for experimental tumors because well-defined, strong, tumor-specific antigens are expressed by most of these tumors, especially virally induced experimental tumors. Tumor-specific antigens—in particular, viral structural or virally coded antigens—are difficult to demonstrate in human tumors. So far, only tumors associated with herpes viruses (Burkitt's lymphoma, nasopharyngeal carcinoma, and possibly, carcinoma of the uterine cervix) have expressed such antigens. The immune response to these tumors varies according to the clinical state of the patient. For example, antibodies to early antigens correlate with persistent or recurrent tumors whereas antibodies to membrane antigens reflect long tumor-free state. It is most disturbing that while immunotherapy, as applied in the form of nonspecific immunostimulation with BCG, augments the immunocompetence of the patients, it fails to provide any clinical benefits for such a highly antigenic and chemotherapy-responsive tumor as African Burkitt's lymphoma (Magrath and Ziegler, 1976).

Many of the human tumor antigens so far isolated appear to be related to normal fetal antigens or to cross-react with Forssman antigens. A good case may be made for virally (oncornavirus) related antigenic expressions in human breast carcinoma (Black *et al.,* 1975), but the true meaning and prognostic value of regional lymph node reactivity is still open to various questions and interpretations (Fisher *et al.,* 1975; Hunter *et al.,* 1975). Thus, the evidence for human tumor-specific antigens is weak, and there is no definite proof that the addition of human tumor antigens to nonspecific immunostimulation significantly improves the effects of the latter modality applied above. In acute myelogenous leukemia (Powles *et al.,* 1977) and malignant melanoma (Newlands *et al.,* 1976), the addition of tumor antigens to nonspecific immunostimulation appeared to result in significant retardation of disease progression, but without significant improvement in survival time upon prolonged observation. The addition of viral oncolysates to immunostimulation with BCG in the early part of the current clinical trials appears to have increased the benefits; i.e., the progression of disease (malignant melanoma, sarcomas) has been retarded in those patients who received both BCG and tumor cell viral oncolysates (Sinkovics *et al.,* 1977a). However, it is too early to make a definite conclusion; the final evaluation should be made after at least two to three years of clinical trials.

In the immunotherapy for human osteosarcoma, the two lymphocyte products, interferon and transfer factor, continue to provide promising leads. Both of these agents appear to act in a nonspecific fashion: interferon as a regulator of cell growth and transfer factor as an amplifier of general immunity.

Many of the controversial results of immune assessment of patients with malignant tumors could be due to overlapping faculties of the human antitumor immune response: various subtypes of nonselective killer cells (null cells, antibody-dependent B lineage cells); selectively cytotoxic lymphocytes (both T and

B lineage cells); various subtypes of suppressor and helper cells and their circulating mediators; and blocking and potentiating serum factors. The wealth of human lymphocyte subpopulations has been paradoxically recognized by identifying the leading cell type in pathologic entities in which clonal proliferation of one particular subtype takes place. The wealth of B lineage subtypes is well known (as different subtypes of B lineage lymphoid cells are preponderant in chronic lymphocytic leukemia, diffuse and nodular malignant lymphomas, "histiocytic" lymphomas, macroglobulinemia, heavy chain diseases, multiple myeloma, and leukemic reticuloendotheliosis or hairy cell leukemia). The null cells and T lineage lymphoid cells of acute lymphocytic leukemia of childhood have not revealed their normal function (except that the natural killer cells resemble null cells), but the pathologic T lineage lymphocytes of Hodgkin's disease are suppressor cells (Twomey *et al.,* 1975) and those in Sezary syndrome are helper cells (Broder *et al.,* 1976).

Molecular mediators of suppressive function circulate in the blood and can be extracted from diseased tissues in Hodgkin's disease (Sinkovics and Thota, in press). The erythroderma of Sezary syndrome well may be consequential to the autonomous release of skin-reactive factor from the neoplastic T-lymphocytes. It has been more than eight years since we first recognized a nonselectively cytotoxic population of lymphocytes in the blood of a patient with lymphosarcoma cell leukemia and preterminal "wasting disease" (Sinkovics *et al.,* 1971a) and suggested that neoplastic lymphocytes continue to autonomously release their molecular mediators that are physiologically produced by their normal counterparts. Thus, we have suggested that there is a "cytotoxic lymphoma," in which autonomously released molecular mediators simulate a chronic delayed hypersensitivity reaction reminiscent of graft versus host disease. It now appears that normal lymphocytic functions are vastly multiple, are in a dynamic state, and overlap extensively.

Tumor cells expressing phase-specific fetal glycoproteins can possibly activate those immune faculties that physiologically protect the allogeneic fetus against maternal rejection; thus, fetal antigens may have a fundamental physiologic role (Sinkovics *et al.,* 1970a). Undifferentiated tumors imitating fetal growth thus induce tolerance and activate suppressor cells. However, if antigens other than those normally expressed in fetal life, such as viral or virally coded antigens, were expressed also in human tumors, these antigens would possibly evoke a strong, defensive immune reaction consisting of nonselectively cytotoxic lymphocytes, B lineage cells producing antibodies potentiating this effect, arming macrophages, or lysing tumor cells in the presence of complement. Thus, a tumor-protective immune mechanism dominated by tolerant lymphoid cells and suppressor cells would compete with a defensive and cytotoxic immune mechanism. Crude assays with nonfractionated lymphoid cell populations would yield contradictory results. Until human tumor antigens become well characterized and the assays for the immune responses adequately refined, the human antitumor immune response can only be envisioned but not clearly documented.

The power of the activated macrophage with which it distinguishes cells growing in a contact-inhibited fashion from those growing in a haphazard, contact-uninhibited fashion provides most, if not all, the benefits that have been achieved in the immunotherapy for human tumors. It is likely that tumor cells are attacked by molecular mediators released from primed and activated macrophages and that bacterial lipopolysaccharides (endotoxin) elicit the release of these factors. The mechanism of action of primed or activated macrophages has been well recognized in the case of experimental tumors. Again, there is strong possibility but no data proving that human macrophages exert their antitumor effect in a similar fashion. Patients with acute leukemia who were immunized against pseudomonas sepsis with a polyvalent pseudomonas vaccine achieved longer remissions than nonimmunized patients; this chance observation remains positive inasmuch as the trend for fewer relapses in the groups of patients treated with the pseudomonas vaccine has been sustained, but the difference in remission duration between the immunized and conventionally treated control patients is not significant (Gee *et al.,* 1978). Probably all current adjuvant chemotherapy protocols should include an immunotherapy regimen to counterbalance oncogenic effects, if any, of the chemotherapy.

One of the most controversial issues of modern medicine concerns the proper evaluation of treatment regimens. In the early 1960s, treatment protocols for malignant diseases were extremely harsh. The treatment often was highly toxic, and control patients were given placebo (less than the best possible treatment known at that time). Sometimes, patients continued to be entered in a failing treatment group to satisfy the statisticians' requirements. While much was learned from this approach, many medical and surgical oncologists (among them, the senior author of this review) exempted themselves from participating in these early clinical trials.

By the early 1970s, treatment protocols greatly improved. Now there is built-in deescalation to reduce toxicity, and control patients always receive the best conventional treatment for sake of comparison; patients are fully informed of the alternatives, toxicities involved, and randomization procedures. The remaining major problem is randomization. The most important factor in determining the value of a comparative trial is the balance of prognostic factors, whether set by randomization or by matching of historical controls. However, historical controls are often from a past treatment era; such differing factors as their supportive care (nutrition, blood products, antibiotics, etc.), diagnostic work-up (e.g., X-ray studies versus scans and echograms), and staff attendance can introduce subtle changes in the clinical course. For example, more attention to the patient may result in the patient's better attitude and nutrition. Refined diagnostic techniques and meticulous care may result in earlier recognition (and earlier treatment) of relapse. Thus, concurrent, adequately randomized controls are now preferred.

Patients with sarcomas are extremely difficult to stratify according to prognostic factors. Even within the same subtype, for example, liposarcoma, there are cell types (pleomorphic and round cell) that are much more malignant than the common myxoid liposarcoma. The malignant fibrous histiocytoma with inflammatory cells may be more malignant than the type without inflammatory cells. Embryonal rhabdomyosarcoma is more malignant than the alveolar type. Synovial sarcoma, clear cell sarcoma of the tendon sheaths, and epithelial sarcoma cover a wide variety of possible clinical courses. Osteosarcoma appears in the classic intramedullary form and in additional subtypes (periosteal, parosteal, those arising in pagetic bone or after irradiation). The prognoses of these tumors differ vastly. Even among the classic intramedullary osteosarcomas, those arising at the proximal femur have much worse prognosis than those arising in the distal femur. Size of the tumor at diagnosis, time elapsed between diagnosis and development of pulmonary metastasis, and age and sex of the patient are all important prognostic factors.

In the M. D. Anderson Hospital series, patients with primary osteosarcoma of the proximal femur or with primary tumors larger than 10 cm all succumbed to the disease rapidly (Uribe-Botero *et al.,* 1977). In other series, the survival rate for female patients at two years after diagnosis was 45.8% versus 16% for male patients (Scranton *et al.,* 1975). Only those who have the opportunity to observe how highly individual the human host-tumor relationship can be can fully appreciate the need for well-designed clinical trials in which large numbers of patients are stratified in the various treatment groups according to well-established prognostic factors.

CONCLUSIONS

Nonspecific immunostimulation appears to have profound effect on macrophages and other participants of the delayed hypersensitivity reaction. Most successful trials of human tumor immunotherapy have been based on locoregional nonspecific (immunologically not tumor-specific) immunostimulation. The additive effect of tumor-specific immunotherapy is suggestive but has not been proved.

Combined nonspecific immunostimulation and sarcoma-directed active immunization appear to delay disease progression in patients with soft tissue sarcomas. Two products of lymphocytes, interferon and transfer factor, appear to exert a suppressive effect on micrometastases of osteosarcoma.

The prognostic factors for patients with sarcomas are so highly variable and so difficult to balance between groups of patients treated with immunotherapy and conventional means that all past clinical trials should be viewed with reservations. Based on promising leads, comparisons of well-stratified groups of patients should be made in future trials.

ACKNOWLEDGMENTS

The authors are grateful to the Kelsey-Leary Foundation of Houston for essential support and to Mrs. Karen Hill and Miss Donna Liling for secretarial assistance.

REFERENCES

Black, M. M., Zachrau, R. E., Shore, B., Moore, D. H., and Leis, H. P., Jr. 1975. Prognostically favorable immunogens of human breast cancer tissue: Antigenic similarity to murine mammary tumor virus. Cancer, 35:121–128.

Broder, S., Edelson, R. L., Lutzner, M. A., Nelson, D. L., MacDermott, R. P., Durm, M. E., Goldman, C. K., Meade, B. D., and Waldman, T. A. 1976. The Sezary syndrome. A malignant proliferation of helper cells. J. Clin. Invest., 58:1297–1306.

Bukowski, R. M., Barna, B., Deodhar, S., and Hewlett, J. S. 1976. Nonspecific lymphocyte cytotoxicity in patients with malignant melanoma, renal cell carcinoma and sarcomas and in nontumor patients. Cancer, 38:1962–1967.

Byers, V. S., Levin, A. S., Hackett, A. J., and Fudenberg, H. H. 1975a. Tumor-specific cell-mediated immunity in household contacts of cancer patients. J. Clin. Invest., 55:500–513.

Byers, V. S., Levin, A. S., Johnston, J. O., and Hackett, A. J. 1975b. Quantitative immunofluorescence studies of the tumor antigen-bearing cell in giant cell tumor of bone and osteogenic sarcoma. Cancer Res., 35:2520–2531.

Byers, V. S., Levin, A. S., LeCam, L., Johnston, J. O., and Hackett, A. J. 1976. Tumor-specific transfer factor therapy in osteogenic sarcoma: A two-year study. Ann. NY Acad. Sci., 277:621–627.

Carswell, E. A., Old, L. J., Kassel, R. L., Green, S., Fiore, N., and Williamson, B. 1975. An endotoxin-induced serum factor that causes necrosis of tumors. Proc. Natl. Acad. Sci. USA, 72:3666–3670.

Coley, W. B. 1893. A preliminary note on the treatment of inoperable sarcoma by the toxin products of erysipelas. Postgrad. Med., 8:278–286.

Coley, W. B. 1898. The treatment of inoperable sarcoma with the mixed toxins of erysipelas and B. prodigiosus. JAMA, 31:389–456.

Coley, W. B. 1908. The treatment of sarcoma by mixed toxins of erysipelas and B. prodigiosus. Boston Med. Surg. J., 158:175–182.

Currie, G. A. 1973. Effect of active immunization with irradiated tumor cells on specific serum inhibitors of cell-mediated immunity in patients with disseminated cancer. Br. J. Cancer, 28:25–35.

Dobozy, A., Husz, S., Hunyadi, J., Bierks, G., and Simon, N. 1973. Immune deficiencies and Kaposi's sarcoma. Lancet, 2:265.

Eilber, F. R., Nizze, J. A., and Morton, D. L. 1975a. Sequential evaluation of general immune competence in cancer patients: Correlation with clinical cancer. Cancer, 35:660–665.

Eilber, F. R., Townsend, C., and Morton, D. T. 1975b. Osteosarcoma. Results of treatment employing adjuvant immunotherapy. Clin. Orthop., 111:94–100.

Fisher, E. R., Gregorio, R. M., Fisher, B., Redmond, C., Vellios, F., and Sommers, S. C. 1975. The pathology of invasive breast cancer. Cancer, 36:1–85.

Fudenberg, H. H. 1976. Dialyzable transfer factor in the treatment of human osteosarcoma: An analytical review. Ann. NY Acad. Sci., 227:545–557.

Gainor, B. J., Forbes, J. T., Enneking, W. P., and Smith, R. T. 1976. Specific antigen stimulated lymphocyte proliferation in osteosarcoma. Cancer, 37:743–750.

Gamblin, J. G., Forbes, J. T., Enneking, W. F., and Smith, R. T. 1977. An immunologic profile of osteosarcoma. Read before the 23rd Annual Conference of the Orthopedic Research Society, Las Vegas, Nevada, February 1–3.

Gee, T. S., Dowling, M. D., Cunningham, I., Oettgen, H. S., Armstrong, D., and Clarkson, B. D. 1978. Evaluation of *Pseudomonas aeruginosa* vaccine for prolongation of remission in adults with acute nonlymphoblastic leukemia treated with the L-12 protocol: A preliminary report. In

Terry, W. D., and Windhorst, D. (eds.): Immunotherapy of Cancer: Present Status of Trials in Man. New York, Raven Press, pp. 415–421.

Giraldo, G., Beth, E., Coeur, P., Vogel, C. L., and Dhru, D. S. 1972. Kaposi's sarcoma: A new model in the search for viruses associated with human malignancies. J. Natl. Cancer Inst., 49:1495–1507.

Giraldo, G., Beth, E., Hirshaut, Y., Aoki, T., Old, L. J., Boyse, E. A., and Chopra, H. C. 1971. Human sarcomas in culture. Foci of altered cells and a common antigen; induction of foci and antigen in human fibroblast cultures by filtrates. J. Exp. Med., 133:454–478.

Golub, S., O'Connel, T. X., and Morton, D. L. 1974. Correlation of *in vivo* and *in vitro* assays of immunocompetence in cancer patients. Cancer Res., 34:1833–1837.

Green, A. A., Pratt, C., Webster, R. G., and Smith, K. 1976. Immunotherapy of osteosarcoma patients with virus-modified tumor cells. Ann. NY Acad. Sci., 277:396–411.

Hardy, M. A., Goldfarb, P., Levine, S., Dattner, A., Muggia, F. M., Levitt, S., and Weinstein, E. 1976. *De novo* Kaposi's sarcoma in renal transplantation. Case report and brief review. Cancer, 38:144–148.

Hirshaut, Y., Pei, D. T., Marcove, R. C., Mukherji, B., Spielvogel, A. R., and Essner, E. 1974. Seroepidemiology of human sarcoma antigen S_1. N. Engl. J. Med., 291:1103–1107.

Hunter, R. L., Ferguson, D. J., and Coppleson, L. W. 1975. Survival with mammary cancer related to the interaction of germinal center hyperplasia and sinus histiocytosis in axillary and internal mammary lymph nodes. Cancer, 36:528–539.

Israël, L., and Edelstein, R. 1975. Nonspecific immunostimulation with *Corynebacterium parvum* in human cancer. In: Immunological Aspects of Neoplasia (The University of Texas System Cancer Center M. D. Anderson Hospital and Tumor Institute 26th Annual Symposium on Fundamental Cancer Research). Baltimore, Williams & Wilkins, pp. 485–504.

Ivins, J. C., Ritts, R. E., Jr., Pritchard, D. J., Gilchrist, G. S., Miller, G. C., and Taylor, W. F. 1976. Transfer factor *versus* combination chemotherapy: A preliminary report of a randomized postsurgical adjuvant treatment study in osteogenic sarcoma. Ann. NY Acad. Sci., 277:558–574.

Kay, H. D., Thota, H., and Sinkovics, J. G. 1976. Reactions of lymphocytes and serum factors from normal donors to cultured tumor cells. Clin. Immunol. Immunopathol., 5:218–233.

Klein, E., Holtermann, O. A., Helm, F., Rosner, D., Milgrom, H., Adler, S., Stoll, H. L., Jr., Case, R. W., Prior, R. L., and Murphy, G. P. 1975. Immunologic approaches to the management of primary and secondary tumors involving the skin and soft tissues: Review of a ten-year program. Transplant. Proc., 7:297–315.

Kotz, R., Rella, W., and Salzer, M. 1976. The immune status in patients with bone and soft tissue sarcomas. In Grundmann, E. (ed.): Malignant Bone Tumors. New York, Springer-Verlag, pp. 197–205.

Krementz, E. T., Mansell, P. W. A., Hornung, M. O., Samuels, M. S., Sutherland, C. A., and Benes, E. N. 1974. Immunotherapy of malignant disease: The use of viable sensitized lymphocytes or transfer factor prepared from sensitized lymphocytes. Cancer, 33:394–401.

Kufe, D., Hehlman, R., and Spiegelman, S. 1972. Human sarcomas contain RNA related to RNA of a mouse leukemia virus. Science, 175:182–185.

Magrath, I. T., and Ziegler, J. L. 1976. Failure of BCG immunostimulation to affect the clinical course of Burkitt's lymphoma. Br. Med. J., 1:615–618.

Marcove, R. C., Mike, V., Huvos, A. C., Southam, C. M., and Levin, A. G. 1973. Vaccine trials for osteogenic sarcoma. CA, 23:74–80.

Marsh, B., Flynn, L., and Enneking, W. 1972. Immunologic aspects of osteosarcoma and their application to therapy. J. Bone Joint Surg., 54A:1367–1397.

Master, S. P., Taylor, J. F., Kyalwazi, S. K., and Ziegler, J. L. 1970. Immunological studies in Kaposi's sarcoma. Br. Med. J., 1:600–602.

McCoy, J. L., Jerome, L. J., Cannon, G. B., Pomeroy, T. C., Conner, R. J., Oldham, R. K., Weese, J. L., and Herberman, R. B. 1977. Leukocyte migration inhibition in patients with Ewing's sarcoma by 3 M potassium chloride extracts of fresh and tissue cultured Ewing's sarcoma. J. Natl. Cancer Inst., 59:1119–1125.

McMaster, J. H., Ferguson, R. J., Weinert, C. R., Jr., and Dickens, D. R. V. 1974. Cellular immunity to human osteosarcoma. J. Bone Joint Surg., 56A:863.

McMaster, J. H., Weinert, C. R., Jr., and Dickens, D. R. V. 1973. Immunocompetence of lymphocytes from osteosarcoma patients. Lancet, 1:781–782.

McMurtrey, M. J., Sinkovics, J. G., Plager, C., Romero, J. J., and Romsdahl, M. M. 1977. Adjuvant chemoimmunotherapy for stage III (regional lymph node metastases) malignant melanoma (Abstract #C-168). In: Proceedings of the American Society of Clinical Oncology 13th Annual Meeting, p. 308.

Mills, B. G., and Singer, F. R. 1976. Nuclear inclusions in Paget's disease of bone. Science, 194:201–202.

Morton, D. L., Malmgren, R. A., Hall, W. T., and Schidlovsky, G. 1969. Immunological and virus studies with human sarcomas. Surgery, 66:152–161.

Mukherji, B., and Hirshaut, Y. 1973. Evidence for fetal antigen in human sarcomas. Science, 181:440–442.

Myers, B. D., Kessler, E., Levi, J., Pick, A., and Rosenfeld, J. B. 1974. Kaposi's sarcoma in kidney transplant recipients. Arch. Intern. Med., 133:307–311.

Nauts, H. C. 1974. Ewing's Sarcoma of Bone: End Results Following Immunotherapy (Bacterial Toxins) Combined with Surgery and/or Radiation. New York, Cancer Research Institute, monograph 14, 108 pp.

Nauts, H. C. 1975a. Osteogenic Sarcoma: End Results Following Immunotherapy with Bacterial Vaccines, 165 Cases or Following Bacterial Infections or Fever, 41 Cases. New York, Cancer Research Institute, monograph 15.

Nauts, H. C. 1975b. Beneficial Effects of Immunotherapy (Bacterial Toxins) on Sarcoma of the Soft Tissues Other Than Lymphosarcoma. New York, Cancer Research Institute, monograph 16, 219 pp.

Nauts, H. C. 1976. Giant Cell Tumor of Bone: End Results Following Immunotherapy (Coley Toxins) Alone or Combined with Surgery and/or Radiation, 66 Cases and Concurrent Infection, 4 Cases, 2nd edition. New York, Cancer Research Institute, monograph 4, 85 pp.

Neff, J. R., and Enneking, W. F. 1975. Adoptive immunotherapy in primary osteosarcoma. In Godden, J. O., and Sinks, L. F. (eds.): Conflicts in Childhood Cancer. New York, Alan R. Liss, pp. 289–296.

Neidhart, J. A., and LoBuglio, A. F. 1974. Transfer factor therapy of malignancy. Semin. Oncol., 1:379–385.

Newlands, E. S., Oon, C. J., Roberts, J. T., Elliott, P., Mould, R. F., Topham, C., Madden, F. J. F., Newton, K. A., and Westbury, G. 1976. Clinical trial of combination chemotherapy and specific active immunotherapy in disseminated melanoma. Br. J. Cancer, 34:174–179.

Pinsky, C. M., Domieri, A. E., Caron, A. S., Knapper, W. H., and Oettgen, H. P. 1974. Delayed hypersensitivity reactions in patients with cancer. In Mathé, G., and Weiner, R. (eds.): Recent Results in Cancer Research: Investigation and Stimulation of Immunity in Cancer Patients. New York, Springer-Verlag, 47:37–41.

Powles, R. L., Russell, J., Lister, T. A., Oliver, T., Whitehouse, J. M. A., Malpas, J., Chapius, B., Crowther, D., and Alexander, P. 1977. Immunotherapy for acute myelogenous leukemia: A controlled clinical study 2½ years after entry of the last patient. Br. J. Cancer, 35:265–272.

Pritchard, D. J., Ivins, J. C., and Ritts, R. E., Jr. 1976. Immunologic aspects of human sarcomas. In Grundmann, E. (ed): Malignant Bone Tumors. New York, Springer-Verlag, pp. 185–196.

Pritchard, D. J., Reilly, C. A., Jr., Finkel, M. P., and Ivins, J. C. 1974. Cytotoxicity of human osteosarcoma sera to hamster sarcoma cells. Cancer, 34:1935–1939.

Rebel, A., Bregeon, C., Basle, M., Malkani, K., LePatezour, A., and Filmon, R. 1975. Les inclusions des osteoclastes dans la maladie osseuse de Paget. Rev. Rhum. Mal. Osteoartic., 42:637–641.

Rosato, F. E., Brown, A. S., Miller, E. E., Rosato, E. F., Mullis, W. F., Johnson, J., and Moskowitz, A. 1974. Neuraminidase immunotherapy of tumors in man. Surg. Gynecol. Obstet., 193:675–682.

Roth, J. A., Silverstein, M. J., Gupta, R. K., and Morton, D. L. 1975. Restoration of immunocompetence by lymphocyte transfusion. J. Surg. Oncol., 7:63–66.

Scranton, P. E., McMaster, J. H., Kenny, F. M., Foley, T. P., Jr., and Taylor, F. H. 1975. Investigation of carbohydrate metabolism and somatomedin in osteosarcoma patients. J. Surg. Oncol., 7:403–409.

Sethi, J., and Hirshaut, Y. 1976. Complement-fixing antigen of human sarcomas. J. Natl. Cancer Inst., 57:489–493.

Singh, I., Tsang, K. Y., and Blakemore, W. S. 1977. Effect of xenogeneic immune RNA on normal human lymphocytes against human osteosarcoma cells *in vitro.* J. Natl. Cancer Inst., 58:505–510.

Sinkovics, J. G. 1976a. Acquisition of resistance by human tumor cells to lymphocyte-mediated cytotoxicity (Abstract #393). In: Proceedings of the 67th Annual Meeting of the American Association for Cancer Research, 17:99.

Sinkovics, J. G. 1976b. Immunology of tumors in experimental animals. In Harris, J. E., and Sinkovics, J. G.: The Immunology of Malignant Disease, 2nd edition. St. Louis, C. V. Mosby Company, pp. 93–282.

Sinkovics, J. G. 1976c. Modalities of immunotherapy for virally induced murine neoplasms. Ann. NY Acad. Sci., 276:557–564.

Sinkovics, J. G. 1977. Immunotherapy with viral oncolysates for sarcoma. JAMA, 237:869.

Sinkovics, J. G., Cabiness, J. R., and Shullenberger, C. C. 1972a. Monitoring *in vitro* of immune reactions to solid tumors. Front. Radiat. Ther. Oncol., 7:141–154.

Sinkovics, J. G., Cabiness, J. R., and Shullenberger, C. C. 1972b. Disappearance after chemotherapy of blocking serum factors as measured *in vitro* with lymphocytes cytotoxic to tumor cells. Cancer, 30:1428–1437.

Sinkovics, J. G., Cabiness, J. R. and Shullenberger, C. C. 1973. *In vitro* cytotoxicity of lymphocytes to human sarcoma cells. Bibl. Haematol., 39:846–851.

Sinkovics, J. G., Campos, L. T., Kay, H. D., Loh, K. K., Gonzalez, F., Cabiness, J. R., Ervin, F., and Gyorkey, F. 1975a. Immunological studies with human sarcomas: Effects of immunization and therapy on cell- and antibody-mediated immune reactions. In: Immunological Aspects of Neoplasia (The University of Texas System Cancer Center M. D. Anderson Hospital and Tumor Institute 26th Annual Symposium on Fundamental Cancer Research). Baltimore, Williams & Wilkins, pp. 367–401.

Sinkovics, J. G., Campos, L. T., Loh, K. K., Cormia, F., Velasquez, W., and Shullenberger, C. C. 1976a. Chemoimmunotherapy for three categories of solid tumors (sarcoma, melanoma, lymphoma): The problem of immunoresistant tumors. In Crispen, R. (ed.): Neoplasm Immunity: Mechanisms (1975 Chicago Symposium). Chicago, ITR, pp. 193–212.

Sinkovics, J. G., DiSaia, P., and Rutledge, F. 1970a. Tumor immunology and evolution of the placenta. Lancet, 2:1190–1191.

Sinkovics, J. G., Dreyer, D., Shirato, E., Cabiness, J. R., and Shullenberger, C. C. 1971a. Cytotoxic lymphocytes. I. Destruction of neoplastic cells by lymphocytes in cultures of human origin. Tex. Rep. Biol. Med., 29:227–242.

Sinkovics, J. G., and Harris, J. E. 1976. The Immunology of Malignant Disease, 2nd edition. St. Louis, C. V. Mosby Company, pp. 410–578.

Sinkovics, J. G., Kay, H. D., and Thota, H. 1976b. Evaluation of chemoimmunotherapy regimens by *in vitro* lymphocyte cytotoxicity directed to cultured human tumor cells. Bibl. Haematol., 43:281–284.

Sinkovics, J. G., and Plager, C. 1977. Bone sarcomas: Clinical experience. Can. J. Surg., 20:542–546.

Sinkovics, J. G., Plager, C., McMurtrey, M. J., Romero, J. J., and Romsdahl, M. M. 1977a. Viral oncolysates for the immunotherapy of human tumors (Abstract #344). In: Proceedings of the 68th Annual Meeting of the American Association for Cancer Research, 18:86.

Sinkovics, J. G., Plager, C., McMurtrey, M. J., Romero, J. J., and Romsdahl, M. M. 1977b. Immunotherapy of human sarcomas. In: Current Concepts in the Management of Primary Bone and Soft Tissue Tumors (The University of Texas System Cancer Center M. D. Anderson Hospital and Tumor Institute 21st Annual Clinical Conference). Chicago, Year Book Medical Publishers, pp. 361–410.

Sinkovics, J. G., Plager, C., and Romero, J. J. 1977c. Immunology and immunotherapy of patients with sarcomas. In Crispen, R. (ed.): Neoplasm Immunity: Solid Tumor Therapy (1977 Chicago Symposium). Philadelphia, Franklin Institute Press, pp. 211–219.

Sinkovics, J. G., Shirato, E., Cabiness, J. R., and Martin, R. G. 1970b. Rhabdomyosarcoma after puberty. Clinical, tissue culture and immunological studies. J. Med., 1:313–326.

Sinkovics, J. G., Shirato, E., Martin, R. G., Cabiness, J. R., and White, E. C. 1971b. Chondrosarcoma. Immune reactions of a patient to autologous tumor. Cancer, 27:782–793.

Sinkovics, J. G., Shirato, E., Martin, R. G., and White, E. C. 1970c. Chondrosarcoma. A brief review of eighty-three patients. J. Med., 1:15–25.

Sinkovics, J. G., and Thota, H. 1978. Project M/16: Immunological studies *in vitro* in Hodgkin's disease. In: Research Report 1978. Houston, M. D. Anderson Hospital and Tumor Institute (in press).

Sinkovics, J. G., Thota, H., Loh, K. K., Gonzalez, F., Campos, L. T., Romero, J. J., Kay, H. D., and King, D. 1975b. Prospectives for immunotherapy of human sarcomas. In: Cancer Chemotherapy: Fundamental Concepts and Recent Advances (The University of Texas System Cancer Center M. D. Anderson Hospital and Tumor Institute 19th Annual Clinical Conference on Cancer). Chicago, Year Book Medical Publishers, Inc., pp. 417–443.

Sinkovics, J. G., Thota, H., Romero, J. J., and Waldinger, R. 1977d. Bone sarcomas: Etiology and immunology. Can. J. Surg., 20:494–503.

Sinkovics, J. G., Williams, D. E., Campos, L. T., Kay, H. D., and Romero, J. J. 1974. Intensification of immune reactions of patients to cultured sarcoma cells: Attempts at monitored immunotherapy. Semin. Oncol., 1:351–365.

Strander, H., and Einhorn, S. 1977. Effect of human leukocyte interferon on the growth of human osteosarcoma cells in tissue culture. Int. J. Cancer, 19:468–473.

Sutherland, C. M., Krementz, E. T., Hornung, M. O., Carter, R. D., and Holmes, J. 1976. Transfer of *in vitro* cytotoxicity against osteogenic sarcoma cells. Surgery, 79:682–685.

Taylor, J. F., Jung, U., Wolfe, L., Deinhardt, F., and Kyalwazi, S. K. 1971. Lymphocyte transformation in patients with Kaposi's sarcoma. Int. J. Cancer, 8:468–474.

Taylor, J. F., and Ziegler, J. L. 1974. Delayed cutaneous hypersensitivity reactions in patients with Kaposi's sarcoma. Br. J. Cancer, 30:312–318.

Townsend, C. M., Eilber, F. R., and Morton, D. L. 1976. Skeletal and soft tissue sarcomas: Treatment with adjuvant immunotherapy. JAMA, 236:2187–2189.

Twomey, J. J., Laughter, A. H., Farrow, S., and Douglas, C. C. 1975. Hodgkin's disease. An immunodepleting and immunosuppressive disorder. J. Clin. Invest., 56:467–475.

Twomey, P. L., and Chretien, P. B. 1975. Impaired lymphocyte responsiveness in osteosarcoma. J. Surg. Res., 18:551–554.

Uribe-Botero, G., Russell, W. O., Sutow, W. W., and Martin, R. G. 1977. Primary osteosarcoma of bone. A clinicopathologic investigation of 243 cases with necropsy studies in 54. Am. J. Clin. Pathol., 67:427–435.

Wang, C. H., Sinkovics, J. G., Kay, H. D., Gyorkey, F., and Shullenberger, C. C. 1975. Growth of permanent lymphoid cell cultures from human source: Tenth anniversary. Tex. Rep. Biol. Med., 33:213–250.

Wood, W. C., and Morton, D. L. 1971. Host immune response to a common cell surface antigen in human sarcomas. N. Engl. J. Med., 284:569–572.

Yonemoto, R. H. 1976. Adoptive immunotherapy utilizing thoracic duct lymphocytes. Ann. NY Acad. Sci., 277:7–19.

Yu, A., Watts, H., Jaffe, N., and Parkman, R. 1977. Concomitant presence of tumor-specific cytotoxic and inhibitor lymphocytes in patients with osteogenic sarcoma. N. Engl. J. Med., 297:121–127.

Immunotherapy of Human Cancer,
The University of Texas System Cancer Center
M. D. Anderson Hospital and Tumor Institute.
Raven Press, New York © 1978.

Immunotherapy for Genitourinary Cancer*

David Eidinger, M.D., Ph.D.

*Department of Microbiology, Faculty of Medicine, University of Saskatchewan,
Saskatoon, Saskatchewan*

Clinical immunotherapeutic trials for the treatment of genitourinary cancer in man have not received wide attention. This is surprising when one considers that genitourinary neoplasms, with the possible exception of some forms of testicular tumors, are particularly resistant to current regimens of chemotherapy (Carter and Wasserman, 1975). Moreover, there is evidence of tumor induction by chemical carcinogens (Miller, 1970; Morrison and Cole, 1976; Kantor *et al.,* 1976), which would likely induce strong, tumor-specific transplantation antigens and thereby facilitate immunotherapy. Currie (1972) has summarized eight decades of experience with immunotherapy for human cancer. It is particularly worthwhile to consider the current trials of immunotherapy for genitourinary cancer in the context of the various potential models of tumor immunotherapy available to the clinician.

ACTIVE-SPECIFIC IMMUNOTHERAPY

Active-specific immunotherapy implies that an augmentation of host immune defense mechanisms can be induced directly in tumor-bearing hosts. Recent trials in which autologous tumor cell vaccines are administered to human hosts with various types of tumors have been evaluated, and the clinical results are varied (Currie *et al.,* 1971; Gutterman *et al.,* 1973; Powles *et al.,* 1976).

Relatively few trials of active-specific immunotherapy for genitourinary tumors have been reported. Helmstein (1972) described the results of treatment of 43 cases of superficial bladder tumors by means of applying hydrostatic pressure to induce necrosis of the superficial tumors. O'Toole and colleagues (1975), using a microcytotoxicity test to appraise the level of cell-mediated immunity, have provided evidence of an antigenic stimulus following application of this treatment in man. However, no consistent increase in microcytotoxicity was observed, nor was there noted a correlation between the response to treatment

---

* Portions of this paper are adapted from Eidinger, D. 1978. Clinical immunotherapy for genitourinary cancer. In LoBuglio, A. F. (ed.): Clinical Immunotherapy. New York, Marcel Dekker, Inc. (in press).

and the levels of microcytotoxicity. Olsson and colleagues (1974) have treated patients with recurrent bladder tumors by immunization with keyhole limpet hemocyanin (KLH) as an integral part of a study of the level of anergy in patients with bladder cancer. The authors speculated that the reduced tumor recurrence rate for immunized patients represented an induced active, but non-specific, immunotherapeutic effect. However, these workers did not attempt to determine if cross-reacting antigens existed between the complex antigen, KLH, and tumor antigens in the bladder tumors. Thus, possible active-specific immunization with KLH secondary to cross-reactivity has not been ruled out. A precedent for such a view is the observed cross-reactivity between bacillus Calmette-Guérin (BCG) and guinea pig hepatoma cells (Borsos and Rapp, 1973) or human malignant melanoma cells (Minden et al., 1974).

Cryosurgery for the destruction of prostatic tumors has been employed by Ablin (1975). Because prostatic tumors have been shown to contain tumor antigens (Ablin et al., 1970), it is likely that such cryostatic surgical procedures could initiate active-specific immunization secondary to tumor cell destruction and release of tumor antigen into the circulation. Although the disappearance of distant metastases after cryosurgery has been described (Gursel et al., 1972), this form of treatment has not received wide acceptance.

ACTIVE-NONSPECIFIC IMMUNOTHERAPY

Active-nonspecific immunotherapy depends on the ability of the host to augment general defense mechanisms versus tumors, without an essential requirement for increased immune reactions directed specifically against tumor antigens. The best-studied example of this form of immunotherapy is administration of the bacterial adjuvants BCG and *Corynebacterium parvum*. Although these materials augment immunologically specific antitumor immunity of both the humoral and cell-mediated types, overwhelming evidence implicates their ability to augment nonspecific immune responses as a primary mechanism for antitumor effects.

Superficial recurrent bladder tumors in man exemplify those features of a human tumor model that may be the essential prerequisites for successful immunotherapy with BCG. In fact, some aspects of the human bladder tumor model are equivalent to the guinea pig hepatoma tumor model of Zbar and colleagues (1971, 1972), which responds to nonspecific adjuvant immunotherapy with BCG. These common aspects are: (1) The tumor burden is small. (2) Direct contact between BCG and tumor, which is of primary importance in generating a favorable response, is readily achieved. (3) It is likely that an antitumor effect mediated by an intense inflammatory reaction is generated. (4) Because bladder cancer in man appears to be carcinogen induced, potent tumor-specific antigens are present in tumor cells. Thus, immunologically specific antitumor immunity may be augmented by means of local BCG therapy. (5) Relatively little BCG need be administered, and side effects are modest.

Successful immunotherapy with BCG for a bladder tumor has been achieved by direct inoculation of the tumor (deKernion *et al.,* 1975a). The inflammatory effects of BCG administration in the dog, which have been documented by Bloomberg and colleagues (1975), indeed may be an essential prerequisite for a therapeutic effect. Hanna and colleagues (1972), using the guinea pig hepatoma model (Zbar *et al.,* 1971), have examined the histopathology of tumor regression after intralesional injection of *Mycobacterium bovis.* The granulomatous reaction that ensued was characterized by an influx of macrophages and activated histiocytes, to which degenerating tumor cells were found in close proximity. Cerottini and Brunner (1974) have reviewed the role of macrophages activated by BCG in relation to the observed antitumor effects.

As mentioned, the possibility that active-specific immunotherapy may be of importance in BCG-induced tumor immunity has not been excluded (Borsos and Rapp, 1973; Minden *et al.,* 1974). Moreover, in view of the widely diverse humoral and cell-mediated immune reactions induced by BCG (Chess *et al.,* 1973; Holm *et al.,* 1973; Hawrylko, 1975), it is difficult to assess which of the immune parameters are of primary importance in inducing antitumor effect. However, my personal bias lies in favor of the nonspecific defense mechanisms secondary to macrophage activation.

Relatively few trials of adjuvant immunotherapy for genitourinary cancer have been carried out in man. Description of our own initial work has been published elsewhere (Eidinger and Morales, 1976a,b; Morales and Eidinger, 1976a,b; Morales *et al.,* 1976a,b; Eidinger, in press). Suffice it to say that the treatment of stage D bladder cancer in man has been disappointing (Morales *et al.,* 1976a). However, Fraley and colleagues (1976) did observe an objective, favorable response in one of three patients with stage D disease.

Laucius *et al.* (personal communication) have treated 15 patients with metastatic renal cell tumors with megestrol and BCG, with no evidence of objective benefit. These workers administered five immunizing doses of BCG every second week for ten weeks, a dosage that may have been ineffective because of its short duration.

BCG immunotherapy has been used also to treat prostatic cancer (Merrin *et al.,* 1975). Of seven patients who had positive reactions to purified protein derivative skin tests, five exhibited a decrease in degree of induration of the prostate. However, there was no evidence of any change in the distant metastatic lesions. It is simply too early to assess if BCG immunotherapy for prostatic cancer will be of any benefit.

PASSIVE-SPECIFIC IMMUNOTHERAPY

Passive-specific immunotherapy refers to systems in which passively administered antibodies of a specificity directed to tumor-specific antigens are injected into tumor-bearing humans. Murray (1958) described a study of 291 patients with metastatic carcinoma of various organs treated by injection of gamma globulin preparations derived from horses immunized with human tumors. Some objective partial remissions were recorded. A corollary to this study has been the use of chemotherapeutic drugs, bacterial toxins, or radionuclides conjugated to the antitumor antibodies (Ghose *et al.,* 1975, 1976; Moolten *et al.,* 1975). In these model systems, the specificity of the antibody for the tumor cell is used to generate the accumulation of cytotoxic agents directed toward tumor target cells. No data focusing on the role of antibodies to genitourinary tumors have been published to date.

PASSIVE-NONSPECIFIC IMMUNOTHERAPY

Passive-nonspecific immunotherapy depends on the transfer of blood-borne activities that subserve an antitumor role. The relationship of many of these factors to specific immunity is not always clear. However, some factors, such as properdin, activation of the alternative complement pathway, and endotoxins, may subserve a nonspecific role of antitumor immunity (Pfordte and Ponsold, 1969; Carswell *et al.,* 1975; Glumac *et al.,* 1976).

ADOPTIVE IMMUNOTHERAPY

Adoptive immunotherapy refers to the passive transfer of immunity by immune lymphocytes, lymphokines or immune RNA, and transfer factors derived from immune lymphocytes. In some of the older studies, two tumor-bearing persons were used in a model system in which tumor cells from each person were cross-implanted in the opposite partner (Nadler and Moore, 1966). Subsequently, blood or circulating lymphocytes were transferred. Unfortunately, little long-term benefit was observed.

Some clinical trials to assess adoptive transfer of immunity in genitourinary cancer have been evaluated. Feneley and associates (1974) treated 25 patients with transitional cell carcinoma of the bladder by infusion of pig lymphocytes obtained from sensitized donors. In agreement with results of the study of Symes and Riddell (1973), most patients exhibited some evidence of tumor necrosis. DeKernion and colleagues (1975b) have tested xenogeneic immune RNA, prepared in sheep following immunization of the animals with human renal cell tumors. In vitro, this material was shown to induce in human lymphocytes cytotoxic responses to autologous tumor cells. Clinically, objective responses were noted in some patients.

CLINICAL EVALUATION OF BCG ADJUVANT IMMUNOTHERAPY

Bladder Cancer

Initial studies of the treatment of superficial recurrent bladder tumors by intracavitary administration of BCG, carried out in collaboration with Alvaro Morales, M.D., have been described (Eidinger and Morales, 1976a,b; Morales and Eidinger, 1976a,b; Morales *et al.,* 1976a,b; Eidinger, in press). It is relevant to consider the circumstances that led to the institution of the clinical trial. In October 1973, Dr. Morales was caring for a patient with a history of recurrent bladder tumors. His treatment had consisted of a partial cystectomy in 1971, and subsequent treatment of recurrences with 5,500 R irradiation and intracavitary instillations of thiotepa. Notwithstanding these treatments, tumor recurrences continued to develop. In view of the patient's serious cardiovascular disease, necessitating a pacemaker, and his strong, cutaneous, delayed response to tuberculin, Dr. Morales decided to treat the patient with intracavitary instillation of purified protein derivative (PPD), in a manner somewhat analogous to that for intracavitary instillations of chemotherapeutic agents, such as thiotepa. During the ensuing months, the patient received three irrigations with 100 mg of PPD contained in sterile neomycin solution. Of possible potential relevance for the future, this patient has remained free of disease for 38 months.

In view of the clamor over the use of BCG as an adjuvant immunotherapeutic treatment, we conducted a clinical trial with BCG rather than PPD. This was warranted further by the need to induce a vigorous delayed response, which could be achieved in PPD-negative patients only by immunization with bacterial suspension. As mentioned in the discussion of active-nonspecific immunotherapy, our initial group of five persons with stage D metastatic transitional cell carcinoma of the bladder failed to respond to BCG administered cutaneously. A second group of patients, with a history of recurrent superficial bladder tumors, was treated for six weeks by weekly instillations of 120 mg of BCG via an indwelling catheter. Each instillation was coupled to a cutaneous immunization with 5 mg of BCG administered by a Heaf gun to the skin of the thigh region. There was early evidence of a favorable response, characterized by a delay in recurrences, in seven patients (Eidinger and Morales, 1976b).

Sixteen patients with superficial recurrent bladder tumors have been treated with BCG. Table 1 summarizes the significant features of the natural history of the disease in this group of patients prior to commencement of BCG treatment. Twelve men and four women, varying in age from 43 to 88 years, have undergone from two to 16 cystoscopic examinations, the results of which were positive for tumor recurrence. The recurrences were either single or multiple. Fifteen patients had transitional cell carcinoma, and one had squamous cell carcinoma. On pathologic examination, five patients exhibited evidence of carcinoma in situ during one or more phases of their illness. Prior treatment of the patients consisted of instillations of thiotepa (triethylenethiophosphoramide) in seven patients and Epodyl (triethylene glycol diglycidyl ether) in six patients; two patients received irradiation treatment. Two of the 16 patients had positive skin tests with PPD in a test dose of 5 IU/ml.

The determination of the recurrence rate in this group presented some difficulty. In the first place, great variability in the rate of recurrence was noted in individual patients during the natural history of their disease. Secondly, for some patients exhibiting multifocal origin of their disease, the tumors were

Table 1. *Tumor Recurrences in Patients with Superficial Recurrent Bladder Tumors Before BCG Treatment*

Patient	Tumor Grade	Treatment	Recurrence Dates (mo/yr)	Remission Duration (mo)
1	3	. . .	6/75, 10/75, 1/76*	5
2	2	thiotepa, Epodyl	3/70, 12/70, 3/71, 9/72, 12/72, 5/73, 10/73, 1/74, 1/75, 5/75, 10/75	5
3	2	thiotepa	6/74, 8/74,* 2/75, 2/76*	12
4	(squamous)	radiation	12/69, 9/72, 1/73, 9/73, 6/74	9
5	2	. . .	5/75, 8/75, 6/76	10
6	2	Epodyl	5/73, 5/74, 9/75*	12
7	3	. . .	11/74, 2/75, 5/75	4
8	. . .†	. . .	4/75, 9/75, 10/75*	6
9	2	thiotepa, Epodyl	4/73, 9/73, 9/74, 11/74	12
10	1–2	thiotepa	5/66, 3/72, 3/74, 3/76	24
11	2	thiotepa	12/68, 9/70, 9/72, 9/73, 9/74, 10/75, 2/76	12
12	2	. . .	7/74, 10/74, 3/75	5
13	3	thiotepa, Epodyl	12/63, 6/70, 9/70, 5/74, 8/74, 1/75	5
14	3	radiation	6/74, 10/75*	16
15	1–2	thiotepa, Epodyl	10/62, 9/63, 1/64, 3/66, 1/69, 4/69, 4/70, 7/70, 10/70, 6/71, 8/71, 1/72, 9/73, 8/74, 10/74, 2/75	11
16	2–3	Epodyl	8/73, 3/74, 7/74	10

* Carcinoma in situ.
† Positive urine cytology following transitional cell carcinoma of the ureter and bladder treated by nephrectomy.

enumerated; for others, the tumors were described as simply single or multiple. In our initial reports, remission duration was determined by the number of tumors observed during a number of months' follow-up (Eidinger and Morales, 1976b). Subsequently, the determination of recurrence was based on results of the initial cystoscopic examination that was performed to diagnose the patients' illness (Eidinger, in press). This generated a figure of the number of cystoscopic examinations with abnormal results, inclusive of the initial diagnostic procedure, during a period of months to years. This was appropriate for patients with a long-standing history of disease. However, for the patients with a short follow-up, inclusion of the diagnostic cystoscopy created an artificially reduced time span for the recurrence rate.

Consequently, in Table 1, I have designated the remission duration as the longest period between the last four cystoscopic examinations, primarily because this retrospective study did not provide for regular cystoscopic examinations at three-month intervals. Moreover, it was difficult to decide what figure to use for those patients who responded to interim treatment with thiotepa and Epodyl. Finally, use of the maximal time interval created a bias, which only could have worked against us in evaluating the efficacy of BCG treatment; hence, if BCG was significantly effective, it was likely to be even more so in a clinical study in which the times of recurrence before BCG treatment were determined on a regular basis comparable to the period after treatment. The mean duration of remission for the group was 10.1 months.

Table 2 summarizes the data for individual patients after BCG treatment. The number of treatments for the entire group varied from the original plan of weekly administrations for six weeks for a reason that is essentially twofold: In some instances, the patients did not tolerate the full course; in other instances, there was evidence of recurrence on initial cystoscopic follow-up, and consequently, a second course of treatment was carried out. Table 2 also summarizes the current status of individual patients. Two patients (no. 12 and 16) never had a period of remission. This left a total of 14 patients who, at some point in their follow-up, did exhibit evidence of remission. For two of these patients, results of initial cystoscopic examination were positive for tumor, but reverted to normal in one or more follow-up studies; these patients are included in the negative follow-up list. Another five patients have once more reverted to a positive tumor incidence after an initial remission period, leaving a total of

Table 2. *BCG Treatment and Patient Response*

Patient	Age (yr)*	Treatments Onset (mo/yr)	Treatments Number	Follow-Up Cystoscopy Results† Negative	Follow-Up Cystoscopy Results† Positive
1	76	2/76	8	16	22
2	70	12/75	12	15	5
3	80	11/75	5	10	14
4	69	7/76	6	10	. . .
5	81	7/74	5	27	31
6	79	11/75	12	12	4
7	72	6/75	6	22	. . .
8	74	11/75	6	12	. . .
9	76	11/74	3	25	. . .
10	55	3/75	6	20	26
11	84	4/76	6	12	. . .
12	52	3/76	9	. . .	4, 10
13	43	4/75	12	5	10, 18
14	88	11/75	6	13	. . .
15	72	4/75	6	19	. . .
16	59	5/75	10	. . .	3, 7

* At onset of treatment.
† Figures refer to time in months.

nine patients (56%) still in remission. The mean duration of remission for all patients is 15.5 months. Four of the nine patients (25%) have exceeded their remission periods prior to BCG treatment by threefold.

The side effects of BCG administration have been described elsewhere (Eidinger, in press). Suffice it to say that in only two patients were there serious side effects to a degree that necessitated immediate cessation of BCG treatment. In one patient, the bladder mucosa exhibited marked edema, which compromised the renal outflow tracts, producing a hydronephrosis. The condition cleared within a few weeks of cessation of treatment. A second patient experienced migratory polyarthralgia and arthritis, primarily involving the hands. The skin of the hands was also edematous and characterized further by scaly, erythematous lesions. This condition also disappeared within several weeks of cessation of treatment. Severe dysuria was experienced by four patients and necessitated cessation of treatment in two. Acute cystitis with *Escherichia coli* developed in four patients and responded to treatment.

In further evaluation of the effects of BCG treatment, patients still in remission after treatment were compared with those who since have had recurrences (Table 3). Among patients who had recurrences, the mean disease-free period was 15.6 months; the mean pretreatment remission duration was seven months. However, it was not until a period approximating three times that of the pretreatment remission had passed that cystoscopic examination showed recurrence of tumor.

Table 3. *Remission Durations for Patients with Superficial Recurrent Bladder Tumors Before and After BCG Treatment**

Patient Group	Remission Duration (mo)		Month of Recurrence† After Treatment
	Pretreatment	Post-Treatment	
With recurring tumor			
1‡	5	16	22
3‡	12	10	14
5	9	27	31
10	3	20	26
13	5	5	10
Mean	7	15.6	20.6
In remission			
2	5	15	. . .
4	10	10	. . .
6‡	12	12	. . .
7	4	22	. . .
8‡	6	12	. . .
9	12	25	. . .
11	24	12	. . .
14‡	16	13	. . .
15	11	19	. . .
Mean	11.7	15.5	. . .

* Two patients (no. 12 and 16) never had a period of remission.
† Shown by cystoscopy.
‡ Patient with carcinoma in situ.

It is important to emphasize that no change was evident in the grade of tumors recurring after treatment. However, the one squamous cell carcinoma recurred as a transitional cell carcinoma 31 months after onset of BCG treatment.

Nine patients are still in remission for a mean of 15.5 months, compared with 11.7 months' remission duration prior to BCG treatment. The latter figure well might be artificially inflated by the addition of one patient with a long natural history of tumor. Nonetheless, the data for the group experiencing post-treatment recurrences suggest that a mean disease-free interval of approximately three times that in the pretreatment period can be expected.

Five patients had carcinoma in situ, which has a particularly ominous prognosis. For two of the patients, follow-up cystoscopies have reverted to positive; three patients are still in remission (see Table 3).

Metastatic Renal Cell Tumors

In the group of patients with metastatic lesions secondary to hypernephromas, BCG was administered initially as has been described, according to the following general format: After an initial, single, intradermal inoculation, 40 mg was administered weekly for four weeks, then twice monthly for two months, and then monthly for an indefinite period or until the patient's condition deteriorated.

Table 4 summarizes the conditions of our initial five patients. Only one patient is alive and well, at 34 months following onset of BCG treatment. This patient is now a young woman, who, at the age of 8, underwent a nephrectomy for removal of a hypernephroma. When she was 16, small metastatic deposits were found in both lung fields on radiologic examination; a thoracotomy confirmed the presence of metastases from the renal tumor. No further surgical intervention has been undertaken. The most recent radiologic examination revealed densities that are difficult to interpret in terms of whether they represent tumor deposits or fibrotic, scarified lesions. The remaining four patients showed evidence of an initial, but short-lived, objective response.

Table 4. *Response of Patients with Metastatic Hypernephroma to BCG Treatment**

Prior Treatment	BCG Effect on Pulmonary Metastases	Patient's Status
Nephrectomy	None initially, then total disappearance	Dead at 28 mo
None	Reduction; improved function on IVP†	Dead at 10 mo
Nephrectomy	Reduction	Dead at 4 mo
Nephrectomy	Reduction	Dead at 17 mo
Nephrectomy	None	Alive and well at 34 mo

* Three additional patients died within months of onset of BCG therapy without objective response or skin test conversion. Two others are alive and well at 18 months.
† Intravenous pyelogram.

Two additional patients, whose clinical histories have been described elsewhere (Eidinger, in press), are alive and well 18 months after initial diagnosis and treatment. One patient is particularly remarkable, in view of the documented multiple secondary lesions in the liver, which were confirmed by a frozen section of biopsy material taken at the time of nephrectomy to be metastatic deposits from the kidney tumor.

The administration of BCG during the second year of treatment for the three patients currently alive and well has differed to a significant degree from the previously established protocol. For these patients, the BCG was titered according to the individual assessment of the patient. If on a given follow-up, the multiple-puncture site of the previous visit was still intensely inflamed, BCG administration was postponed until a significant decrease of cutaneous reactivity to the bacterial vaccine was visually evident. Thus, 40 mg of BCG was administered by Heaf gun every six to ten weeks. The actual skin regions punctured with the multiple-puncture apparatus were restricted to an area measuring approximately 1 inch square on the upper arm. None of the patients exhibited significant side effects more serious than slight elevations of temperature and a feeling of malaise for one or two days.

CURRENT PHILOSOPHY OF TREATMENT

Bladder Tumors

A short course of BCG treatment may induce remissions in patients with superficial recurrent bladder tumors for an interval three times that attainable prior to treatment. A diagnosis of carcinoma in situ or squamous cell carcinoma does not preclude successful treatment.

Increased doses and more frequent administration of BCG are not beneficial and, in fact, may be harmful in terms of incidence and severity of side effects. Most of the serious side effects in our study were experienced by patients during the second course of BCG and by the two patients who were PPD-reactive prior to onset of treatment. Moreover, in one of the two PPD-reactive patients, the tumor recurred early after onset of treatment. That too much BCG is harmful has been suggested by results of studies in an animal model by Lamoureux *et al.* (1976) and in humans by Sokal and colleagues (1976). This viewpoint should be temporized perhaps to the extent that BCG probably should be administered at three-month intervals for initially responsive patients to further delay recurrence. In that event, I suggest that the actual dose of BCG should be one third of the initial dose, namely, 40 mg administered via intracavitary instillation, and that the cutaneous immunization be omitted.

The inflammatory response induced by cell-mediated reactions may be partly responsible for the antitumor effect. Thus, the fact that the strongly PPD-reactive patient in our study responded, after PPD treatment, with a prolonged recurrence-free interval may indicate the need to develop model systems that have fewer biologic side effects but generate strong, cell-mediated immune reactions with all of the concomitant, inflammatory, antitumor effects.

During our studies, we found no evidence that it was essential to commence BCG instillations into the bladder shortly after the previous cystoscopy had been performed. Based on the work of Bloomberg *et al.* (1975), it is likely that inflammatory responses cannot occur in the intact bladder. If this is true, the current philosophy of treatment would be to commence BCG treatment within one to two weeks after fulguration and biopsy of the bladder epithelial tumors. In general, this was the protocol employed in the present study.

Renal Tumors

I suggest that the BCG be titered according to the individual needs of the patient, based on the degree of skin-test reactivity on prior immunization. As I have mentioned, patients should receive weekly immunizations with 40 mg of BCG, followed by monthly applications via a Heaf gun, until they begin to exhibit intense reactivity at a monthly follow-up visit. Then, the patients should be seen twice a month, and the BCG administered only at the time of waning prior response. Thereby, it is hoped that the initial period of objective response may be prolonged far more significantly than has been possible with a schedule of more frequent BCG administrations.

The current philosophy on the use of minimal amounts of BCG is strengthened by a general knowledge of immune regulation. In the literature are numerous examples of failure to augment immune responses that are already stimulated to maximum levels. Indeed, there is evidence that further attempts to enhance immune responses generate the development of suppressor cells, such as suppressor T-lymphocytes, which may be detrimental to the host. Moreover, there is evidence that T-lymphocytes are long-lived, and that activated macrophages may be functionally active for considerable periods. Consequently, there is little to be gained from attempting to augment immune responses by overzealous use of bacterial adjuvants.

Finally, the failure to convert to PPD-positive skin reactivity within three months after onset of BCG immunization signals a treatment failure and the necessity to cease treatment. In such cases, the number of circulating E-rosettes, which increases with favorable BCG responses (Morales and Eidinger, 1976b), may be used as a measure of clinical response.

ACKNOWLEDGMENTS

I have enjoyed my association with Dr. Alvaro Morales, who collaborated with me in this project during my tenure at Queen's University in Kingston, Ontario. I thank Mrs. Marilyn Haskins for her assistance in preparing the manuscript.

This work was supported by a grant from the Ontario Cancer Treatment Research Foundation.

REFERENCES

Ablin, R. J. 1975. Immunotherapy for prostatic cancer. Previous and prospective considerations. Oncology, 31:177–202.

Ablin, R. J., Bronson, P., Soanes, W. A., and Witebsky, E. 1970. Tissue- and species-specific antigens of normal human prostatic tissue. J. Immunol., 104:1329–1339.

Bloomberg, S. D., Brosman, S. A., Hausman, M. S., Cohen, A., and Battenberg, J. D. 1975. The effects of BCG on the dog bladder. Invest. Urol., 12:423–427.

Borsos, T., and Rapp, H. J. 1973. Antigenic relationship between Mycobacterium bovis (BCG) and a guinea pig hepatoma. J. Natl. Cancer Inst., 51:1085–1086.

Carswell, E. A., Old, L. J., Kassel, R. L., Green, S., Fiore, N., and Williamson, B. 1975. An endotoxin-induced serum factor that causes necrosis of tumors. Proc. Natl. Acad. Sci. USA, 72:3666–3670.

Carter, S. K., and Wasserman, T. H. 1975. The chemotherapy of urologic cancer. Cancer, 36:729–747.

Cerottini, J.-C., and Brunner, K. T. 1974. Cell-mediated cytotoxicity, allograft rejection and tumor immunity. Adv. Immunol., 18:67–132.

Chess, L., Bock, G. N., Ungaro, P. C., Buchholz, D. H., and Mardiney, M. R., Jr. 1973. Immunologic effects of BCG in patients with malignant melanoma: Specific evidence for stimulation of the "secondary" immune response. J. Natl. Cancer Inst., 51:57–65.

Currie, G. A. 1972. Eighty years of immunotherapy: A review of immunological methods used for the treatment of human cancer. Br. J. Cancer, 26:141–153.

Currie, G. A., LeJeune, F., and Hamilton-Fairley, G. 1971. Immunization with irradiated tumour cells and specific lymphocyte cytotoxicity in malignant melanoma. Br. Med. J., 2:305–310.

deKernion, J. B., Golub, S. H., Gupta, R. K., Silverstein, M., and Morton, D. L. 1975a. Successful transurethral intralesional BCG therapy of bladder melanoma. Cancer, 36:1662.

deKernion, J. B., Ramming, K. P., Brower, P., Skinner, D. G., and Pilch, Y. H. 1975b. Immunotherapy for malignant lesions in man using immunogenic ribonucleic acid. Am. J. Surg., 130:575–578.

Eidinger, D. 1978. Clinical immunotherapy for genitourinary cancer. In LoBuglio, A. F. (ed.): Clinical Immunotherapy, New York, Marcel Dekker, Inc. (in press).

Eidinger, D., and Morales, A. 1976a. BCG immunotherapy of adenocarcinoma of the kidney. In Lamoureux, G., Turcotte, R., and Portelance, V. (eds.): BCG in Cancer Immunotherapy. New York, Grune and Stratton, pp. 242–245.

Eidinger, D., and Morales, A. 1976b. Discussion paper: Treatment of superficial bladder cancer in man. Ann. NY Acad. Sci., 277:239–240.

Feneley, R. C. L., Eckert, H., Roddell, A. G., Symes, M. O., and Tribe, C. R. 1974. The treatment of advanced bladder cancer with sensitized pig lymphocytes. Br. J. Surg., 61:825–827.

Fraley, E. E., Lange, P. H., and Hakala, T. R. 1976. Recent studies on the immunobiology and virology of human urothelial tumors. Urol. Clin. North Am., 3:31–51.

Ghose, T., Tai, J., Aquino, J., Guclu, A., Norvell, T., and MacDonald, A. 1975. Tumor localization of ^{131}I-labelled antibodies by radionuclide imaging. Radiology, 116:445–448.

Ghose, T., Tai, J., Guclu, A., Norvell, S. T., Bodurtha, A., Aquino, J., and MacDonald, A. S. 1976. Antibodies as carriers of radionuclides and cytotoxic drugs in the treatment and diagnosis of cancer. Ann. NY Acad. Sci., 277:671–689.

Glumac, G., Mates, A., and Eidinger, D. 1976. The heterocytotoxicity of human serum. III. Studies of the serum levels and distribution of activity in human populations. Clin. Exp. Immunol., 26:601–608.

Gursel, E., Roberts, M., and Veenema, R. J. 1972. Regression of prostatic cancer following sequential cryotherapy to the prostate. J. Urol., 108:928–932.

Gutterman, J. U., Mavligit, G. M., McCredie, K. B., Freireich, E. J, and Hersh, E. M. 1973. Autoimmunization with acute leukemia cells: Demonstration of increased lymphocyte responsiveness. Int. J. Cancer, 11:521–526.

Hanna, M. G., Jr., Zbar, B., and Rapp, H. J. 1972. Histopathology of tumor regression after intralesional injection of Mycobacterium bovis. I. Tumor growth and metastasis. J. Natl. Cancer Inst., 48:1441–1455.

Hawrylko, E. 1975. BCG immunopotentiation of an antitumor response: Evidence for a cell-mediated mechanism. J. Natl. Cancer Inst., 55:413–423.

Helmstein, K. 1972. Treatment of bladder carcinoma by a hydrostatic pressure technique. Report on 43 cases. Br. J. Urol., 44:434–450.

Holm, G., Stejskal, V., and Perlmann, P. 1973. Cytotoxic effects of activated lymphocytes and their supernatants. Clin. Exp. Immunol., 14:169–179.

Kantor, A. L. F., Meigs, J. W., Heston, J. F., and Flannery, J. T. 1976. Epidemiology of renal cell carcinoma in Connecticut, 1935–1973. J. Natl. Cancer Inst., 57:495–500.

Lamoureux, G., Poisson, R., and Desrosiers, M. 1976. An antagonistic side-effect of BCG immunotherapy: Induction of immunological anergy. In Lamoureux, G., Turcotte, R., and Portelance, V. (eds.): BCG in Cancer Immunotherapy. New York, Grune and Stratton, pp. 167–178.

Merrin, C., Han, T., Klein, E., Wajsman, Z., and Murphy, G. P. 1975. Immunotherapy of prostatic carcinoma with bacillus Calmette-Guerin. Cancer Chemother. Rep., 59:157–163.

Miller, J. A. 1970. Carcinogenesis by chemicals: An overview. C. J. A. Clowes Memorial Lecture. Cancer Res., 30:559–576.

Minden, P., McClatchy, J. K., Wainberg, M., and Weiss, D. W. 1974. Shared antigens between Mycobacterium bovis (BCG) and neoplastic cells. J. Natl. Cancer Inst., 53:1325–1331.

Moolten, F. L., Capparell, N. J., Zajdel, S. H., and Cooperband, S. R. 1975. Antitumor effects of antibody-diphtheria toxin conjugates. II. Immunotherapy with conjugates directed against tumor antigens induced by simian virus. J. Natl. Cancer Inst., 55:473–477.

Morales, A., and Eidinger, D. 1976a. Bacillus Calmette-Guerin in the treatment of adenocarcinoma of the kidney. J. Urol., 115:377–380.

Morales, A., and Eidinger, D. 1976b. Immune reactivity in renal cancer: A sequential study. J. Urol., 115:510–513.

Morales, A., Eidinger, D., and Bruce, A. W. 1976a. Intracavitary bacillus Calmette-Guerin in the treatment of superficial bladder tumours. J. Urol., 116:180–183.

Morales, A., Eidinger, D., and Bruce, A. W. 1976b. Adjuvant immunotherapy with BCG in recurrent superficial bladder cancer. In Lamoureux, G., Turcotte, R., and Portelance, V. (eds.): BCG in Cancer Immunotherapy. New York, Grune and Stratton, pp. 247–262.

Morrison, A. S., and Cole, P. 1976. Epidemiology of bladder cancer. Urol. Clin. North Am., 3:13–29.

Murray, G. 1958. Experiments in immunity in cancer. Can. Med. Assoc. J., 79:249–259.

Nadler, S. H., and Moore, G. E. 1966. Clinical immunologic study of malignant disease. Response to tumor transplants and transfer of leukocytes. Ann. Surg., 164:482–490.

Olsson, C. A., Chute, R., and Rao, C. N. 1974. Immunologic reduction of bladder cancer recurrence rate. J. Urol., 111:173–176.

O'Toole, C., Helmstein, K., Perlmann, P., and Moberger, G. 1975. Cellular immunity to transitional cell carcinoma of the urinary bladder. III. Effects of hydrostatic pressure therapy. Int. J. Cancer, 16:413–426.

Pfordte, K., and Ponsold, W. 1969. The tumor inhibiting effect of properdin. Neoplasma, 16:609–612.

Powles, R. L., Russell, J. A., Toy, J. L., and Chapuis, B. 1976. New methods of assessing treatment-success in acute myelogenous leukemia. In Lamoureux, G., Turcotte, R., and Portelance, V. (eds.): BCG in Cancer Immunotherapy. New York, Grune and Stratton, pp. 279–284.

Sokal, J. E., Moayeri, H., and Aungst, C. W. 1976. BCG immunotherapy in malignant lymphoma. In Lamoureux, G., Turcotte, R., and Portelance, V. (eds.): BCG in Cancer Immunotherapy. New York, Grune and Stratton, pp. 287–294.

Symes, M. O., and Riddell, A. G. 1973. The use of immunized pig lymph-node cells in the treatment of patients with advanced malignant disease. Br. J. Surg., 60:176–180.

Zbar, B., Bernstein, I. D., Bartlett, G. L., Hanna, M. G., Jr., and Rapp, H. J. 1972. Immunotherapy of cancer: Regression of intradermal tumors and prevention of growth of lymph node metastases after intralesional injection of living Mycobacterium bovis. J. Natl. Cancer Inst., 49:119–130.

Zbar, B., Bernstein, I. D., and Rapp, H. J. 1971. Suppression of tumor growth at the site of infection with living bacillus Calmette-Guerin. J. Natl. Cancer Inst., 46:831–839.

Immunotherapy of Human Cancer,
The University of Texas System Cancer Center
M. D. Anderson Hospital and Tumor Institute.
Raven Press, New York © 1978.

Immunotherapy for Gynecologic Malignancies

Stanley A. Gall, M.D.

*Department of Obstetrics and Gynecology, Duke University Medical Center,
Durham, North Carolina*

Immunotherapy for gynecologic malignancies is in an early stage of development. The fifth volume of the compendium of tumor immunotherapy protocols, published by the National Cancer Institute in September 1977, lists only seven protocols by which gynecologic malignancies are treated. These include two protocols for the treatment of cervical cancer, three for ovarian cancer, and two for advanced (stages III and IV) cervical and ovarian carcinoma. The same compendium lists 88 protocols for treatment of malignant melanoma and 68 for various leukemias and lymphomas. There is a similar lack of published data on results of immunotherapy for gynecologic malignancies. The current, published data and preliminary results of ongoing studies will form the basis of this report.

The principles of immunology relevant to immunotherapy, host mechanisms for the control of tumor growth that can be modulated by immunotherapy, and clinical rationale for immunotherapy and its role in cancer treatment have been thoroughly discussed in earlier sections of this volume. There is no evidence that the principles of immunology applicable to nongenital tumors cannot be applied to genital tumors.

Both genital and nongenital malignancies exhibit tumor-associated antigens. The work by investigators in the mid-1950s (Foley, 1953; Prehn and Main, 1957) demonstrated antigenic properties peculiar to methylcholanthrene-induced murine tumor cells. The presence of tumor-specific or tumor-associated antigens on human neoplasms is strongly suggested by four clinical and laboratory observations. First, spontaneous and dramatic regressions of metastatic malignancies may indicate a possible host immune response to these antigens. Documented cases of spontaneous regression have been collected (Everson and Cole, 1966). Included in the 176 documented cases are 29 neuroblastomas and 19 malignant melanomas. A second line of clinical evidence for the existence of tumor-associated antigens and a host response to these antigens is the favorable prognosis that is associated with tumors that are infiltrated by lymphocytes (Thomas,

---

Abbreviation used in this chapter: FIGO—International Federation of Gynecology and Obstetrics.

1973). Thirdly, the studies of patients with primary immunodeficiency disorders and those whose immune systems are iatrogenically depressed have revealed a substantial increase in the incidence of malignancy (Penn and Starzl, 1972). The fourth line of evidence comes from the laboratory demonstration of the presence of these antigens. Tumor-associated antigens in genital cancers include a carcinoembryonic antigen (Gold and Freedman, 1965) and α-fetoprotein (Abelev, 1968), and have been demonstrated in studies of neuroblastoma (Hellström and Hellström, 1968), melanoma (Jehn *et al.*, 1970), and Hodgkin's disease (Order *et al.*, 1971). Tumor-associated antigens have been observed in ovarian (Chen *et al.*, 1973; Bhattacharya and Barlow, 1973) as well as cervical cancer (Levi *et al.*, 1969; Levi, 1971; DiSaia *et al.*, 1972; Gall *et al.*, 1973; Wells *et al.*, 1973), and more recently, in advanced ovarian malignancy (Knauf and Urbach, 1977). The premise that human cancers produce tumor-associated or specific antigens is central to any discussion of immunotherapy. Unless the immune system is stimulated by a tumor antigen, then in all probability, any attempt to manipulate the immune system will be futile.

Gynecologic malignancies possess unique features. Each gynecologic tumor has its own natural course, including etiology; symptomatology; spread pattern, local and distant; and manifestations when far advanced. The pattern of metastasis and lymph node involvement is an important consideration when planning therapy. Thus, a multidisciplinary approach to treatment of gynecologic malignancies is necessary. No single approach will suffice in the proper evaluation, treatment, and continuing care of the patient with gynecologic cancer.

Gynecologic malignancies continue to be a threat to women and rank third, after cancers of the breast and colon, in magnitude. The main sites of malignancy are the endometrium, cervix, and ovary. The numbers of newly diagnosed cancers of these sites and the yearly mortality for each are shown in Table 1. Obviously, the main problem is ovarian cancer, more than 80% of which is epithelial. More than 10,000 women die of ovarian cancer each year, and there has been no improvement in mortality for two decades (Graber, 1969).

Ovarian carcinoma presents vague signs in its early stages, and when the diagnosis is made, 60% of patients have disease outside the true pelvis (FIGO stages III and IV). Of equal concern is the fact that after resection of what appears to be localized disease (FIGO stages I and II), recurrent disease necessitating further therapy will develop in 20% to 50% of women (Munnell, 1968; Bagley *et al.*, 1972). Therefore, some form of systemic therapy is required for

Table 1. *Incidence of Genital Cancer in 1977*

Site	Number of Cases	Mortality
Endometrium	27,000	8,000
Cervix (invasive)	20,000	3,000
Ovary	17,000	10,000

primary management of localized as well as advanced disease or for subsequent management of recurrent disease. Consequently, interest has arisen in the systemic use of alkylating agents. The initial response rates with adjuvant alkylating agent therapy range from 45% to 65%, with 5% to 15% of treated patients continuing to respond two years after initiation of therapy (Masterson and Nelson, 1965; Smith and Rutledge, 1970; Wallach *et al.,* 1970), but the five-year survival rate for patients with stage III disease is only 5% (Tobias and Griffiths, 1976).

The best five-year survival rate reported in the literature for stage IIB cancer of the cervix is 66%; for stage IIIB, 36%; and for stage IV, 14% (Fletcher, 1973). There are two general causes of failures in treatment. First, the large, bulky, central lesion is difficult to sterilize, and a small percentage of patients have central or regional treatment failures. The other failures result from distant disease and are probably more difficult to manage. For patients with distant disease, adjuvant therapy in addition to primary surgery or radiotherapy is essential. Through the use of screening techniques, the incidence of invasive cervical cancer has decreased.

Adenocarcinoma of the endometrium is the most common gynecologic malignancy in the United States owing to a decreased incidence of invasive cervical carcinoma combined with a rise in incidence of endometrial carcinoma since 1970 (Christopherson *et al.,* 1971; Cramer *et al.,* 1974). Whether this increased frequency of adenocarcinoma of the endometrium is due to usage of estrogens and oral contraceptives or other etiologic agents associated with improved standards of living, such as better nutrition, decreased parity, delayed menopause, or increased longevity, has yet to be determined. Unfortunately, this malignancy has been given insufficient attention, and survival rates have been less than optimal. Although results of some studies indicate a survival rate of 90% with simple surgery (total abdominal hysterectomy, bilateral salpingo-oophorectomy) (Keller *et al.,* 1974), the annual report of treatment results for gynecologic cancers (Kottmeier, 1973) as well as a review of a collected series (Morrow *et al.,* 1973) note a five-year survival rate in the range of 70% to 76% for stage I carcinoma of the endometrium. The lack of improvement in the cure rate is due largely to lymph node involvement: In one study, there was an 11% incidence of involved pelvic lymph nodes and a 7% incidence of involved para-aortic lymph nodes in 102 patients with stage IA or IB adenocarcinoma of the endometrium (Creasman *et al.,* 1976). Lymph node involvement necessitates the use of adjuvant therapy, as routine hysterectomy and pelvic radiotherapy will not control all of stage I disease, much less the advanced stages.

The remaining cancers of the genital tract, i.e., vulva, vagina, and fallopian tube, and trophoblastic tumors do not occur frequently and consequently, have attracted little attention in immunotherapy protocols. Trophoblastic tumors would be logical cancers to treat with immunotherapy; however, there is the ethical problem of exposing patients with these tumors to unproved therapy when the cure rate is excellent with relatively simple chemotherapy.

In each gynecologic malignancy described, there is a stage, or stages, of disease that fits the criteria for the use of immunotherapy. Unfortunately, the vast majority of effort has been limited to therapy for ovarian cancer, although one report focuses on immunotherapy for vaginal cancer (Guthrie and Way, 1975) and there are several older reports of serotherapy for trophoblastic disease. As a result, the majority of studies on immune monitoring, immune reactivity, and differing approaches to immunotherapy have involved ovarian carcinoma patients.

IMMUNE STATUS OF GYNECOLOGIC CANCER PATIENTS PRIOR TO THERAPY

Determination of the immune status of patients with gynecologic malignancies has been attempted unsuccessfully many times. It is not possible at this time to measure the status of humoral immunity, cell-mediated immunity, macrophage immunity, antibody-dependent cellular cytotoxicity, or natural antibody killing as related to the patient with clinical gynecologic cancer. Many of the investigators using immune function tests have relied on delayed hypersensitivity (Wells *et al.,* 1973; Nalick *et al.,* 1974) or on indirect or direct measurement of lymphokine function (Chen *et al.,* 1973; Levin *et al.,* 1975; Chatterjee *et al.,* 1975; Yamagata and Green, 1976) and attempted to correlate their findings with prognosis or clinical status. These findings have been suggestive of immunologic defects in gynecologic cancer patients but have not offered the degree of reliability or specificity desired.

The correlation of the ability of cancer patients to develop delayed hypersensitivity reactions with prognosis was popularized by Eilber and Morton and Lee *et al.* in 1970. They described an almost perfect correlation between dinitrochlorobenzene (DNCB) reactivity and successful control of the cancer. Nalick *et al.* (1974), using a battery of skin test antigens and dinitrofluorobenzene (DNFB), studied 125 patients with various gynecologic cancers (see Table 2).

Table 2. *Relation of Delayed Hypersensitivity and Clinical Status**

Carcinoma	No. of Patients	Antigen-Positive (%)	DNFB-Positive (%)	Clinical Status†
Control	96	96.0	90.0	. . .
Cervical	81	81.5	47.9	NED
		22.2	19.2	Dead
Ovarian	24	60.0	75.0	NED
		36.8	25.0	Dead
Endometrial	20	72.7	72.7	NED
		66.7	33.3	Dead

* Adapted from Nalick *et al.,* 1974.
† Patients with no evidence of disease (NED) had good response to therapy. Deaths were caused by progressive or recurrent malignancy.

They found that patients who had a delayed hypersensitivity reaction to one of a battery of skin test antigens and responded to DNFB had an improved prognosis. Despite these observations, the correlation cannot be extended to all patients, thereby limiting its clinical usefulness. The lack of response in some patients is not understood. In another study of skin test antigens, evaluations were paired on 30 patients prior to and during *Corynebacterium parvum* immunotherapy. Seventy-six percent of the initial testing elicited no responses (Fisher *et al.,* 1976), indicating a depression of cell-mediated immunity, but it is impossible to equate the lack of response to prognosis.

The ability of ovarian carcinomas to induce an immune response in the host is accepted. However, induction of a cell-mediated response does not necessarily predict the clinical course of disease. Mitchell and Kohorn (1976), using short-term culture of tumor cells, measured lymphocyte-mediated cytotoxicity in 24 patients with ovarian cancer. Three patients with low cytotoxicity on the initial testing showed greater cytotoxicity as their disease progressed. Of equal importance was the demonstration of blocking factor in 14 of 16 patients who had shown progressive disease. Other investigators (Levin *et al.,* 1975) demonstrated a blastogenic response of peripheral blood lymphocytes from patients with ovarian cancer to ovarian cancer and fetal ovary cell extracts. The responses were significantly greater in patients in remission. This work suggests a common ovarian origin of epithelial tumors because of the blastogenic response to fetal cell extracts. Cytotoxicity of peripheral blood lymphocytes from ovarian carcinoma patients to allogeneic tumor cells in culture was demonstrated also by DiSaia *et al.* (1972). However, these investigators were unable to demonstrate blocking antibody in 22 patients with progressive disease. Nonspecific blocking was demonstrated in the cell-mediated, tumor-specific cytotoxicity reaction to cultured ovarian carcinoma cells (Saksela *et al.,* 1974). These results suggested that effector cells are Fc-receptor-carrying cells and that their cytotoxic activity can be nonspecifically blocked by saturating the Fc receptors with aggregated IgG or unrelated immunocomplexes.

Thus, it appears that ovarian carcinoma induces a cell-mediated response and that some form of blocking exists. No data exists in the literature regarding suppressor T cells or the presence of natural antibody in ovarian carcinoma. Additional laboratory evaluation will delineate the impact of suppression and methods to abrogate its effect.

Yamagata and Green (1976) studied the effect of therapeutic irradiation on the immune capacity of patients with cervical cancer, as evaluated by lymphocyte counts and lymphocyte response to phytohemagglutinin. They found that lymphocyte counts were depressed to 20% to 50% of pretreatment values and lymphocyte responses depressed to 10% to 33% of pretreatment values. The highest values for both lymphocyte counts and reactivities were found in patients with good clinical responses to radiotherapy. Of equal importance was the finding that the immunodepressive effect of patients' sera on lymphocyte reactivity decreased and disappeared in patients showing a good response, whereas it remained unchanged or increased in patients with a poor clinical response. The finding of a significantly higher incidence of "nonspecific" lymphocytotoxic antibodies in serum from cancer patients strengthens the evidence for humoral as well as cell-mediated factors responding to in vivo sensitization (Vos *et al.,* 1972).

It may be concluded that cervical carcinomas have tumor-associated antigen(s) and evoke an immune response. The exact nature and the control mechanisms of the response are unknown, but both cell-mediated and humoral immunity are involved. Depression of the response seems to be proportional to the extent of the tumor, and the response apparently returns to normal as the tumor is controlled.

EXPERIMENTAL IMMUNOTHERAPY FOR CLINICAL GYNECOLOGIC CANCER

The possible approaches to immunotherapy have been outlined in this volume by Drs. Fahey, Weiss, and Hersh, and previously by Morton (1972) (Table 3). Various combinations of immunotherapy for gynecologic cancer have been reported, but nonspecific immunotherapy with either bacillus Calmette-Guérin (BCG) or *C. parvum* and a chemotherapeutic agent has been used to the greatest extent.

Active-Specific Immunotherapy

Protocols with active-specific immunotherapy for ovarian and cervical carcinomas have been reported (Imperato, 1974; Pattillo, 1976; Hudson *et al.,* 1976). Pattillo (1976) treated 17 patients with advanced, recurrent cervical cancer and ten patients with recurrent or persistent ovarian cancer with BCG or BCG plus tumor antigens. Unfortunately, the therapy program presented is confusing, but apparently, 6×10^8 viable BCG organisms (Tice strain) was administered weekly, after which 0.6 mg/kg of Adriamycin was administered intravenously on a weekly basis to induce a remission. After induction of remission, 10 mg/kg of actinomycin D and 0.3 mg/kg of methotrexate were administered intravenously once a week for maintenance. Melphalan, 0.125 mg/kg, was given on three consecutive days per week after the first year of therapy. The results of Pattillo's therapy program cannot be determined from the data given. Several anecdotal cases are presented with impressive results, but no conclusion can be drawn from this publication.

Hudson *et al.* (1976) treated ten patients with advanced or recurrent ovarian cancer with a combination of chemotherapy and active-specific immunotherapy consisting of intradermal inoculation of 2×10^6 live BCG organisms (Glaxo strain) with 10^7 allogeneic irradiated tumor cells into four adjacent sites. Chemotherapy of an unspecified type was given between the inoculations of BCG and tumor cells. The frequency of vaccine administration was not reported. Control patients had been treated with different chemotherapeutic regimens at

Table 3. *Approaches to Immunotherapy**

Active Immunotherapy
  Whole tumor cell vaccines
    Living tumor cells—autologous, allogeneic
    Tumor cells inactivated by irradiation, mitomycin C, freezing and thawing, heat
    Tumor cells modified to increase antigenicity by addition of carrier proteins, chemical
      modification, neuraminidase treatment, concanavalin A
  Vaccines composed of subcellular components
    Crude cell extracts
    Isolated cell membranes
    Purified, solubilized, cell-surface tumor antigens
  Immune adjuvants
    Freund's adjuvant
    Bacterial—BCG, MER, *C. parvum*
Passive Immunotherapy
  Antitumor sera—xenogeneic, allogeneic
  Lymphocytes
    Nonactivated—from allogeneic cancer patients, normal identical twins or HLA-matched
      sibling, autologous lymphocytes grown in culture
    Activated in vitro—stimulated with PHA, specifically sensitized by tumor antigens
    Sensitized by cross-transplantation of tumors
  Extracts from sensitized lymphoid cells—transfer factor, immune RNA
Nonspecific Immunotherapy
  Local—BCG, DNCB
  Systemic—BCG, MER, *C. parvum,* levamisole

---

* Adapted from Morton, 1972.

other cancer treatment centers. The authors presented evidence that the survival rates for the chemoimmunotherapy group were significant at the 0.5% level. The results of this study are encouraging for a pilot study and should warrant a prospective controlled protocol.

Nonspecific Immunotherapy for Vaginal Cancer

In one report, immunotherapy for nonclinical vaginal cancer has been described (Guthrie and Way, 1975). The series consisted of seven patients who had had a hysterectomy and subsequently had three or more vaginal Papanicolaou smears positive for malignant cells. Colposcopy was not done. These patients were treated with 0.1% DNCB in aqueous cream base applied daily to the vaginal vault until an intense local reaction occurred. The patients previously had been sensitized with DNCB. Six of the seven patients treated have normal Papanicolaou smears and no evidence of disease, with follow-ups of two to 35 months. No evaluation of local or systemic immunity was reported.

Nonspecific Immunotherapy for Ovarian Carcinoma

Nonspecific immunotherapy for ovarian cancer also has been used (Creasman *et al.,* unpublished data) because of continuously suboptimal results with chemotherapy. Our interest in the gram-positive anaerobic bacterium *C. parvum,* an immunostimulating agent, was aroused after demonstration of its stimulatory effect on the reticuloendothelial system (Halpern *et al.,* 1973). Subsequent work demonstrating its antitumor properties in animals (Scott, 1974) has led to the clinical interest in *C. parvum* as a potent anticancer agent in humans. Laboratory evaluation of the efficacy of *C. parvum* and chemotherapy in murine fibrosarcomas (Currie and Bagshawe, 1970) was extremely encouraging. In that study, the importance of the sequence of administration of the agents, i.e., chemotherapy prior to immunotherapy, also was demonstrated.

The purpose of our study was to evaluate the effectiveness of melphalan plus *C. parvum* therapy as an adjunct to total abdominal hysterectomy, bilateral salpingo-oophorectomy, and/or debulking of tumor with omentectomy, if technically feasible, for stages II, III, and IV epithelial tumors of the ovary (Creasman *et al.,* unpublished data). Patients with proven stage II, III, or IV epithelial carcinoma of the ovary were eligible for the study. Each patient had undergone exploratory laparotomy. Total abdominal hysterectomy, bilateral salpingo-oophorectomy, omentectomy, and the debulking of as much tumor as possible were highly desirable; however, on occasion, only a biopsy of the tumor had been done. After a complete blood count and platelet count were obtained, the first course of melphalan was initiated, usually nine days after surgery, and *C. parvum* was administered on day 7 of the treatment cycle (see Fig. 1). The courses of therapy were administered monthly. A minimum of 12 courses in 18 months was required. Immunologic testing included responses to the skin test antigens dermatophytin, purified protein derivative, and streptokinase-streptodornase; T cell determinations; and response of peripheral blood lymphocytes to phytohemagglutinin, concanavalin A, and pokeweed mitogen.

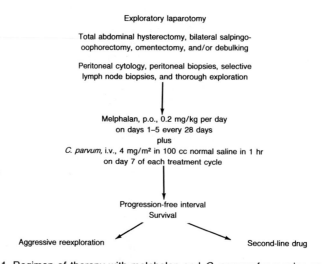

Figure 1. Regimen of therapy with melphalan and *C. parvum* for ovarian carcinoma.

Table 4. *Epithelial Carcinoma Treated with Melphalan and C. parvum (24-Month Interval)*

Tumor Characteristics	Number	Percent
Stage		
I	1	1.5
II	6	8.8
III	56	82.3
IV	3	4.4
Recurrent	2	3.0
Differentiation		
Good	7	10.3
Moderate	27	39.7
Poor	34	50.0

Sixty-eight patients were admitted to the study during the 24 months from July 1, 1975 to June 30, 1977. Ten patients could not be evaluated, as they had received less than three courses of therapy when the evaluation period closed. The stages and differentiation of the tumors are listed in Table 4. When first seen, 59/68 (86.7%) of the patients had advanced disease; thus, complete surgical resection of the tumor was often impossible, and many patients had ascites at the time of the initial surgery and suboptimal residual disease (nodules larger than 2 cm) at the conclusion of the operative procedure (Table 5). The incidence of various histologic types of the cancers is not unusual (Table 6). The initial 35 patients were hospitalized for their first course of *C. parvum* and carefully observed for toxicity. All subsequent patients were treated as outpatients. Patients' temperature, pulse, and blood pressure were monitored every 15 minutes during *C. parvum* infusion and hourly for at least six hours after infusion. Patients were encouraged to drink hot liquids throughout the infusion,

Table 5. *Initial Operative Procedures and Findings in Patients with Ovarian Carcinoma*

	Number of Patients
Procedure*	
TAH, BSO, omentectomy	29
TAH, BSO	5
BSO, omentectomy	14
TAH	1
BSO	7
Biopsy only	12
Findings	
Ascites	58
No ascites	10
Optimal disease	18
Suboptimal disease	50

* BSO, bilateral salpingo-oophorectomy; TAH, total abdominal hysterectomy.

Table 6. *Histologic Types of Ovarian Carcinoma*

Type	No. (%)
Serous cystadenocarcinoma	31 (45.6)
Undifferentiated carcinoma	27 (39.7)
Mucinous cystadenocarcinoma	6 (8.8)
Endometrial carcinoma	4 (5.9)

as suggested by Chen *et al.* (1976). An aggressive program of surgical reexploration was incorporated into the protocol. Twenty patients have undergone reexploration within the 24-month period of observation.

Patients were examined monthly or more frequently. Clinical responses to the melphalan plus *C. parvum* therapy were classified as follows: optimal response, all disease resected at time of initial surgery and no evidence of disease at three months; complete response, disappearance of all gross evidence of disease for at least three months; partial response, 50% or greater reduction in tumor size or regression of ascites or pleural effusion for at least three months; stable disease, status quo with less than 50% reduction in tumor size or regression of ascites or pleural effusion for at least three months; and progressive disease, 50% or greater increase in tumor size documented on two separate examinations, or appearance of new lesions, or development of ascites or pleural effusion.

During the 24-month period, 507 courses of melphalan and *C. parvum* were administered. Toxic manifestations of *C. parvum* were considered minimal (Gall *et al.,* in press). The responses of patients to therapy are listed in Table 7. The partial response and stable disease categories are important because of the large, bulky tumors involved in ovarian carcinoma; it is not unusual to find a tumor that has decreased to less than 50% of the original size but has not disappeared by three months. The 60.3% response rate at three months compares favorably with previously published data, which determined response after one month of therapy. Another determinant of therapeutic efficacy is the progression-free interval (Table 7). Patients in the stable disease and partial response categories had similar, relatively short progression-free intervals, reflecting the large tumor burdens remaining in these patients.

The survival data are presented in Table 7 also. Overall, 38/58 (65.5%) patients were alive at two years; obviously, however, not all patients were followed two years. An assessment of survival and progression-free interval was generated by the Kaplan and Meier (1958) approach, in which the product limit (PL) estimate P(t) is used. This life table analysis for 55 patients is shown in Figure 2. Two patients with recurrent cancer and the one patient with stage I disease were excluded. The survival rates, as assessed by life table analysis, for patients with optimal versus suboptimal disease are shown in Figure 3. The differences are striking, as only two of 18 patients with optimal disease have died (Table 5).

Aggressive reexploration has been an important aspect of therapy. Of 20 patients who underwent reexploration (Table 8), ten had an initial complete

Table 7. *Effect of Melphalan and* C. parvum *Therapy on Progression-Free Interval and Survival Rates for Responding Patients*

Response	Progression-Free Interval		Survival	
	No. (%) Progression Free*	Months' Duration/ Total Months (%)†	No. (%) Alive*	Months' Duration/ Total Months (%)‡
Progressive disease (n = 8)	0 (0)	20/136 (14.7)	0 (0.0)	54/136 (39.7)
Stable disease (n = 15)	6 (40.0)	96/229 (41.9)	9 (60.0)	114/229 (49.8)
Partial response (n = 11)	4 (36.3)	108/177 (61.0)	8 (72.7)	151/177 (85.3)
Complete response (n = 14)	12 (85.7)	170/191 (89.0)	12 (85.7)	182/191 (95.3)
Optimal (n = 10)	8 (80.0)	147/160 (91.8)	9 (90.0)	156/160 (97.5)

* At 24 months.
† Cumulative number of months patients had no tumor progression/total time of observation (cumulative), from initial examination to June 30, 1977.
‡ Cumulative number of months' survival (until death of patient or end of observation period)/total observation time (cumulative).

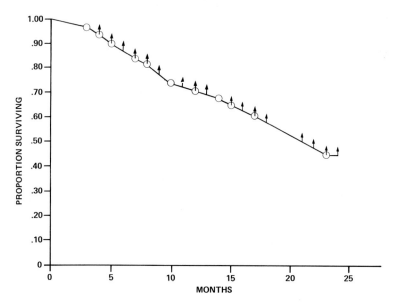

Figure 2. Estimated survival rates for 55 patients with ovarian carcinoma (life table analysis).

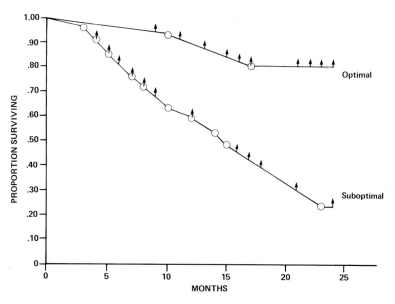

Figure 3. Estimated survival rates for patients with optimal versus suboptimal ovarian carcinoma (life table analysis). Evaluated were 18/18 patients with optimal disease and 37/50 with suboptimal disease.

Table 8. *Reexploration Experience in Patients with Epithelial Ovarian Carcinoma Treated with Melphalan and C. parvum*

ient	Therapy		Initial Response	Findings at Reexploration	Subsequent Therapy	Patient Status
	No. of Courses	Duration (mo)				
1	12	12	Optimal	Ascites positive; peritoneal implants	CIT	Vaginal nodule, 12 mo
2	9	12	Optimal	Ascites negative; PA node, nodule in cul-de-sac positive	XRT to ncde; CIT	NED, 4 mo
3	12	14	Stable	PA node, diaphragm positive; washings negative	XRT to ncde; CIT	Pelvic nodule, 9 mo
4	6	6	Stable	(TAH, sigmoid resection) Washings negative	CIT	NED, 6 mo
5	7	9	CR	Ascites positive; multiple nodules	CIT; ADR + CTX	Dead, 15 mo
6	12	13	CR	Washings negative; right obturator node positive (Peritoneal biopsy)	XRT to pelvis; CIT	NED, 2 mo
7	3	4	CR	(TAH, BSO, omentectomy) Nodes, washings negative	CIT	NED, 6 mo
8	8	11	CR	(TAH, BSO, omentectomy) Nodes, washings negative	CIT	NED, 15 mo
9	3	3	CR	(TAH, BSO, omentectomy) Nodes, washings negative; omentum, right tube positive	CIT	Dead, 12 mo
10*	7	7	CR	(TAH, omentectomy) Nodule on uterus positive	CIT	...
11	17	19	CR	Nodes, washings negative	None	NED, 4 mo
11	12	15	CR	Washings, pelvic nodes negative; PA node positive	XRT to PA node; CIT	NED, 6 mo

(continued)

Table 8. *Continued*

Patient	Therapy		Initial Response	Findings at Reexploration	Subsequent Therapy	Patient Status
	No. of Courses	Duration (mo)				
12	12	12	Stable	(TAH, sigmoid resection) Ascites, diaphragm positive	CIT	NED, 6 mo
13	6	6	CR	Washings, omentectomy positive; small peritoneal implants	CIT	NED, 4 mo
14	11	13	PR	Tumor on bowel surface; washings positive	CIT	Progressive disease, 7 mo
15	12	19	PR	Nodes negative; washings positive	CIT	NED, 4 mo
16	12	13	PR	Washings negative; no intraperitoneal disease (Resection of retroperitoneal mass)	XRT; none further	NED, 4 mo
17	10	13	CR	Small peritoneal implants	Cis-Pt + ADR × 1; further therapy refused	NED, 5 mo
18	12	13	PR	Washings positive; peritoneal implants	CIT	NED, 8 mo
19	9	12	CR	Ascites, diaphragm positive	Cis-Pt + ADR	NED, 1 mo
20	12	13	Optimal	Washings negative; NED	None	NED, 10 mo

Abbreviations: ADR, Adriamycin; BSO, bilateral salpingo-oophorectomy; cis-Pt, cis-platinum; CIT, chemoimmunotherapy (melphalan + *C. parvum*); CR, complete response; CTX, cyclophosphamide; NED, no evidence of disease; PA, para-aortic; PR, partial response; TAH, total abdominal hysterectomy; XRT, radiotherapy.
* Patient 10 had two reexplorations.

response: three from the optimal response category, three from the group with stable disease, and four from the partial response category. Small amounts of disease in the peritoneal cavity or on remaining pelvic organs were present in 12/20 patients. Lymph nodes were involved in 4/20, and the involved lymph node beds subsequently were treated with radiotherapy. After reexploration, 15 of the 20 patients continued to receive chemoimmunotherapy (one of these patients had a second reexploration, after which therapy was discontinued); three were switched to a regimen of Adriamycin and cyclophosphamide or cis-platinum; one, in whom the only finding at reexploration was a retriperitoneal mass, received radiotherapy; and one received no further therapy. Two patients died of disease 15 and 12 months after reexploration. The policy of aggressive reexploration and resection of tumor burden with continuing chemoimmunotherapy is in keeping with the finding of Rao *et al.* (1977), in whose study of advanced, recurrent ovarian carcinoma, the only patients who responded to chemoimmunotherapy were those who had undergone tumor-reductive surgery at the time of reexploration.

The data from immunologic testing have been disappointing. Extensive use of T cell and mitogen assays have produced little, if any, helpful data. Blastogenic responses tended to be more depressed as the disease progressed, but it was not possible to use this test in a prognostic manner. Results of skin tests were almost identical to those reported by Fisher *et al.* (1976). Use of assay procedures currently in the testing phase to measure levels of ovarian carcinoma antigens should be a great asset in monitoring a patient's clinical course.

SUMMARY

The use of immunologic technique in the therapy for gynecologic malignancies is a new experience for oncologists. Only a few studies have been completed, but results of these studies hold promise of improved clinical results. The Gynecologic Oncology Group has a current protocol for stage III optimal ovarian epithelial carcinoma comparing melphalan alone versus melphalan plus *C. parvum*. Utilization of this protocol in a randomized, prospective study should provide important information. In other studies, allogeneic or autologous cells plus immunotherapy continue to be used. Therefore, recent studies have provided evidence of benefit from adjuvant immunotherapy, and it can be expected that future studies will show even better results.

ACKNOWLEDGMENTS

The author gratefully acknowledges the expert secretarial help of Mrs. Ann Robinette and Mrs. Linda Woodlief. Clinical *C. parvum* and statistical assistance was provided by the Immunology and Clinical Statistics Sections of Burroughs Wellcome Co.

The work was supported in part by grants 2-RIO-CA 12534–06 and CA 13641–05 from the National Cancer Institute, National Institutes of Health.

REFERENCES

Abelev, G. I. 1968. Production of embryonal serum globulin by hepatomas: Review of experimental and clinical data. Cancer Res., 28:1344–1350.

Bagley, C. M., Young, R. C., Canellos, G. P., and DeVita, V. T. 1972. Treatment of ovarian carcinoma: Possibilities for progress. N. Engl. J. Med., 287:856–862.

Bhattacharya, M., and Barlow, J. J. 1973. Immunologic studies of human serous cystadenocarcinoma of ovary. Demonstration of tumor-associated antigens. Cancer, 31:588–595.

Chatterjee, M., Barlow, J. J., Allen, H. J., Chung, W. S., and Piver, M. S. 1975. Lymphocytes response to autologous tumor antigen(s) and phytohemagglutinin in ovarian cancer patients. Cancer, 36:956–962.

Chen, S. Y., Koffler, D., and Cohen, C. J. 1973. Cell-mediated immunity in patients with ovarian carcinoma. Am. J. Obstet. Gynecol., 115:467–470.

Chen, V. S. T., Suit, H. D., Wang, C. C., and Cummings, C. 1976. Non-specific immunotherapy by Corynebacterium parvum. Cancer, 37:1687–1695.

Christopherson, W. M., Mendez, W. M., Parker, J. E., Aundin, F. E., and Ahuja, E. M. 1971. Carcinoma of the endometrium: A study of the change in race over a 15 year period. Cancer, 27:1005.

Cramer, D., Cutler, S. J., and Christine, B. 1974. Trends in the incidence of endometrial cancer in the United States. Gynecol. Oncol., 2:130–143.

Creasman, W. T., Boronow, R. C., Morrow, C. P., DiSaia, P. J., and Blessing, J. 1976. Adenocarcinoma of the endometrium: Its metastatic lymph node potential. Gynecol. Oncol., 4:239–243.

Currie, G. A., and Bagshawe, K. P. 1970. Active immunotherapy with Corynebacterium parvum and chemotherapy in murine fibrosarcomas. Br. Med. J., 1:541.

DiSaia, P. J., Sinkovics, J. G., Rutledge, F. N., and Smith, J. P. 1972. Cell-mediated immunity to human malignant cells. Am. J. Obstet. Gynecol., 114:979–989.

Eilber, F. R., and Morton, D. L. 1970. Impaired immunologic reactivity and recurrence following cancer surgery. Cancer, 25:362.

Everson, T. C., and Cole, W. H. 1966. Spontaneous Regression of Cancer. Philadelphia, W. B. Saunders, pp. 1–10.

Fisher, B. F., Rubin, H., Sartiano, G., Ennis, L., and Wolmark, N. 1976. Observations following Corynebacterium parvum administration to patients with advanced malignancy. Cancer, 38:119–130.

Fletcher, G. H. 1973. Textbook of Radiotherapy. Philadelphia, Lea & Febiger, pp. 620–625.

Foley, E. J. 1953. Antigenic properties of methylcholanthrene induced tumors in mice of the strain of origin. Cancer Res., 13:835.

Gall, S. A., DiSaia, P. J., Schmidt, W. T., Mittelstaedt, L., Neuman, P., and Creasman, W. T. 1978. Toxicity manifestations following intravenous Corynebacterium parvum administration to patients with ovarian and cervical carcinoma. Am. J. Obstet. Gynecol. (in press).

Gall, S. A., Walling, J., and Pearl, J. 1973. Demonstration of tumor-associated antigens in human gynecological malignancies. Am. J. Obstet. Gynecol., 115:387–393.

Gold, P., and Freedman, S. O. 1965. Demonstration of tumor specific antigens in human colonic carcinoma by immunologic tolerance and absorption techniques. J. Exp. Med., 121:439–462.

Graber, E. A. 1969. Early diagnosis of ovarian cancer. Clin. Obstet. Gynecol., 12:958–971.

Guthrie, D., and Way, S. 1975. Immunotherapy of non-clinical vaginal cancer. Lancet, 2:1242–1243.

Halpern, B., Fray, A., Crepin, Y., Platica, O., Lorinet, A. M., Rabourdin, A., Sparros, L., and Isac, R. 1973. Corynebacterium parvum, a potent immunostimulant in experimental infections and in malignancies. Ciba Found. Symp., 18:217.

Hellström, I. E., and Hellström, K. E. 1968. Demonstration of cell-bound and humoral immunity against neuroblastoma cells. Proc. Natl. Acad. Sci. USA, 60:1341–1348.

Hudson, C. N., McHardy, J. E., Curling, O. M., English, P. E., Levin, L., Poulton, T. A., Crowther, M., and Leighton, M. 1976. Active specific immunotherapy for ovarian cancer. Lancet, 2:877–879.

Imperato, S., Rossi, R., Ermiglia, G., DeMarini, M., and Cassolino, A. 1974. Active specific and non-specific immunotherapy with immunological monitoring in late stage ovarian cancers. Acta Eur. Fertil., 5:25–39.

Jehn, U. W., Nathanson, L., and Schwartz, R. S. 1970. In-vitro lymphocyte stimulation by a soluble antigen from malignant melanoma. N. Engl. J. Med., 283:329–333.

Kaplan, E. L., and Meier, P. 1958. Non-parametric estimation from incomplete observations. Am. Statist. Assoc. J., 53:457–481.

Keller, D., Kempson, R. L., Levine, G., and McLennan, C. 1974. Management of the patient with early endometrial carcinoma. Cancer, 33:1108–1116.

Knauf, S., and Urbach, G. I. 1977. Purification of human ovarian tumor-associated antigen in patients with advanced ovarian malignancy. Am. J. Obstet. Gynecol., 127:705–710.

Kottmeier, H. L. (ed.) 1973. Annual report of the results of treatment in carcinoma of the uterus, vagina and ovary. Stockholm, Sweden, Radium Hemmet, vol. 15.

Lee, A. K., Rowley, M., and MacKay, I. R. 1970. Antibody-producing capacity in human cancer. Br. J. Cancer, 24:454.

Levi, M. M. 1971. Antigenicity of ovarian and cervical malignancies with a view toward possible immuno-diagnosis. Am. J. Obstet. Gynecol., 109:689–698.

Levi, M. M., Keller, S., and Mandl, I. 1969. Antigenicity of a papillary serous cystadenocarcinoma tissue homogenate and its fractions. Am. J. Obstet. Gynecol., 105:856–861.

Levin, L., McHardy, J. E., Curling, O. M., and Hudson, C. N. 1975. Tumor antigenicity in ovarian cancer. Br. J. Cancer, 32:152–159.

Masterson, J. G., and Nelson, J. H. 1965. The role of chemotherapy in treatment of gynecological malignancy. Am. J. Obstet. Gynecol., 93:1102–1111.

Mitchell, M. S., and Kohorn, E. I. 1976. Cell-mediated immunity and blocking factor in ovarian carcinoma. Obstet. Gynecol., 48:590–597.

Morrow, C. P., DiSaia, P. J., and Townsend, D. E. 1973. Current management of endometrial carcinoma. Obstet. Gynecol., 42:399–406.

Morton, D. L. 1972. Immunotherapy of cancer. Cancer, 30:1647–1655.

Munnell, E. W. 1968. The changing prognosis and treatment in cancer of the ovary. Am. J. Obstet. Gynecol., 100:790–806.

Nalick, R. H., DiSaia, P. J., Rea, T. H., and Morrow, C. P. 1974. Immuno-competence and prognosis in patients with gynecological cancer. Gynecol. Oncol., 2:81–92.

Order, S. E., Porter, M., and Hellman, S. 1971. Hodgkin's disease, evidence for a tumor associated antigen. N. Engl. J. Med., 285:471–474.

Pattillo, R. A. 1976. Immunotherapy and chemotherapy of gynecological cancers. Am. J. Obstet. Gynecol., 124:808–817.

Penn, I., and Starzl, T. E. 1972. Malignant tumors arising de novo in immunosuppressed organ transplant recipients. Transplantation, 14:407–417.

Prehn, R. T., and Main, J. M. 1957. Immunity to methylcholanthrene induced sarcomas. J. Natl. Cancer Inst., 18:769.

Rao, B., Wanebo, H. J., Ochoa, M., Lewis, J. F., and Oettgen, H. F. 1977. Intravenous Corynebacterium parvum. Cancer, 39:514–526.

Saksela, E., Penttinen, K., and Pyrhonen, S. 1974. "Non-specific" blocking of human ovarian carcinoma-associated cellular cytotoxicity in vitro. Scand. J. Immunol., 3:781–788.

Scott, M. T. 1974. Corynebacterium parvum as an immunotherapeutic anti-cancer agent. Semin. Oncol., 1:367–378.

Smith, J. P., and Rutledge, F. N. 1970. Chemotherapy in treatment of cancer of the ovary. Am. J. Obstet. Gynecol., 107:691–703.

Thomas, E. 1973. Current thoughts on facts that influence prognosis of gastric cancer. Med. J. Aust., 2:821.

Tobias, J. S., and Griffiths, C. T. 1976. Management of ovarian carcinoma. N. Engl. J. Med., 294:818–823.

Wallach, R. C., Kabakow, B., Blinick, G., and Antopol, W. 1970. Thio-tepa chemotherapy for ovarian carcinoma. Obstet. Gynecol., 35:278–286.

Wells, S. A., Jr., Melewicz, F. C., Christianse, C., and Ketcham, A. S. 1973. Delayed cutaneous hypersensitivity reactions to membrane extracts of carcinomatosis cells of the cervix uteri. Surg. Gynecol. Obstet., 136:717–720.

Vos, G. H., Hammond, M. D., Vos, D., Grobbelaar, B. G., Auslander, H. P., and Marescotti, G. 1972. An evaluation of humoral antibody responses in patients with carcinoma of the cervix. J. Obstet. Gynaecol. Br. Commonw., 79:1040–1046.

Yamagata, S., and Green, G. H. 1976. Radiation-induced immune changes in patients with cancer of the cervix. Br. J. Obstet. Gynecol., 83:400–408.

Immunotherapy of Human Cancer,
The University of Texas System Cancer Center
M. D. Anderson Hospital and Tumor Institute.
Raven Press, New York © 1978.

Immunotherapy and Chemoimmunotherapy for Human Breast Cancer

G. N. Hortobagyi, M.D., J. U. Gutterman, M.D.,*
G. R. Blumenschein, M.D., A. U. Buzdar, M.D., S. P. Richman,
M.D.,* C. Wiseman, M.D., and E. M. Hersh, M.D.*

*Medical Breast Service, Department of Medicine, and * Department of Developmental Therapeutics, The University of Texas System Cancer Center M. D. Anderson Hospital and Tumor Institute, Houston, Texas*

Immunotherapy is the newest and certainly the most exciting development in the often frustrating field of cancer treatment. Since the turn of the century, experimental and clinical information supporting the importance of host defense mechanisms in the development and prognosis of malignant tumors has accumulated. Consequently, tumor immunology and, more recently, immunotherapy have become important and incredibly complex. Studies on well-defined experimental tumor systems have demonstrated the existence of specific tumor-associated antigens and the ability of the host to respond to the presence of such antigens and reject the tumor by immunologic means. Clinical investigation of human tumors has proved more difficult, in part for ethical reasons, and although considerable information has been accrued, a multitude of important questions remain unanswered. Although an exhaustive review of breast cancer immunology is beyond the scope of this paper, a summary relevant to the rationale and design of clinical immunotherapy trials will be presented.

EVIDENCE FOR HOST IMMUNE RESPONSES

Breast cancer is a tumor or group of tumors with marked variations in clinical behavior. Analysis of patients with untreated breast cancer shows that although the median survival time from onset of symptoms to death is 2.7 years (Bloom *et al.,* 1962), 20% of the patients are still alive at five years and 4% at ten years. The prognostic significance of lymphocytic infiltration of the primary tumor was first described by Moore and Foote in 1949. These authors and others (Bloom *et al.,* 1970) suggested that recurrence rate is much lower and survival rate much higher for medullary breast carcinoma than for breast tumors of other histology, and attributed this to the extensive lymphoid infiltrate. The importance of lymphocytic infiltration of the tumor was emphasized by Black *et al.* in 1955. They reported that the pathologic examination of the regional lymph nodes in breast cancer patients shows a variety of reactive changes. A specific lymph node pattern called sinus histiocytosis, described by Black *et al.* in 1953, indicates a favorable prognosis. The lymphoreticuloendothelial response within the primary tumor also correlates with a favorable clinical course. It also has been suggested that breast cancers with lymphocytic infiltrates have fewer axillary nodal metastases, with less frequent involvement of apical lymph nodes when metastases are present, and a higher cure rate (Berg, 1963). Berg (1959) also reported that plasma cell infiltrate surrounding the primary tumor was associated with improved survival; however, this could not be confirmed by other investigators (Champion *et al.,* 1972). Subsequent analyses of immunologic and histologic factors have become more complex but tend to confirm the initial observation that the presence or absence of inflammatory cells within primary or metastatic tumor correlates with prognosis (Hamlin, 1968; Zelen, 1968).

The basic theoretical requirement for host defense to respond to neoplastic tissue is the presence of a characteristic antigen not present on the normal host cells. Although these tumor-associated antigens have been isolated regularly in experimental tumor systems, they have been elusive in human tumors. By applying a cryostat section of autologous breast cancer tissue to a "skin window," Black and Leis (1973) found evidence of cell-mediated immunity in 40% of breast cancer patients. Irradiated tumor cells, or crude extracts of the same, have been used for skin testing by a number of investigators. Stewart (1969) reported that 20% of breast cancer patients were reactive to crude, autologous tumor extracts in skin tests; survival duration was inversely proportional to the degree of reactivity. Skin test reactivity was observed with crude membrane extracts and partially separated, soluble, sonicated extracts of breast tissue (Alford *et al.,* 1973). However, this reactivity appeared to be organ-specific because reactivity to tumoral as well as normal breast tissue extracts was observed. Further purification of a soluble membrane antigen by polyacrylamide gel electrophoresis (PAGE) and chromatography on Sephadex G-200 resulted in the production of an antigen that evoked reactivity to both autologous and allogeneic tumor fractions. Other authors, utilizing various technologies, have provided further evidence of the existence of tumor-associated breast cancer antigen (Gentil and Flickinger, 1972; Mavligit *et al.,* 1973; Maluish and Halliday, 1974; Roberts and Bass, 1975).

IMMUNOCOMPETENCE AND PROGNOSIS

The ability of a host to mount an immune response has been measured by delayed cutaneous hypersensitivity testing with recall or established antigens or primary antigens, enumeration of lymphocyte subpopulations, and measurement of in vitro blastogenic response of lymphocytes to mitogens or common antigens. Anergy, or inability to mount an immune response, has been shown in patients with a variety of malignant and nonmalignant diseases. Compared with that in patients with other solid tumors, the degree of immunosuppression detected in breast cancer patients is less pronounced (Eilber *et al.*, 1975).

In a group of patients with miscellaneous solid tumors, Eilber and Morton (1970) found a strong, positive correlation between pretreatment reactivity to dinitrochlorobenzene (DNCB) and disease-free survival rate. In contrast, 90% of the patients unable to respond to DNCB were found to be inoperable or had recurrence of tumor promptly after surgery. Minimal to moderate impairment of DNCB responsiveness in patients with operable or recurrent tumors was noted by other authors (Golub *et al.*, 1974; Bolton *et al.*, 1975; Pinsky *et al.*, 1976; Wanebo *et al.*, 1976; Cunningham *et al.*, 1976).

Batteries of recall antigens also have been used to measure immunocompetence of breast cancer patients. Most investigators have shown none or only minimal suppression of reactivity to recall antigens in patients with early or localized breast cancer, whereas immunosuppression is usually moderately severe to severe in patients with advanced or disseminated tumors (Roberts and Jones-Williams, 1968, 1974; Nemoto *et al.*, 1974; Bolton *et al.*, 1975, 1976).

It has been suggested that an inverse correlation exists between the stage of disease and the preteatment peripheral lymphocyte count (Papatestas and Kark, 1974); a low pretreatment absolute lymphocyte count correlated well with a high incidence of relapse in the first five years after mastectomy (Glas *et al.*, 1976), although this latter correlation could not be confirmed by others (Wanebo *et al.*, 1976; Bolton *et al.*, 1976). Further analysis of absolute lymphocyte count by enumeration of T- and B-lymphocyte subpopulations has offered conflicting results. Some investigators have found an inverse relationship between stage of disease and T-lymphocyte levels (Weese *et al.*, 1977; Lamoureux and Poisson, 1977), whereas no such abnormality was observed by others (Wanebo *et al.*, 1976). There is evidence, on the other hand, that complement receptor-bearing B cells are fewer in advanced breast cancer patients (Wanebo *et al.*, 1976).

A number of in vitro tests to measure immunocompetence have been performed and analyzed for potential prognostic value. These have been reviewed extensively (Gutterman *et al.*, 1977). Although several investigators have reported conflicting results, there appears to be a trend suggesting that lymphocyte blastogenic response to mitogens is inversely related to the stage of disease.

INFLUENCE OF THERAPEUTIC MANEUVERS ON IMMUNE SYSTEM

There is strong evidence that breast cancer is immunosuppressive to the host, the degree of immunosuppression parallels the extent of disease, and, compared with other malignant tumors, breast cancer has a less marked immunosuppressive effect than, for instance, squamous cell carcinoma. There is also strong evidence, however, that the different modalities of treatment greatly affect the immune response of the host.

Recent reports have shown that major surgery (and/or anesthesia) produces a transient but definite immunosuppression in normal and tumor-bearing patients (Howard and Simmons, 1974; Slade *et al.,* 1975; Turnbull and Cooper, 1975; Vose and Moudgil, 1975; Roth *et al.,* 1976). Recovery from surgery-induced immunosuppression is usually rapid, averaging four weeks. Although the long-term effect of this transient immunosuppression has not been well defined, Crile (1974) suggests that minimal surgery be performed in breast cancer patients to decrease the extent of surgical trauma.

Radiation therapy has definite immunosuppressive activity in the host. The absolute peripheral lymphocyte count has been shown to be depressed shortly after radiation therapy is started, and this effect has persisted for as long as 60 months (McCredie *et al.,* 1972; Stjernsward *et al.,* 1972; Blomgren *et al.,* 1976; Order, 1977). Data related to the irradiation effect on lymphocyte subpopulations are somewhat more conflicting. Anderson *et al.* (1975) and Stjernsward and collaborators (1972) have reported a sharp decrease in both B- and T-lymphocyte populations. T lymphopenia persists longer and may be noticeable for as long as four years. Other investigators, however, have not found T cell depression following radiation therapy (Blomgren *et al.,* 1976). McCredie and colleagues (1972) showed that in vitro lymphocyte blastogenic response to phyto-hemagglutinin was decreased for as long as 12 months following radiation therapy. However, their results were not confirmed by others (Blomgren *et al.,* 1976). Stjernsward (1974) suggested that postoperative irradiation might actually shorten the survival of breast cancer patients and attributed this to the immuno-suppressive effect of radiation. His results have not been confirmed by others, and the controversy over the clinical relevance of radiation-induced immunosuppression continues.

Immunosuppression is one of the well-known effects of most chemotherapeutic agents used in the treatment of breast cancer. In particular, the alkylating agents Adriamycin and methotrexate are known for their strong immunosuppressing effect. This subject has been reviewed (Berenbaum, 1974; Hersh, 1974; Schein and Winokur, 1975). Chemotherapy administered on an intermittent, cyclic schedule has a much less marked immunosuppressive effect than when given on a continuous, daily schedule.

Estrogens have been shown to be important stimulators of the reticuloendothelial system (Biozzi *et al.,* 1957; Halpern *et al.,* 1960; Magarey and Baum, 1971; Pentycross *et al.,* 1973). Administration of stilbestrol prevents surgery- and radiation-induced immunosuppression (Magarey and Baum, 1971; Pentycross *et al.,* 1973); other estrogenic compounds lack this protective effect.

Corticosteroids are known to be immunosuppressive; it is no surprise that a similar action is observed when breast cancer patients are treated with these compounds, especially with daily, continuous administration (Iversen, 1957; Sherlock and Hartman, 1962; Thompson and Van Furth, 1970).

IMMUNOTHERAPY

In light of the information described, it is clear that the immune response of the host can modify the clinical course of breast carcinoma; the degree of immunocompetence existing prior to local or systemic therapy might influence the outcome; and all therapeutic maneuvers for breast carcinoma have, in turn, pronounced effects on the host immune reaction. The first attempts to use immunotherapy for malignant neoplasms were the result of empiricism. During the last few decades, with increasing knowledge of tumor immunology, the rationale of immune manipulation has been better defined. The theoretical background, the pretreatment requirements, and the potential and limitations of multiple modalities of immune modulation have been described in numerous review articles (Currie, 1972; Holmes *et al.*, 1975; Pilch *et al.*, 1975; Gutterman *et al.*, 1976b).

The goals of immunotherapy, at this point, are reversal or correction of tumor-induced immunosuppression, correction or prevention of immunosuppression secondary to antineoplastic treatment, and restoration or enhancement of tumor-specific immune responses. The different approaches currently available to achieve these goals include nonspecific immunotherapy with agents that stimulate general immunologic reactivity (bacillus Calmette-Guérin (BCG), *Corynebacterium parvum*, mixed bacterial vaccine, endotoxin, levamisole); active-specific immunization with inactivated tumor cells or tumor cell extracts from the patient (autologous) or from other patients with the same type of tumor (allogeneic); adoptive immunotherapy by transfer of lymphocyte extracts (immune RNA, transfer factor) from immunocompetent donors; and passive immunotherapy with serum, plasma, or specific antibody from donors known to have a specific immunity to the type of tumor concerned.

Local Immunotherapy

Coley's observations of objective tumor regressions following spontaneous or iatrogenic infections within or around the tumor often have been credited as the beginning of local immunotherapy (Nauts, 1969). A few patients with carcinoma of the breast, responding to local immunotherapy, were included in Coley's case series. Despite this early documentation of the efficacy of local nonspecific immunotherapy, it was not until the early 1950s that human immunotherapy was applied systematically and according to modern scientific methods.

Dr. Edmund Klein (1968a,b, 1969) was one of the first to administer locally a variety of antigens (triaziquone, DNCB) or bacterial organisms (BCG) for the treatment of basal or squamous cell carcinoma of the skin and cutaneous lesions of melanoma. He later reported that seven of 14 breast cancer patients with tumor recurrences in the chest wall responded to local administration of a variety of immunogenic materials that induced a delayed-type hypersensitivity reaction (Klein and Holtermann, 1972). Materials utilized were BCG and purified protein derivative (PPD). Smith and co-workers (1973) administered BCG (Tice strain) intralesionally to breast cancer and melanoma patients with cutaneous recurrences. All eight breast cancer patients treated with intralesional BCG experienced sloughing of the tumor nodules. These same authors treated six breast cancer patients by injecting a leukocyte extract prepared by cross-immunization of the same patients. One of the five evaluable patients had objective regression of chest wall lesions (Smith *et al.,* 1973). In a similar trial, Garas *et al.* (1975) confirmed these results. Another interesting clinical trial was reported by Stjernsward and Levin (1971). They induced delayed hypersensitivity reactions by applying DNCB on the skin overlying cutaneous lesions of breast carcinoma. Seven of eight patients were sensitized to DNCB; three exhibited objective tumor regression and two had stabilization of the treated lesions. Partridge and collaborators (1977) have reported their experience in treating ten breast cancer patients with tumor recurrence in the chest wall: BCG (Glaxo strain) was inoculated intralesionally every two weeks until complete response or progressive disease was noted. Six of the ten patients had a complete regression of chest wall lesions, and five have remained free of disease in the chest wall for 9 to 14 months since intralesional BCG treatment was begun. Rosenberg and Powell (1973) reported an objective remission in one breast cancer patient with chest wall tumor recurrence injected with BCG. Mastrangelo *et al.* (1976) reported objective regressions in six of seven breast cancer patients treated with intratumoral injection of BCG. In all of the mentioned reports, only the injected lesions regressed; uninjected lesions failed to show objective regression. This has been our experience at M. D. Anderson Hospital, where we have employed, instead of intralesional injection, epilesional scarification with BCG, as described by Richman *et al.* (1975). We also have used BCG cell wall skeleton with P3 for intralesional injection of chest wall lesions. Objective regression of injected nodules was observed in three of five patients so treated.

Another nonspecific immunostimulant, *C. parvum,* has been used in local therapy for metastatic breast cancer. Dimitrov *et al.* (1977) administered *C. parvum* intralesionally at a dose of 2.8 to 4.2 mg once a week. They reported that in all nine patients treated in this fashion, the injected lesions completely regressed, and no local recurrences were observed up to one year after initiation of treatment.

Glucan, a synthetic polymer shown to be a strong reticuloendothelial stimulant, has had limited clinical trials. Mansell *et al.* (1976) reported objective improvement in two patients treated with intralesional glucan administration. (See Table 1 for summarized results of studies with local immunotherapy for breast cancer.)

Active-Nonspecific Immunotherapy

As in trials for other hematologic malignancies and solid tumors, nonspecific immunotherapy has been used in most clinical immunotherapy trials for breast

Table 1. *Results of Local Immunotherapy for Breast Cancer*

Investigators	Agent	No. Responding/ No. Treated
Stjernsward and Levin, 1971	DNCB	3/8
Klein *et al.,* 1975	PPD	
	BCG	
	DNCB	7/14
	Triaziquone (Trenimon)	
	Others	
Smith *et al.,* 1973	BCG	8/8
	Leukocyte extract	1/6
Rosenberg and Powell, 1973	BCG	1/1
Partridge *et al.,* 1977	BCG	6/10
Mastrangelo *et al.,* 1976	BCG	6/7
Garas *et al.,* 1975	BCG	3/20
Dimitrov *et al.,* 1977	*C. parvum*	9/9
Mansell *et al.,* 1976	Glucan	2/2

cancer. The agents most commonly used have been BCG and *C. parvum,* although the methanol extraction residue (MER) of BCG, BCG cell wall skeleton preparations, and levamisole also have been used to a limited extent. All these agents have been used for the treatment of advanced breast cancer as well as in adjuvant immunotherapy for minimal residual (micrometastatic) disease. In both circumstances, nonspecific immunostimulants have been administered systemically by intradermal, subcutaneous, and intravenous routes. Immunotherapy has been given alone and in combination with chemotherapy. The basic principles of clinical immunotherapy and chemoimmunotherapy were developed in the treatment of acute leukemia and malignant melanoma. These subjects have been reviewed by a number of investigators (Seminars in Oncology, 1974; Holmes *et al.,* 1975; Gutterman *et al.,* 1976b).

Immunotherapy and Chemoimmunotherapy for Advanced Breast Cancer

BCG was the first nonspecific immunostimulant used in the systemic treatment of advanced breast cancer. Following the extensive experience acquired at our institution and elsewhere with the use of this agent in acute leukemia and malignant melanoma, it became clear that the addition of BCG to combination chemotherapy did not alter the objective response rate; however, remissions achieved by chemotherapy were significantly prolonged, as was the survival of patients achieving an objective response. Based on this information, we added nonspecific immunotherapy with BCG by scarification to our best combination chemotherapy regimen (5-fluorouracil + Adriamycin + cyclophosphamide: FAC) for disseminated breast cancer. Preliminary results of this study have been published elsewhere (Hortobagyi *et al.,* 1978b). Lyophilized Tice or Connaught strain BCG was administered by the scarification technique interspersed between courses of high-dose intermittent chemotherapy (FAC). The results of this

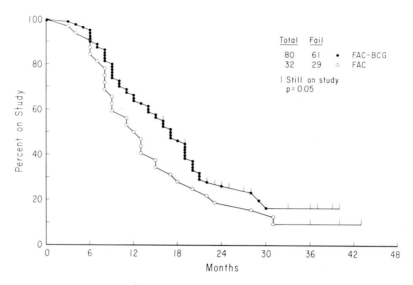

Figure 1. Duration on study (from beginning of chemotherapy until progressive disease was detected) for patients responding to chemotherapy with FAC (5-fluorouracil, Adriamycin, cyclophosphamide) and chemoimmunotherapy (FAC + BCG).

chemoimmunotherapy were compared with those obtained previously with chemotherapy alone.

The objective response rates for the two groups were essentially identical (FAC, 73%; FAC-BCG, 76%). However, the median duration of remission for patients who received chemoimmunotherapy was significantly longer than that for those treated with chemotherapy alone (Gutterman *et al.,* 1976a,c): nine months with FAC alone and 14 months with FAC-BCG ($p = 0.008$). The duration on study (from the beginning of chemotherapy until progressive disease was detected) for responding patients was 12 months for the chemotherapy group and 17 months for the chemoimmunotherapy group ($p = 0.05$) (Fig. 1). The greatest difference between these two groups, however, was the survival rate: 42 of 80 responders treated with FAC-BCG have died (median survival, 23.8 months), whereas 23 of 32 responders to FAC alone have died (median survival, 15 months). This difference is highly significant ($p = 0.01$) (Fig. 2). Nonresponders did not appear to benefit from the addition of immunotherapy, and the durations of stability and survival were identical in both groups of patients. These two groups have been followed for more than 40 months now, and the above-described differences have remained apparent at every analysis.

Subsequent to this study, we have entered 250 additional patients in the trial of the FAC-BCG chemoimmunotherapy protocol or minor modifications of it. The preliminary results for this larger group are identical to our previous results (Hortobagyi *et al.,* unpublished data).

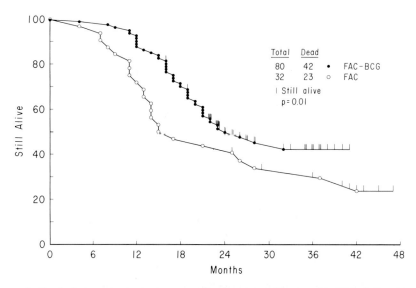

Figure 2. Survival rates for patients responding to chemotherapy with FAC (5-fluorouracil, Adriamycin, cyclophosphamide) and chemoimmunotherapy (FAC + BCG).

In an attempt to isolate the most effective antigenic components of heterogeneous materials such as BCG, and also in view of the potentially life-threatening toxicity of BCG (Sparks *et al.,* 1973; Bast *et al.,* 1974), a number of investigators have undertaken the task of separating the different, biologically active components of these organisms (Yamamura *et al.,* 1974; Lederer *et al.,* 1975; Ribi *et al.,* 1976; Weiss, 1976). Several antigenic subcomponents have been identified. Of these nonviable fractions of BCG, MER has been utilized the most extensively.

After our initial studies with BCG showed the benefits of nonspecific immunotherapy in prolonging remission and survival, we compared MER with BCG in a comparative, sequential trial, combining either agent with the same type of combination chemotherapy, designated VAC-FUM (vincristine, Adriamycin, cyclophosphamide—5-fluorouracil, methotrexate) (Tashima *et al.,* 1976). Whereas BCG was administered by scarification, MER was given subcutaneously, initially at a dose of 0.5 mg/m^2 and later, because of excessive toxicity, at a dose of 0.1 mg/m^2. Even with this lower dose, we observed excessive local and systemic toxicity with persistent ulceration at the injection site, which precluded administration of MER according to protocol. Preliminary analysis of this comparative trial showed that MER and BCG probably have equivalent immunostimulating properties. Although the duration of response in the MER group was slightly shorter than for patients treated with BCG, this difference was not statistically significant and was attributed, in part, to the fact that MER could not be administered regularly owing to local toxicity (Fig. 3). However, those patients who achieved complete remissions and remained on MER therapy had durations of remission and survival similar to or greater than those

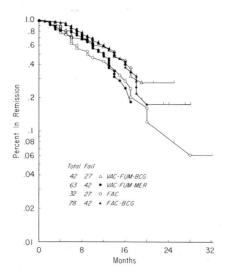

Figure 3. Remission duration for stage IV breast cancer patients receiving chemoimmunotherapy. A, Adriamycin; BCG, bacillus Calmette-Guérin; C, cyclophosphamide; FU, 5-fluorouracil; M, methotrexate; MER, methanol extraction residue of BCG; V, vincristine.

for patients treated with the same combination chemotherapy and BCG (Hortobagyi *et al.*, unpublished data) (Fig. 4). On the basis of these preliminary results, we have changed the route of administration of MER to intradermal, and tolerance has improved substantially.

Perloff and collaborators (1976) have reported results with the use of MER combined with chemotherapy (cyclophosphamide, methotrexate, 5-fluorouracil) and concluded that compared with results for historical controls, overall remission rates and duration improved. However, because of the small number of patients involved in the trial, additional patients were still being entered and their results were considered preliminary. This lead is being pursued in a prospective, controlled trial by the Cancer and Leukemia Group B.

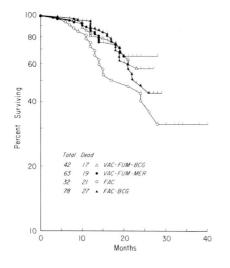

Figure 4. Survival rates for stage IV breast cancer patients receiving chemoimmunotherapy. See Figure 3 legend for definition of abbreviations.

In a small study, Hadziev *et al.* (1975) injected intradermally a water-salt extract from BCG into two patients with advanced breast cancer. The extract was administered as the only modality of treatment. In both patients, objective regression of the lesions reportedly was achieved. An extension of this approach (Hadziev, personal communication, 1977) showed six objective responses in nine patients treated with immunotherapy alone.

Song and Choi (1977) reported the results of a small, randomized trial with Adriamycin, vincristine, methotrexate, 5-fluorouracil (5-FU), and cyclophosphamide, with and without BCG. Their preliminary results show that the duration of remission for the patients who received chemoimmunotherapy is slightly longer than for those who received chemotherapy alone, although this difference does not appear to be significant.

A number of investigators have evaluated the role of *C. parvum* alone or combined with chemotherapy in the treatment of breast cancer. In a broad phase II study, Israël *et al.* (1975) administered *C. parvum* by the intravenous route daily to patients with a variety of solid tumors. Nine of 33 patients achieved partial regression of disease. Of two breast cancer patients included in this group, one had an objective response. In a second broad phase II study, Band *et al.* (1975) reported a partial response in one of four breast cancer patients treated daily with intravenous *C. parvum*.

In a prospective, randomized study, Israël (1976) incorporated combination chemotherapy with or without *C. parvum*. Although the comparability of the two groups is not well described, Israël's results show a statistically significant difference in survival rate at one, two, and three years following onset of treatment, favorable to the group treated with chemoimmunotherapy (Table 2).

Similar results were reported by Pinsky and collaborators (1978). In their prospective randomized study, combination chemotherapy was administered with or without *C. parvum*. The durations of response and survival were almost twice as long in the chemoimmunotherapy-treated group as in the group receiving chemotherapy alone. An additional study with *C. parvum* and combination chemotherapy was reported by Haskell and collaborators (1977). In a small, randomized study designed to detect the protective effect of *C. parvum* on the bone marrow, no differences were noted in durations of remission and survival between the group treated with chemotherapy alone and the group treated with chemoimmunotherapy.

A number of ongoing studies with BCG or *C. parvum* in the treatment of metastatic breast cancer are summarized in Table 3. Due to the short follow-up time, results are not yet available.

Another interesting agent used in nonspecific immunotherapy is levamisole, a synthetic compound with strong antihelminthic activity. It has been shown to restore cell-mediated immune responsiveness in anergic patients, and is known to be a potent stimulator of the reticuloendothelial system. The first clinical trial of levamisole for breast cancer was reported by Rojas and collaborators (1976). In a small, randomized study, breast cancer patients with locally ad-

Table 2. Results of Studies of Immunotherapy and Chemoimmunotherapy for Advanced Breast Cancer

Investigator (Institution)*	Treatment Regimen†	No. of Patients	Response Rate (%)	Remission Duration (mo)	Median Survival (mo)	Comments
Hortobagyi et al. (MDAH)	FAC	44	73	8.5	15	...
	FAC + BCG	105	76	13.5	22	
	FAC + levamisole	111	72	14	21	
Pinsky et al.	CAMF	23	48	ND‡	ND	...
	CAMF + C. parvum	24	58	ND	ND	
Haskell et al. (UCLA)	CMF	8	ND	ND	ND	No difference noted
	CMF + C. parvum	6	ND	ND	ND	
Song et al. (Mercy Hosp.)	AVMFC	9	ND	ND	ND	Remission longer in BCG group
	AVMFC + BCG	24	ND	ND	ND	
Israël	CMFVbST	43	60	ND	37§	...
	CMFVbST + C. parvum (s.c.)	45	71	ND	68§	

* MDAH, M. D. Anderson Hospital; UCLA, University of California at Los Angeles.
† A, Adriamycin; BCG, bacillus Calmette-Guérin; C, cyclophosphamide; F, 5-fluorouracil; M, methotrexate; ST, streptonigrin; V, vincristine; Vb, vinblastine.
‡ No data.
§ One-year survival.

Table 3. *Ongoing Studies of Immunotherapy and Chemoimmunotherapy for Advanced Breast Cancer*

Investigator (Institution)*	Treatment Regimen†	No. of Patients
Hadziev *et al.* (Bulgaria)	BCG-F70 BCG-F70 + Retabolil	Unknown
Lipton *et al.* (Horshoy Mod. Center)	FAC FAC + *C. parvum* FAC + *C. parvum* + BCG	37
Mayr *et al.* (OSAKO)	AVCMF AVCMF + *C. parvum*	100
Haskell *et al.* (UCLA)	AC AC + *C. parvum*	Unknown
Margolese *et al.* (Jewish Gen. Hosp.)	CMF CMF + levamisole	< 20
McCulloch *et al.* (Ontario Cancer Fdn.)	FAC FAC + BCG	30 since 8/76
Blumenschein *et al.* (MDAH)	FAC FAC + *C. parvum* (i.v.) FACM + L-asparaginase FACM + L-asparaginase + PV	60 since 7/77

* MDAH, M. D. Anderson Hospital; OSAKO, Cooperative Oncology Group of Eastern Switzerland; UCLA, University of California at Los Angeles.

† A, Adriamycin; BCG, bacillus Calmette-Guérin; C, cyclophosphamide; F, 5-fluorouracil; M, methotrexate; PV, pseudomonas vaccine; Retabolil, nandrolone decanoate; V, vincristine.

vanced, inoperable (stage III) tumors were treated with radical radiation therapy; half of the group was randomized to receive adjuvant treatment with levamisole (150 mg orally for three days every 14 days). At 30 months, 90% of levamisole-treated patients and 35% of control patients were alive; a similar difference in disease-free interval was observed (25 months and 9 months, respectively). Encouraged by these and our own results with BCG, we initiated a study in which levamisole was added to our FAC combination chemotherapy regimen. As we had observed previously with BCG, there was no change in the complete and partial remission rates (Table 4); however, compared with our previous results

Table 4. *Response Rates for Breast Cancer Patients Receiving Chemoimmunotherapy*

	No. (%) Responding		
Response	FAC* (n = 44)	FAC-BCG (n = 105)	FAC-Levamisole (n = 111)
Complete remission	6 (14)	20 (19)	11 (10)
Partial remission	26 (59)	60 (57)	69 (62)
Stabilization	12 (27)	21 (20)	27 (24)
Progressive disease	...	6 (5.7)	4 (3.6)

* FAC, 5-fluorouracil, Adriamycin, cyclophosphamide.

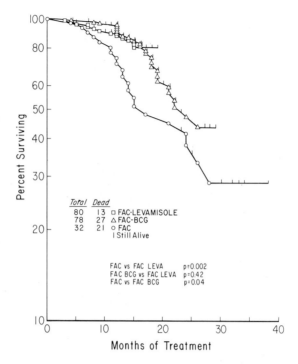

Figure 5. Survival rates for patients with metastatic breast cancer responding to chemoimmunotherapy. BCG, bacillus Calmette-Guérin; FAC, 5-fluorouracil, Adriamycin, cyclophosphamide; LEVA, levamisole.

with FAC alone, the addition of levamisole produced a significant prolongation of remission as well as survival among responding patients. The results, in general, appear identical to those achieved with chemotherapy and BCG or MER (Hortobagyi *et al.,* 1978a). The survival curves for this group of patients are shown in Figure 5.

Interferon is a natural substance intimately involved in the host's natural defense against viral infections. In addition, it has a variety of effects on healthy and deficient immune systems. Some preliminary work has been done with interferon (Habif, 1974) and interferon inducers (Regelson, 1976) in a variety of solid tumors, including breast cancer. Although some evidence of improvement was observed in both trials, more extensive work with these agents is needed before their exact role in the treatment of breast cancer is defined.

Many other natural substances have had limited trials or currently are being evaluated in the treatment of breast cancer. Asada (1974) reported on the use of mumps virus in the treatment of a variety of human solid tumors. Of two patients with advanced breast cancer, both experienced benefits after treatment was administered. Zymosan, a fungal extract (Martin *et al.,* 1964), and glucan have had some limited clinical evaluation.

Thus, a number of nonspecific immunostimulants have produced encouraging preliminary results (see Tables 2 and 4 for summaries). BCG, its subcellular fractions, *C. parvum,* and levamisole appear to have modest, but definite, therapeutic actions against breast cancer when administered alone or, preferably, in combination with chemotherapy. The other agents mentioned have not had adequate trials, but their use should be further explored in the clinic.

Immunotherapy and Chemoimmunotherapy for Micrometastases

The results of treatment of metastatic disease, with the exception of hematologic malignancies, lymphomas, and a few solid tumors (choriocarcinoma and testicular neoplasms), have been disappointing. Although with the advent of combination chemotherapy programs as well as the more frequent use of multidisciplinary forms of treatment, the remission rate has increased for most tumors, systemic treatment remains palliative at best. For this reason and because of the encouraging results of systemic treatment of micrometastases in animal models, aggressive systemic therapy for micrometastases (postoperative adjuvant treatment) has become widely accepted. This has been especially true in breast cancer, as subgroups at high risk of tumor recurrence following surgery can be identified readily. It has been demonstrated that combination chemotherapy prolongs the disease-free interval and survival of breast cancer patients with stages II and III disease (Fisher *et al.,* 1975; Bonadonna *et al.,* 1976). In the experimental model, nonspecific immunotherapy alone prolongs survival and eliminates a small number of tumor cells in a fraction of patients. However, maximum benefits can be obtained by the combination of optimal cytoreductive chemotherapy and immunotherapy (Table 5).

In 1974, after evaluating the preliminary results of our FAC-BCG regimen in patients with metastatic breast cancer, we started a postoperative adjuvant chemoimmunotherapy program with the same combination of drugs and BCG for patients with stages II and III breast cancer. Therapy was started after mastectomy and radiation therapy. Preliminary results of this study have been reported (Buzdar *et al.,* 1977a,b). During the past 45 months, 190 patients have been entered in the study. Of these, 131 patients have been followed for more than 12 months. Seventeen (13%) of 131 patients have relapsed; in contrast, 56 (37%) of 151 historical controls have relapsed ($p < 0.01$). The regimen has significantly prolonged the disease-free interval for all patients, irrespective of menopausal status or nodal involvement, and similarly, has prolonged the survival of treated patients. Sparks *et al.* (1977) have reported the results of the second analysis of their adjuvant chemoimmunotherapy program for breast cancer. They used the same chemotherapy regimen, CMF (cyclophosphamide, methotrexate, 5-FU), as did Bonadonna (1976), but added BCG or BCG and allogeneic tumor cells to the treatment of two subgroups of patients. Their report confirms the benefit of adjuvant chemotherapy, but as of the last analysis, the role of immunotherapy was uncertain. Sparks suggested that a longer follow-

Table 5. *Results of Adjuvant Therapy for Breast Cancer*

Investigator (Institution)*	Treatment†	No. of Patients	Median Follow-up (mo)	No. (%) Relapses
Sparks (UCLA)	CMF	23	13	NS‡
	CMF + BCG	53	21	9 (17)
	CMF + BCG + Tc	40	21	4 (10)
Buzdar (MDAH)	Historical control	151	31	59 (39)
	FAC + BCG	186	17	16 (9)
Scanlon (Evanston Hosp.)	L	33	NS	8 (24)
	CFP	33	NS	2 (6)
	CFP + BCG	33	NS	1 (3)
Rojas	Placebo	23	>30	21 (91)
	Levamisole	20	>30	11 (57)
Senn (OSAKO)	Control ⎫	206 (open since 6/74)	NS	(15)
	LMF + BCG ⎭		NS	(2.3)§

* MDAH, M. D. Anderson Hospital; OSAKO, Cooperative Oncology Group of Eastern Switzerland; UCLA, University of California at Los Angeles.

† A, Adriamycin; BCG, bacillus Calmette-Guérin; C, cyclophosphamide; F, 5-fluorouracil; L, L-phenylalanine mustard; M, methotrexate; P, prednisone; Tc, tumor cells.

‡ Not stated.

§ No difference for N+ patients.

up was needed to detect any additional benefit of the combination of immunotherapy and chemotherapy.

Another report, by Perloff *et al.* (1977), suggests no advantage with the addition of MER to combination chemotherapy. However, the noncomparability of the chemotherapy and chemoimmunotherapy groups is well described, and the validity of their conclusion is questionable. Two additional adjuvant chemoimmunotherapy trials have been reported. Scanlon (personal communication, 1977) reported a postoperative adjuvant study comparing chemotherapy with L-phenylalanine mustard (L-PAM) versus cyclophosphamide, 5-FU, and prednisone, versus this same combination chemotherapy plus Tice strain BCG administered by the Tine multipuncture method. More than 100 patients have been entered in this study within two years. At the most recent evaluation, both combination chemotherapy regimens were superior to L-PAM, but no additional benefit was detectable with the chemoimmunotherapy regimen.

Senn (1977) reported the results of the adjuvant trial by the Eastern Switzerland Co-operative Oncology Group. They compared combination chemotherapy with methotrexate, L-PAM, 5-FU, and BCG to no further treatment. Their preliminary results show significant protection by the chemoimmunotherapy for patients with uninvolved axillary lymph nodes, regardless of their menopausal status. No clear-cut protective effect was noticed in patients with involved axillary nodes. Because of the design of their trial, it is impossible to assess the role of immunotherapy in this program (Table 5).

The French Cancer Immunology and Immunotherapy Group, under the direction of Dr. Serrou, recently completed a clinical trial comparing the results of adjuvant immunotherapy with BCG and adjuvant chemotherapy with vincristine, cyclophosphamide, and 5-FU for patients with locally advanced (T3, T4, N+) breast cancer following radiation therapy with or without surgery (Serrou, personal communication, 1977). The relapse rate for the group of patients treated with adjuvant BCG was no different from that for untreated controls, whereas significantly fewer patients relapsed in the group treated with combination chemotherapy.

A list of adjuvant immunotherapy and chemoimmunotherapy trials currently being undertaken is shown in Table 6 (Compendium of Tumor Immunotherapy Protocols, 1977), but results are not yet available.

There is insufficient information on the role of adjuvant immunotherapy for breast cancer; however, many ongoing clinical trials will define the contribution of this modality within the next few years. Theoretically, the adjuvant setting is where the maximum benefit of immunotherapy can be observed.

Active-Specific Immunotherapy

Remarkably little work has been done with active-specific immunotherapy for breast cancer. As with other types of tumors, technical difficulties have delayed the availability of a purified, strongly antigenic fraction. Furthermore, the administration of unmodified cancer cells has been precluded for ethical reasons. Experience with this modality has been limited to small numbers of patients in uncontrolled trials.

Cunningham *et al.* (1969) used autologous tumor cells coupled to rabbit gamma globulin with bisdiazobenzidine and incomplete Freund's adjuvant to treat 42 patients with a variety of solid tumors. One of six breast cancer patients achieved an objective regression. Homogenates of allogeneic breast cancer cells or purified subcellular fractions of these homogenates, with or without exchange of allogeneic peripheral leukocyte preparations, were used by Humphrey *et al.* (1974) to treat breast cancer patients. Three of 19 patients treated with the vaccine alone and 12 of 42 treated with the vaccine plus allogeneic leukocyte preparation showed evidence of response.

Pattillo (1976) reported his experience with combination chemotherapy and immunotherapy with BCG and autologous and allogeneic tumor-associated antigens for patients with a variety of gynecologic cancers, including 15 patients with breast cancer. Although the patients receiving immunotherapy exhibited a stronger in vitro blastogenic response to mitogens compared with control subjects, the study design precludes assessment of the value of immunotherapy.

Injection of irradiated autologous cancer cells was used by Anderson *et al.* (1974) as adjuvant treatment following simple mastectomy and irradiation. The small group in this study was thought to have unfavorable prognostic characteristics, but 11 of the 16 are alive and free of disease four to seven years after

Table 6. *Ongoing Studies of Adjuvant Therapy for Breast Cancer**

Investigator (Institution)*	Treatment Regiment	Disease Stage	No. of Patients
Buzdar *et al.* (MDAH)	S + RT + FAC S + RT + FAC + BCG	II, III	(Study open since 6/77)
Serron *et al.* (Centre Paul Lamarque)	S ± RT S ± RT + VFC S ± RT + BCG	III	150
Oettgen *et al.* (MSKI)	S + L S + CAF S + levamisole	II, III	100–150
Tormey *et al.* (CALGB)	S + CMFVP S + CMF S + CMF + MER		>100/regimen
Hermon-Taylor *et al.* (St. George's Hosp. Med. School)	S S + BCG	I, II	75
Araujo *et al.* (NCI-Brazil)	S + Um + BCG	I, II	Unknown
Anderson (Royal Infirmary)	S + Tc (irradiated) S + LFM	I, II	<50
Retsas *et al.* (KCWAHA)	RT + levamisole	III	Unknown
Kerry (Univ. of Illinois)	S + BCG S + CMF S + RT S + CMF + BCG S + CMF + RT + BCG	II, III	<10
Lacour *et al.* (Gustave-Roussy)	S + RT S + RT + polyA : U S + polyA : U	I, II, III	Unknown
DeCarli *et al.* (Oncologic Hosp. of Buenos Aires)	S (historical)	I, II, III	~100
Fisher (NSABP)	S + LF S + LF + Cp (i.v.)	II, III	(Study open since 10/76)

* CALGB, Cancer and Leukemia Group B; KCWAHA, Kensington and Chelsea and Westminster Area Health Authority; MDAH, M. D. Anderson Hospital; MSKI, Memorial Sloan-Kettering Institute; NCI, National Cancer Institute; NSABP, National Surgical Adjuvant Breast Program.

† A, Adriamycin; BCG, bacillus Calmette-Guérin; C, cyclophosphamide; Cp, *C. parvum;* F, 5-fluorouracil; L, L-phenylalanine mustard; M, methotrexate; MER, methanol extraction residue of BCG; P, prednisone; RT, radiotherapy; S, surgery; Tc, tumor cells; Um, uracil mustard; V, vincristine.

initiation of therapy. No control subjects were used in this study, but comparison with surgical or radiotherapeutic trials is favorable.

Clearly, more work with active-specific immunotherapy is necessary. Technical developments have made purified tumor-associated antigens more available for clinical use; we hope this will stimulate the planning and execution of large clinical trials aimed at defining the influence of active-specific immunotherapy in the prognosis of breast cancer.

Passive Immunotherapy

Experience with passive immunotherapy is scarce. Small studies with limited numbers of patients have been conducted to explore this therapeutic modality. Oettgen *et al.* (1974) treated five patients with advanced breast cancer with pooled, dialyzable transfer factor from healthy adult donors. They noted that immune responsiveness was restored in three of these patients, one of whom experienced a dramatic partial remission lasting six months. A limited trial with immune RNA failed to elicit benefits in breast cancer patients (Kern and Pilch, 1975).

It was reported recently that tumor-specific cell-mediated immunity exists among close relatives (Yonemoto *et al.,* 1976) and household contacts (Byers *et al.,* in press) of breast cancer patients. A similar tumor-specific cellular immunity appears to exist in breast carcinoma patients clinically free of disease (Avis *et al.,* 1974; Yonemoto *et al.,* 1976; Brandes and Goldenberg, 1976). This information could help identify an ideal population of donors of transfer factor, which would facilitate larger clinical studies to confirm the efficacy of this subcellular fraction in the treatment of breast cancer.

CONCLUSIONS

During the last few years, a number of immunomodulating agents—crude bacterial organisms as well as purified fractions of such organisms—have been developed. These agents have been administered by a variety of routes and schedules, although their administration by the intravenous (presumably the most efficacious) route remains largely unexplored. The initial immunotherapy and chemoimmunotherapy trials have given us experience in repeated administration of immunomodulators combined with chemotherapy, surgery, and/or radiation therapy. However, more experimental and clinical work is needed to define optimal ways to combine these different therapeutic modalities to avoid therapeutic interference and to produce optimal clinical benefit. Furthermore, we need to develop methods to quantitate the effect of immunotherapy and the interaction of this modality with other forms of treatment.

The combination of different modalities of immunotherapy is a promising perspective. The use of combined active-specific and active-nonspecific or adoptive immunotherapy seems well within reason. Techniques for the more systemic application of local immunotherapy also must be developed. As these empiric approaches are coupled with progress in basic immunology, cell kinetics, and pharmacology, inevitable progress will be made in cancer immunotherapy. While immunotherapy remains an experimental tool, well-designed trials will be needed to define the role of each modality of immune manipulation in the therapy for breast cancer.

ACKNOWLEDGMENTS

This work was supported in part by contract NO1-CB-33888, and grants CA-05831 and CA-11430 from the National Cancer Institute.

Dr. Gutterman is a recipient of a Research Career Development Award (CA-71001-03) from the National Cancer Institute.

The authors would like to thank Audrey Faye Grubbs and Clarice Riewe for preparation of the manuscript.

REFERENCES

Alford, C., Hollinshead, A., and Herberman, R. 1973. Delayed cutaneous hypersensitivity reactions to extracts of malignant and normal human breast cells. Ann. Surg., 178:20–24.

Anderson, J. M., Campbell, J. B., Wood, S. E., Boyd, J. E., and Kelly, F. 1975. Lymphocyte subpopulations in mammary cancer after radiotherapy. Clin. Oncol., 1:201–206.

Anderson, J. M., Kelly, F., Wood, S. E., and Halnan, K. E. 1974. Stimulatory immunotherapy in mammary cancer. Br. J. Surg., 61:778–784.

Asada, T. 1974. Treatment of human cancer with mumps virus. Cancer, 34:1907–1911.

Avis, F., Mosonov, I., and Haughton, G. 1974. Antigenic cross reactivity between benign and malignant neoplasms of the human breast. J. Natl. Cancer Inst., 52:1041–1049.

Band, P. K., Jao-King, C., Urtasun, R., and Haraphongse, M. 1975. A phase I study of intravenous C. parvum in solid tumors. Proc. Am. Assoc. Cancer Res., 16:9.

Bast, R. C., Jr., Zbar, B., Borsos, T., and Rapp, H. J. 1974. BCG and cancer. N. Engl. J. Med., 290:1413–1420, 1458–1469.

Berenbaum, M. C. 1974. Effects of cytotoxic drugs and ionizing radiation on immune responses. In Stoll, B. A. (ed.): Host Defense in Breast Cancer. Chicago, Yearbook Medical Publishers, pp. 147–171.

Berg, J. W. 1959. Inflammation and prognosis in breast cancer: A search for host resistance. Cancer, 12:714–720.

Berg, J. W. 1963. Active host resistance to breast cancer. Rev. UICC, 18:823.

Biozzi, G., Halpern, B. N., Bilbey, D., Stiffel, C., Benacerraf, B., and Mouton, D. 1957. Estrogenes et fonction phagocytaire du system reticulo endothelial (SRE). C. R. Soc. Biol. (Paris), 151:1326–1331.

Black, M. M., Kerpe, S., and Speer, F. D. 1953. Lymph node structure in patients with cancer of the breast. Am. J. Pathol., 29:505–510.

Black, M. M., and Leis, H. P., Jr. 1973. Cellular responses to autologous breast tissue: Sequential observations. Cancer, 32:384–391.

Black, M. M., Oplier, S. R., and Speer, F. D. 1955. Survival in breast cancer cases in relation to the structure of the primary tumor and regional lymph nodes. Surg. Gynecol. Obstet., 100:543–552.

Blomgren, H., Burke, R., Wasserman, J., and Glas, U. 1976. Effect of radiotherapy on blood lymphocyte population in mammary carcinoma. Int. J. Radiat. Oncol. Biol. Phys., 1:177–188.

Bloom, H. J. G., Richardson, W. W., and Field, J. R. 1970. Host resistance and survival in carcinoma of breast: A study of 104 cases of medullary carcinoma in a series of 1411 cases of breast cancer followed for 20 years. Br. Med. J., 1:181–188.

Bloom, H. J. G., Richardson, W. W., and Harries, E. J. 1962. Natural history of untreated breast cancer (1805–1933). Comparison of untreated and treated cases according to histological grade of malignancy. Br. Med. J., 2:213–221.

Bolton, P. M., Mander, A. M., Davidson, J. M., James, S. L., Newcomb, R. G., and Hughes, L. E. 1975. Cellular immunity in cancer: Comparison of delayed hypersensitivity skin tests in three common cancers. Br. Med. J., 3:18–20.

Bolton, P. M., Teasdale, C., Mander, A. M., James, S. L., Davidson, J. M., Whitehead, R. H., Newcomb, R. G., and Hughes, L. E. 1976. Immune competence in breast cancer—Relationship of pretreatment immunologic tests to diagnosis and tumor stage. Cancer Immunol. Immunother., 1:251–258.

Bonadonna, G., Brusamolino, E., Valagussa, P., Rossi, A., Brugnatelli, L., Brambilla, C., DeLena, M., Tancini, G., Begatta, E., Musumeci, R., and Veronesi, U. 1976. Combination chemotherapy as adjuvant treatment in operable breast cancer. N. Engl. J. Med., 294:405–411.

Brandes, L. J., and Goldenberg, G. J. 1976. Peripheral leukocyte migration inhibition reactivity to breast cancer antigens in patients with breast cancer and normal control. Cancer Res., 36:3707–3710.

Buzdar, A. U., Blumenschein, G. R., Gutterman, J. U., Tashima, C. K., Hortobagyi, G. N., Wheeler, W., Gehan, E., Freireich, E. J, and Hersh, E. M. 1977a. Adjuvant chemoimmunotherapy following regional therapy in breast cancer. In Salmon, S. E., and Jones, S. E. (eds.): Adjuvant Therapy of Cancer. Amsterdam, Elsevier/North-Holland Biomedical Press, pp. 139–152.

Buzdar, A. U., Gutterman, J. U., Blumenschein, G. R., Hersh, E. M., Tashima, C. K., Gehan, E., and Freireich, E. J. 1977b. An intensive new adjuvant chemoimmunotherapy program containing 5-fluorouracil (5-FU), Adriamycin (AD), cyclophosphamide (CYT), and BCG (FAC-BCG) for operable breast cancer (Abstract C-187). Proc. Am. Soc. Clin. Oncol., 18:313.

Byers, V. S., Lecam, L., Levin, A. S., Stone, W. H., and Hackett, A. J. 1978. Identification of human populations with a high incidence of cellular immunity against breast carcinoma: Use in transfer factor immunotherapy. Cancer Immunol. Immunother. (in press).

Champion, H. R., Wallace, I. W., and Prescott, R. J. 1972. Histology in breast cancer prognosis. Br. J. Cancer, 26:129–138.

Compendium of Tumor Immunotherapy Protocols from the International Registry of Tumor Immunotherapy. 1977. Bethesda, Maryland, National Institutes of Health.

Crile, G., Jr. 1974. Effect of surgery on host resistance to cancer. In Stoll, B. A. (ed.): Host Defense in Breast Cancer. Chicago, Yearbook Medical Publishers, pp. 121–129.

Cunningham, T. J., Daut, D., Wolfgang, P., Mellyn, M., Maciolek, S., Sponzo, R., and Horton, J. 1976. A correlation of DNCB induced delayed hypersensitivity reactions and the course of disease in patients with recurrent breast cancer. Cancer, 37:1696–1700.

Cunningham, T. J., Olson, K. B., Laffin, R., Horton, J., and Sullivan, J. 1969. Treatment of advanced cancer with active immunization. Cancer, 24:932–937.

Currie, E. 1972. Eighty years of immunotherapy: A review of immunological methods used for the treatment of human cancer. Br. J. Cancer, 26:141–153.

Dimitrov, N. V., Singh, T., and Balcueva, E. 1977. Intralesional injections of *C. parvum* in local skin recurrence of breast cancer. Proc. ASCO, 18:270, C-15.

Eilber, F. R., and Morton, D. L. 1970. Impaired immunologic reactivity and recurrence following cancer surgery. Cancer, 25:362–367.

Eilber, F. R., Nizze, J. A., and Morton, D. L. 1975. Sequential evaluation of general immune competence in cancer patients: Correlation with clinical course. Cancer, 35:660–665.

Fisher, B., Carbone, P., Economou, S. G., Frelick, R., Glass, A., Lerner, H., Redmond, C., Zelen, M., Band, P., Katrych, B. L., Wolmark, N., Fisher, E. R., and other cooperating investigators. 1975. L-phenylalanine mustard (L-PAM) in the management of primary breast cancer. A report of early findings. N. Engl. J. Med., 292:117–122.

Garas, J., Besbeas, S., Papamatheakis, J., Gropas, G., Maragoudakis, S., Katsenis, A., Kiparissiadis, P., Konstadakos, P., and Georgaka, A. 1975. Attempt with immunotherapy to control metastatic skin nodules from breast cancer by BCG. Panminerva Med., 17:193–195.

Gentil, J. M., and Flickinger, J. T. 1972. Isolation of a tumor specific antigen from adenocarcinoma of the breast. Surg. Gynecol. Obstet., 135:69–74.

Glas, U., Wasserman, J., Blomgren, H., de Schryver, A. 1976. Lymphopenia and metastatic breast cancer patients with and without radiation therapy. Int. J. Radiat. Oncol. Biol. Phys., 1:189–195.

Golub, S., O'Connell, D. X., and Morton, D. L. 1974. Correlation in *in vivo* and *in vitro* assays of immunocompetence in cancer patients. Cancer Res., 34:1833–1839.

Gutterman, J. U., Cardenas, J. O., Blumenschein, G. R., Hortobagyi, G. N., Livingston, R. B., Mavligit, G. M., Freireich, E. J, Gottlieb, J. A., and Hersh, E. M. 1976a. Chemoimmunotherapy of disseminated breast cancer: Prolongation of remission and survival. Br. Med. J., 2:1222–1225.

Gutterman, J. U., Mavligit, G. M., and Hersh, E. M. 1976b. Chemotherapy of human solid tumors. Med. Clin. North Am., 60:441–461.

Gutterman, J. U., Mavligit, G. M., Hersh, E. M., Hortobagyi, G. N., and Blumenschein, G. R. 1977. Immunology and immunotherapy of human breast cancer: Recent developments and prospects for the future. In McGuire, W. (ed.): Breast Cancer: Advances in Research and Treatment. New York, Plenum Medical Books, pp. 313–373.

Gutterman, J. U., Mavligit, G. M., Hortobagyi, G. N., Blumenschein, G. R., Burgess, M. A., Jubert, A. D., and Hersh, E. M. 1976c. BCG immunotherapy of disseminated breast cancer and colorectal cancer: Prolongation of remission and survival. In Lamoureux, G., Turcotte, R., and Portelance, V. (eds.): BCG in Cancer Immunotherapy. New York, Grune and Stratton, pp. 227–238.

Habif, D. 1974. Report summary. In: Proceedings of International Workshop of Interferon in the Treatment of Cancer. pp. 49–50.

Hadziev, S., Kavaklieva-Dimitrova, J., and Mandulova, T. 1975. Therapeutic effect of a water-salt extract from BCG in two patients with advanced breast cancer. Neoplasma, 22:269–272.

Halpern, B. N., Stiffel, C., Biozzi, G., and Mouton, D. 1960. Influence des hormones sexuelles sur la stimulation de la fonction phagocytaire du system reticulo endothelial provoquee par l'inoculation du Bacille de Calmette-Guerin (BCG) chez la souris. R. Soc. Biol., 157:1994–2001.

Hamlin, I. M. E. 1968. Possible host resistance in carcinoma of the breast: A histological study. Br. J. Cancer, 22:383–401.

Haskell, C., Ossorio, R. C., and Sarna, G. 1977. Cyclophosphamide, methotrexate and 5 fluorouracil with and without *Corynebacterium parvum* in the treatment of metastatic breast cancer. In Crispen, R. G. (ed.): Neoplasm Immunity: Solid Tumor Therapy. Philadelphia, Franklin Institute Press, pp. 153–160.

Hersh, E. M. 1974. Immunosuppressive agents. In: Handbuch der Experimentellen Pharmakologie. Berlin, Springer-Verlag, vol. 38/1, pp. 577–617.

Holmes, E. C., Eilber, F. R., and Morton, D. L. 1975. Immunotherapy of malignancy in humans— Current status. JAMA, 232:1052–1055.

Hortobagyi, G. N., Gutterman, J. U., Blumenschein, G. R., Tashima, C. K., Buzdar, A. U., and Hersh, E. M. 1978a. Levamisole in the treatment of breast cancer. In Chirigos, M. A. (ed.): Immune Modulation and Control of Neoplasia by Adjuvant Therapy. New York, Raven Press, pp. 131–140.

Hortobagyi, G. N., Gutterman, J. U., Blumenschein, G. R., Tashima, C. K., Schwartz, M., Burgess, M. A., and Hersh, E. M. 1978b. The use of BCG and MER plus chemotherapy in the management of patients with disseminated breast carcinoma. In Terry, W. D., and Windhorst, D. (eds.): Immunotherapy of Cancer: Present Status of Trials in Man. New York, Raven Press, pp. 655–664.

Howard, R. J., and Simmons, R. L. 1974. Acquired immunologic deficiencies after trauma and surgical procedures. Surg. Gynecol. Obstet., 139:771–782.

Humphrey, L. J. 1974. Approaches to immunotherapy in cancer. In Stoll, B. A. (ed.): Host Defense in Breast Cancer. Chicago, Yearbook Medical Publishers, pp. 191–198.

Israël, L. 1976. Immunochemotherapy with Corynebacterium parvum in disseminated cancer. Ann. NY Acad. Sci., 277:241–251.

Israël, L., Edelstein, R., Depierre, A., and Dimitrov, N. V. 1975. Daily intravenous infusions of Corynebacterium parvum in 20 patients with disseminated cancer: A preliminary report of clinical and biological findings. J. Natl. Cancer Inst., 55:29–33.

Iversen, H. G. 1957. Influence of cortisone on frequency of tumor metastasis. Acta Pathol. Microbiol. Scand., 41:273–280.

Kern, B. H., and Pilch, Y. H. 1975. Immunity to human tumor associated antigens mediated by "immune" RNA. Proc. Am. Assoc. Cancer Res., 16:152.

Klein, E. 1968a. Tumors of the skin. IX. Local cytostatic therapy of cutaneous and mucosal premalignant and malignant lesions. NY State J. Med., 68:886–899.

Klein, E. 1968b. Tumors of the skin. X. Immunotherapy of cutaneous and mucosal neoplasms. NY State J. Med., 68:900–911.

Klein, E. 1969. Hypersensitivity reactions at tumor sites. Cancer Res., 29:2351–2362.

Klein, E., and Holtermann, O. A. 1972. Immunotherapeutic approaches to the management of neoplasms. Natl. Cancer Inst. Monogr., 35:379–499.

Klein, E., Holtermann, O. A., Helm, F., Rosner, D., Milgrom, H., Adler, S., Stoll, H. L., Chase, R. W., Prior, R. L., and Murphy, G. P. 1975. Immunologic approaches to the management of primary and secondary tumors involving the skin and soft tissues: Review of a ten year program. Transplant. Proc., 7:297–315.

Lamoureux, G., and Poisson, R. 1977. Evaluation de l'immunite cellulaire specifique au cours de l'evolution du cancer du sein. Ann. Immunol. (Paris), 128c:107–108.

Lederer, E., Adam, A., Clorbaru, R., Petit, J. F., and Wietzermin, J. 1975. Cell walls of mycobacteria and related organisms. Chemistry and immunostimulant properties. Mol. Cell. Biochem., 7:104.

Magarey, C. J., and Baum, M. 1971. Estrogen as a reticuloendothelial stimulant in patients with cancer. Br. Med. J., 2:367–370.

Maluish, A., and Halliday, W. J. 1974. Cell mediated immunity in specific serum factors in human cancer: The leukocyte adherence inhibition tests. J. Natl. Cancer Inst., 52:1415–1420.

Mansell, P. W. A., Diluzio, N. R., McNamee, R., Rowden, G., and Proctor, J. W. 1976. Recognition factors and nonspecific macrophage activation in the treatment of neoplastic disease. Ann. NY Acad. Sci., 277:20 43.

Martin, D. S., Hayworth, P., Fugmann, R. A., English, R., and McNeill, H. W. 1964. Combination therapy with cyclophosphamide and zymosan on a spontaneous mammary cancer in mice. Cancer Res., 24:652–654.

Mastrangelo, M. J., Berd, D., and Bellet, R. E. 1976. Critical review of previously reported clinical trials of cancer immunotherapy with nonspecific immunostimulants. Ann. NY Acad. Sci., 277:94–122.

Mavligit, G. M., Ambus, U., Gutterman, J. U., Hersh, E. M., and McBride, C. M. 1973. Antigens solubilized from human solid tumors: Lymphocyte stimulation and cutaneous delayed hypersensitivity. Nature (London) [New Biol.], 243:188–190.

McCredie, J. A., Inch, W. R., and Sutherland, R. M. 1972. Effect of post-operative radiotherapy on peripheral blood lymphocytes in patients with carcinoma of the breast. Cancer, 29:349–356.

Moore, O. S., and Foote, F. W. 1949. The relatively favorable prognosis of medullary carcinoma of the breast. Cancer, 2:635–641.

Nauts, H. C. 1969. The Apparently Beneficial Effects of Bacterial Infection on Host Resistance to Cancer. New York, Cancer Research Institute, monograph 8, pp. 1–116.

Nemoto, T., Han, P., Minowada, J., Angkur, V., Chamberlain, A., and Daot, L. 1974. Cell mediated immune status of breast cancer patients: Evaluation by skin tests, lymphocyte stimulation, and count of rosette forming cells. J. Natl. Cancer Inst., 53:641–645.

Oettgen, H. F., Old, L. J., Farrow, J. H., Valentine, F. T., Lawrence, H. S., and Thomas, L. 1974. Effects of dialyzable transfer factor in patients with breast cancer. Proc. Natl. Acad. Sci. USA, 71:2319–2323.

Order, S. E. 1977. Beneficial and detrimental effects of therapy on immunity in breast cancer. Int. J. Radiat. Oncol. Biol. Phys., 2:377–380.

Papatestas, A. E., and Kark, A. E. 1974. Peripheral lymphocyte counts in breast carcinoma. An index of immune competence. Cancer, 34:2014–2017.

Partridge, D. H., Sparks, F. C., Wile, A. G., and Morton, D. L. 1977. Intratumor injection of BCG for chest wall recurrence of breast carcinoma (Abstract #C-238). Proc. Am. Soc. Clin. Oncol., 18:325.

Pattillo, R. A. 1976. Immunotherapy and chemotherapy of gynecologic cancers. Am. J. Obstet. Gynecol., 124:808–817.

Pentycross, C. R., Toussis, D., McKinna, J. A., Lawler, S. D., and Greening, W. P. 1973. Effect of hormone therapy on mitogenic responses of lymphocytes on patients with cancer of the breast. Lancet, 2:177–179.

Perloff, M., Holland, J. F., and Bekesi, J. G. 1976. Chemoimmunotherapy of breast cancer (Abstract #C-288). Proc. Am. Soc. Clin. Oncol., 17:308.

Perloff, M., Holland, J. S., Lesnick, G. J., and Bekesi, J. G. 1977. MER chemoimmunotherapy of stage II breast carcinoma. In Salmon, S. E., and Jones, S. E. (eds.): Adjuvant Therapy of Cancer. Amsterdam, Elsevier/North-Holland Biomedical Press, pp. 177–182.

Pilch, Y. H., Myers, G. H., Sparks, F. C., and Golub, S. H. 1975. Prospects for the immunotherapy of cancer. Curr. Probl. Surg., January (pp. 1–46) and February (pp. 1–6).

Pinsky, C. M., DeJager, R. L., Kaufman, R. J., Mike, V., Hansen, J. A., Oettgen, H. F., and Krakoff, I. H. 1978. Corynebacterium parvum as adjuvant to combination chemotherapy in patients with advanced breast cancer. Preliminary results of a prospective, randomized trial. In Terry, W. D., and Windhorst, D. (eds.): Immunotherapy of Cancer: Present Status of Trials in Man. New York, Raven Press, pp. 647–654.

Pinsky, C. M., Wanebo, H., Mike, V., and Oettgen, H. 1976. Delayed cutaneous hypersensitivity reactions and prognosis in patients with cancer. Ann. NY Acad. Sci., 276:407–410.

Regelson, W. 1976. Clnical immunoadjuvant studies with Tyleron, DEAA, fluorene, and Corynebacterium parvum and some observations on the role of host resistance in herpes-like lesions in tumor growth. Ann. NY Acad. Sci., 277:269–287.

Ribi, E., Milner, K. D., Granger, D. L., Kelly, M. T., Yamamoto, K. I., Grehmer, W., Parker, R., Smith, R. F., and Strain, S. M. 1976. Immunotherapy with non-viable microbial components. Ann. NY Acad. Sci., 277:228–238.

Richman, S. P., Mavligit, G. M., Wolk, R., Gutterman, J. U., and Hersh, E. M. 1975. Epilesional scarification: Preliminary report of a new approach to local immunotherapy with BCG. JAMA, 234:1233–1235.

Roberts, M. M., and Bass, E. M. 1975. The immune reaction of human breast cancer tissue. Br. J. Surg., 62:660–668.

Roberts, M. M., and Jones-Williams, W. 1968. Delayed hypersensitivity in breast cancer (Abstract #53). Br. J. Surg., 55:869.

Roberts, M. M., and Jones-Williams, W. 1974. The delayed hypersensitivity reaction in breast cancer. Br. J. Surg., 61:649–652.

Rojas, A., Feierstein, J., Mickiewicz, E., and Glait, H. 1976. Levamisole in advanced human breast cancer. Lancet, 1:211–214.

Rosenberg, E., and Powell, R. 1973. Active tumor immunotherapy with BCG. South. Med. J., 66:1359–1363.

Roth, J. A., Golub, S. H., Grimm, E. A., Eilber, F. R., and Morton, E. L. 1976. Effects of operation on immune response in cancer patients: Sequential evaluation of *in vitro* lymphocyte function. Surgery, 79:46–51.

Schein, P. S., and Winokur, S. H. 1975. Immunosuppressive and cytotoxic chemotherapy: Long term complications. Ann. Intern. Med., 82:84–95.

Seminars in Oncology. 1974. 1:291–432.

Senn, H. J. (Co-operative Oncology Group of Eastern Switzerland—OSAKO). 1977. Chemoimmunoprophylaxis in early resected breast cancer (BCG). In: Compendium of Tumor Immunotherapy Protocols. International Registry of Tumor Immunotherapy, #5. Bethesda, Maryland, National Institutes of Health.

Sherlock, P., and Hartman, W. H. 1962. Adrenal steroids in the pattern of metastasis of breast cancer. JAMA, 181:313–317.

Slade, M. S., Simmons, R. L., Unice, E., and Greenberg, L. J. 1975. Immunodepression after major surgery in normal patients. Surgery, 78:363–372.

Smith, G. V., Morse, P. A., Deraps, G. D., Raju, S., and Hardy, J. D. 1973. Immunotherapy of patients with cancer. Surgery, 74:59–68.

Song, J., and Choi, C. 1977. Immunochemotherapy on patients with advanced breast cancer. In Crispen, R. C. (ed.): Neoplasm Immunity: Solid Tumor Therapy. Philadelphia, Franklin Institute Press, pp. 161–168.

Sparks, F. C., Meyerowitz, B. E., Ramming, K. P., Wolk, R. W., Goldsmith, M. H., Lemkin, S. R., Spears, I. K., and Morton, D. L. 1977. Adjuvant chemotherapy and chemoimmunotherapy for breast cancer. In Salmon, S. E., and Jones, S. E. (eds.): Adjuvant Therapy of Cancer. Amsterdam, Elsevier/North-Holland Publishing Co., pp. 157–161.

Sparks, F. C., Silverstein, M. J., Hunt, J. S., Haskell, C. M., Pilch, Y. H., and Morton, B. L. 1973. Complications of BCG immunotherapy in patients with cancer. N. Engl. J. Med., 289:827–830.

Stewart, T. H. M. 1969. The presence of delayed hypersensitivity reactions in patients toward cellular extracts of their malignant tumors. 2. A correlation between the histologic picture of lymphocyte infiltration of the tumor stroma, the presence of such a reaction and a discussion of the significance of the phenomenon. Cancer, 23:1380–1387.

Stjernsward, J. 1974. Decreased survival related to irradiation postoperatively in early operable breast cancer. Lancet, 2:1285–1286.

Stjernsward, J., Jondal, M., Vanky, F., Wigzell, H., and Sealy, R. 1972. Lymphopenia and change in distribution of human B and T lymphocytes in peripheral blood induced by irradiation for mammary carcinoma. Lancet, 1:1352–1356.

Stjernsward, J., and Levin, A. 1971. Delayed hypersensitivity-induced regression of human neoplasms. Cancer, 28:628–640.

Tashima, C. K., Blumenschein, G. R., and Gutterman, J. U. 1976. Comparison of Adriamycin combination drug program with BCG immunotherapy vs. MER immunotherapy for metastatic breast cancer (Abstract C-207). Proc. Am. Soc. Clin. Oncol., 17:288.

Thompson, J., and Van Furth, R. 1970. The effect of gluco-corticoid steroids on the kinetics of mononuclear phagocytes. J. Exp. Med., 131:429–442.

Turnbull, A. R., and Cooper, A. J. 1975. Depressed immunological responses following surgery— Its possible relevance in the treatment of patients with cancer. Clin. Oncol., 1:53–57.

Vose, B. M., and Moudgil, G. C. 1975. Effect of surgery on tumor-directed leukocyte responses. Br. Med. J., 1:56–58.

Wanebo, H. J., Rosen, T. P., Thaler, T., Urban, J. A., and Oettgen, H. F. 1976. Immunobiology of operable breast cancer: An assessment of biologic risks by immunoparameters. Ann. Surg., 184:258–266.

Weese, J. L., Oldham, R. K., Tormey, D. C., Barlock, A. L., Morales, A., Cohen, M. H., West, W. H., Herberman, R. B., Alford, T. C., Shorb, P. E., Tsangaris, N. T., Cannon, G. B., Dean, J. H., Djeu, J., and McCoy, J. L. 1977. Immunologic monitoring in carcinoma of the breast. Surg. Gynecol. Obstet., 145:209–218.

Weiss, D. W. 1976. MER and other mycobacterial fractions in the immunotherapy of cancer. Med. Clin. North Am., 60:473–497.

Yamamura, Y., Azuma, I., Taniyama, T., Ribi, E., and Zbar, B. 1974. Suppression of tumor growth and regression of established tumor with oil attached mycobacterial fractions. Gann, 65:179–181.

Yonemoto, R. H., Fujisawa, T., and Waldman, S. R. 1976. Selection of donors for transfer factor immunotherapy. Proc. Am. Assoc. Cancer Res., 17:150.

Zelen, M. 1968. A hypothesis of the natural time history of breast cancer. Cancer Res., 28:207–216.

Immunotherapy of Human Cancer,
The University of Texas System Cancer Center
M. D. Anderson Hospital and Tumor Institute.
Raven Press, New York © 1978.

Nonspecific Immunotherapy for Lung Cancer

Martin F. McKneally, M.D., Ph.D.

*Department of Surgery, Albany Medical College, and the Kidney Disease Institute of
the New York State Department of Health, Albany, New York*

Laboratory experiments with animal cancers have provided a sound basis for the conclusion that the immune response may be effectively invoked to reduce or prevent progressive neoplastic growth. Excitation of the immune response by sensitization with tumor antigens or nonspecific potentiators of the immune response, such as bacillus Calmette-Guérin (BCG), *Corynebacterium parvum,* and other bacterial products, can reduce or prevent the establishment and progressive growth of small numbers of tumor cells subsequently injected (Yashphe, 1971).

As in all of medicine, it is easier to prevent than to cure. Experimental demonstrations of elimination of established tumors solely by the immune response are relatively few. Zbar and co-workers have demonstrated that established tumors with known metastases to regional nodes respond to stimulation of the immune response by local injection of BCG (Zbar and Tanaka, 1971). In this example, excitation of the immune response is the sole mode of therapy, and treatment is not applied until after the onset of progressive tumor growth. Direct intralesional injection of BCG into the growing tumor nodule is a reliable method of evoking this response. Paralesional administration of BCG in the field of lymphatic drainage with the tumor has been demonstrated to reduce or eliminate tumor growth, presumably by a similar mechanism (Smith *et al.,* 1975).

Our first trial of nonspecific, active immunotherapy was unintentional (Ruckdeschel *et al.,* 1972). Among 472 patients who underwent pulmonary resection for lung cancer, 18 developed postoperative empyema, a chronic, draining, purulent process that is a highly unacceptable complication of surgical treatment. Nine of these patients survived five years, suggesting that the microbial antigens in the field of lymphatic drainage previously occupied by the tumor might stimulate some form of cross-protective immune response. Several clinical experiences with coincident infection in cancer patients supported this interpretation (Nauts, 1975).

A decade of outstanding experimental work by Old and Boyse, Rapp, Mackaness, and others (reviewed in Bast *et al.,* 1974) pointed to BCG as an effective bacterial potentiator of the immune response that could be introduced as a controlled equivalent of postoperative empyema. In the laboratory, we investigated the optimum dose (Codish and McKneally, 1972) and the safety of introducing BCG into the pleural space following surgical resection (Codish *et al.,* 1973). We compared the intrapleural route of administration with others to determine its efficacy in eradicating tumor nodules colonizing the lungs of mice after intravenous administration of tumor cells (McKneally *et al.,* 1975). Moderate increases over the minimal immunizing dose were found to be well tolerated intrapleurally, especially if a subsequent course of antituberculous treatment was given. A series of patients with malignant effusions was treated with BCG followed by isoniazid in a phase I trial of intrapleural BCG. There were no significant complications of this treatment.

In 1973, a prospective randomized trial was initiated to evaluate intrapleural BCG immunotherapy after pulmonary resection of lung cancer. Postoperative intrapleural administration of 10^7 colony-forming units of Tice strain BCG was followed in two weeks by a 90-day course of isoniazid. Control patients received no BCG, but were given a 90-day course of isoniazid. The preliminary results of our study have been reported (McKneally *et al.,* 1976a,b).

The tuberculin test converted to positive for most tuberculin-negative patients. Failure to convert was associated with recurrence in five of seven BCG-treated patients who previously had negative tuberculin tests. Patients with preoperatively negative phytohemagglutinin skin tests had somewhat lower survival rates than those who had positive tests (Maver *et al.,* unpublished data). The test was not predictive of outcome in individual cases. Randomization resulted in an equal distribution of known and measurable risk factors (Shields *et al.,* 1972) in both control and test groups.

Stage of disease is the most critical determinant of survival in lung cancer. Dr. Mountain's outstanding work at M. D. Anderson Hospital and Tumor Institute has provided a sound basis for predicting the outcome after surgical resection of stages I, II, and III resectable tumors (Mountain, 1977). The outcome for stages II and III patients treated with surgery alone is unfavorable. In our experience, the prognosis for patients with stages II and III resectable tumors was not improved by the introduction of single-dose, intrapleural BCG immunostimulation. However, there has been an encouraging reduction in cancer recurrence in stage I patients treated with intrapleural BCG (Fig. 1). I believe this is a biologically significant observation, indicating that stimulation of the immune response with an appropriate dose of a nonspecific potentiator in the field of lymphatic drainage with the tumor may contribute to the ultimate control of tumor growth.

The results of this study should be reviewed in the perspective of the usual distribution by stage of lung cancer patients at the time of presentation. Of 200 patients admitted to the Albany Medical Center and affiliated hospitals each year, only 35 are treatable by curative surgical resection. Of these, 25 have stage I disease. The remaining 165 patients have advanced or disseminated disease beyond treatment with surgical resection and adjuvant immunotherapy.

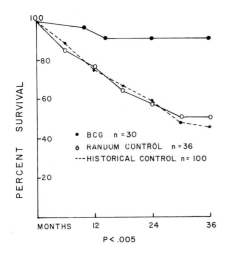

Figure 1. Effect of intrapleural BCG treatment on survival of patients with stage I lung cancer.

This points up the need for developing effective systemic chemotherapy for this disease.

Possibly, the benefit of BCG immunotherapy perceived in this trial may be an artifact related to a maldistribution of unknown risk factors, principally cryptic distant metastases, which are frequent in lung cancer patients (Matthews *et al.,* 1973). Among the control subjects, the survival rate for stage I lung cancer patients in the Albany trial is somewhat lower than that for the stage I patients at M. D. Anderson Hospital (Mountain, 1977). For this reason, a number of larger cooperative trials are under way in an attempt to confirm the apparently beneficial effect of intrapleural BCG.

Baldwin and colleagues (unpublished data) have conducted a trial of the efficacy of a single, intrapleural, low dose of 10^7 organisms of Glaxo strain BCG in the immediate postoperative period. Forty-two stage I patients have been entered in the trial. No conclusions can be drawn from the data at this time. Wright and Hill and their colleagues (1977) have treated patients by surgery alone, intrapleural BCG alone, or intrapleural BCG plus levamisole. The results of the study are preliminary, but no treatment benefit is yet detectable in any treatment group.

Yamamura (1978) has found that intrapleural administration of BCG cell wall skeletons is beneficial to patients with stage III lung cancer, as compared with historical control subjects. Trials of intrapleural *C. parvum* are under way in several centers in North America and Europe. Holmes and co-workers (1977) have injected BCG through a long, transthoracic needle into lung tumors in 15 patients prior to pulmonary resection. Because of the success of intralesional immunotherapy in the guinea pig hepatoma model (Zbar and Tanaka, 1971) and because of the somewhat optimistic results of regional immunotherapy with intrapleural BCG reported here, the results of this enterprising treatment program will be of great interest.

Taking the more systemic and less regional approach to immunostimulation, Edwards and Whitwell (1974) administered Glaxo strain BCG subdermally to 60 consecutive patients recovered from surgical resection of lung cancer. They could discern no statistically significant improvement in patients so treated when compared with historical control patients, although there was a trend toward higher survival rates for the immunotherapy group. Pouillart and co-workers (1977) gave cutaneous inoculations to approximately half of a randomized series of 80 patients following pulmonary resection. A difference "at the limit of statistical significance" was evident at 24 months, when 41 patients had entered the trial. Pines (1976) administered Glaxo BCG cutaneously to a randomized group of advanced lung cancer patients treated with radiotherapy. A significant therapeutic advantage was demonstrable transiently one year after treatment. Khadzhiev and Kavaklieva-Dimitrova (1971) reported that the survival rate among 52 patients with advanced lung cancer treated cutaneously with a water-saline extract of the Russian strain of BCG was improved, compared with that for an untreated group of patients.

In several important trials in progress, immunostimulants, such as BCG or Freund's adjuvant, in combination with tumor antigen are being applied cutaneously. Although those conducting the trials might correctly reject the viewpoint that these are trials of nonspecific immunostimulation, they are susceptible to that interpretation. The results of Herberman's trial of cutaneous BCG and tumor antigen are as yet indeterminate, as there are too few recurrences in any group to draw conclusions (Herberman, in press). Stewart and co-workers (1976) have designed and executed an outstanding study with Freund's adjuvant and purified lung tumor antigens. This positive trial supports the hypothesis that systemic stimulation of the immune response may be a helpful adjunct to resection for treatment of lung cancer. Takita and colleagues (1978) have observed a definable effect of immunologic manipulation using antigenic extracts of lung tumors in combination with Freund's adjuvant. These results are encouraging because they demonstrate a beneficial effect of immunotherapy in patients with more advanced disease.

A number of other important studies of nonspecific active stimulation of the immune response are under way. Dr. Mori in Osaka, Japan, has found that regular administration of 230 ml of fresh whole blood at monthly intervals prolongs the survival of lung cancer patients (unpublished data). Whether this is an exclusively immunologic effect is undetermined, but the approach is intriguing. Israël and Halpern (1972) have observed the beneficial effect of intravenously injected *C. parvum* on patients with advanced lung cancer. Aerosolization of Tice strain BCG failed to alter the course of patients with advanced lung cancer in the experience of Garner and his colleagues (1975) and of Cusumano and co-workers (1975). Severe side effects of BCG by this route of administration precluded evaluation for less advanced disease.

In 1975, Amery (1975) reported a remarkable, randomized, prospective trial with levamisole, 150 mg per day, given orally to patients with resectable lung cancer. In a recent summary (1977), Dr. Amery stated that reduction in tumor recurrence was clearly demonstrable only in patients weighing 70 kg or less, that is, patients who received at least 2 mg/kg body weight. These patients constituted only 40% of the test group, so the conclusions of the study are not as clear as they might be if all patients had been treated adequately. Nevertheless, there were nine recurrences among 39 adequately treated patients (23%) and 22 recurrences among 51 comparable control patients (43%). These results are provocative because the incidence of recurrence at distant sites seemed to be reduced in the levamisole-treated patients.

In view of the fact that most experimental attempts to reduce tumor growth in animals by immunologic means fail when applied in a therapeutic mode after the establishment of tumor growth, it is not surprising that the therapeutic use of immunostimulation in cancer treatment in man is often ineffective. Apart from cancer, therapeutic stimulation of the immune response has few convincing and successful applications in human disease. If healthy effector cells of the immune system or their molecular products are introduced into a congenitally immunodeficient host, a small but definable advantage in the contest with an infectious agent may be conferred. The results are far more often unsuccessful when the infectious process is established and progressing. Definitive chemotherapy is the most important factor in arresting infection in this circumstance, and I suspect that this will prove true in the control of lung cancer growth as well, as this tumor is so frequently far advanced at the time of initial diagnosis. If the minor degrees of immunodeficiency demonstrable in lung cancer patients contribute significantly to progressive growth, then restoration of the immune response may prove a partially effective remedy for this tumor. If the antigenicity of lung cancers can be exploited to secure a measure of selective toxicity in therapy, there is further reason for hope that stimulation of the immune response will provide a unique and significant benefit.

ACKNOWLEDGMENTS

This work was supported in part by grants RO1-CA-17346, MO1-RR00749, and NO1-CB-53940 from the National Institutes of Health, U.S. Public Health Service, and by the New York State Kidney Disease Institute (unit of New York State Department of Health).

REFERENCES

Amery, W. 1975. Immunopotentiation with levamisole in resectable bronchogenic carcinoma: A double-blind controlled trial. Br. Med. J., 3:461–464.

Amery, W. 1977. Levamisole in resectable lung cancer. Read before the Symposium on Immunotherapy of Malignant Diseases, Vienna.

Bast, R. C., Zbar, B., Borsos, T., and Rapp, H. J. 1974. BCG and cancer. N. Engl. J. Med., 290:1413–1420.

Codish, S. D., and McKneally, M. F. 1972. Dynamics and control of intrapleural BCG infection (Abstract). Fed. Proc., 31:658.

Codish, S. D., Ratnam, M., and McKneally, M. F. 1973. Intrapleural BCG infection: Studies in dogs and humans (Abstract). Fed. Proc., 32:847.

Cusumano, C. L., Jernigan, J. A., and Waldman, R. H. 1975. Aerosolized BCG (Tice strain) treatment of bronchogenic carcinoma: Phase I study. J. Natl. Cancer Inst., 55:275–279.

Edwards, F. R., and Whitwell, F. 1974. Use of BCG as an immunostimulant in the surgical treatment of carcinoma of the lung. Thorax, 29:654–658.

Garner, F. B., Meyer, C. A., White, D. S., and Lipton, A. 1975. Aerosol BCG treatment of carcinoma metastatic to the lung: A phase I study. Cancer, 35:1088–1094.

Herberman, R. B. 1978. Prospects for specific immunotherapy of lung cancer. In Rozencweig, M., and Muggia, F. (eds.): Treatment of Lung Cancer (Progress in Cancer Research and Therapy, vol. 11). New York, Raven Press (in press).

Holmes, E. C., Mink, J., Ramming, K. P., Coulson, W. F., and Morton, D. L. 1977. New method of immunotherapy for lung cancer. Lancet, 1:586–587.

Israël, L., and Halpern, B. 1972. Le Corynebacterium parvum dans les cancers avancés. Nouv. Presse Med., 1:19–23.

Khadzhiev, S., and Kavaklieva-Dimitrova, Y. 1971. The treatment of patients with bronchial cancer with water-saline extracts of BCG. Vopr. Onkol., 17:51–57.

Matthews, M. J., Kanhouwa, S., Pickren, J., and Robinette, D. 1973. Frequency of residual and metastatic tumor in patients undergoing curative surgical resection for lung cancer. Cancer Chemother. Rep., 4:63–67.

McKneally, M. F., Maver, C., Civerchia, L., Codish, S. D., Kausel, H. W., and Alley, R. D. 1975. Regional immunotherapy for lung cancer using intrapleural BCG. In Crispen, R. G. (ed.): Neoplasm Immunity: Theory and Application. Chicago, ITR, pp. 153–158.

McKneally, M. F., Maver, C. M., and Kausel, H. W. 1976a. Regional immunotherapy of lung cancer with intrapleural BCG. Lancet, 1:377–379.

McKneally, M. F., Maver, C. M., Kausel, H. W., and Alley, R. D. 1976b. Regional immunotherapy with intrapleural BCG for lung cancer. J. Thorac. Cardiovasc. Surg., 72:333–338.

Mountain, C. F. 1977. Assessment of the role of surgery for control of lung cancer. Ann. Thorac. Surg., 24:365–373.

Nauts, H. C. 1975. Immunotherapy of cancer by microbial products. In Mizuno, D. (ed.): Host Defense Against Cancer and Its Potentiation (Fifth International Symposium of the Princess Takamatsu Cancer Research Fund, Tokyo, 1975). Baltimore, University Park Press, pp. 337–349.

Pines, A. 1976. A five year controlled study of BCG and radiotherapy for inoperable lung cancer. Lancet, 1:380–381.

Pouillart, P., Palangie, P., Huguenin, P., Morin, H., Gautier, H., Lededente, A., Baron, A., and Mathé, G. 1977. Attempt at immunotherapy with BCG of patients with bronchus carcinoma: Preliminary results. In Salmon, S. E., and Jones, S. E. (eds.): Adjuvant Therapy of Cancer. Amsterdam, North-Holland Publishing Co., pp. 225–235.

Ruckdeschel, J. C., Codish, S. D., Stranahan, A., and McKneally, M. F. 1972. Postoperative empyema improves survival in lung cancer: Documentation and analysis of a natural experiment. N. Engl. J. Med., 287:1013–1017.

Shields, T. W., Higgins, G. A., and Keehan, R. J. 1972. Factors influencing survival after resection for bronchial carcinoma. J. Thorac. Cardiovasc. Surg., 64:391–399.

Smith, H. G., Bast, R. C., Jr., Zbar, B., and Rapp, H. J. 1975. Eradication of microscopic lymph node metastases after injection of living BCG adjacent to the primary tumor. J. Natl. Cancer Inst., 55:1345–1352.

Stewart, T. H. M., Hollinshead, A. C., Harris, J. E., Belanger, R., Crepeau, A., Hooper, G. D., Sachs, H. J., Klaassen, D. J., Hirte, W., Rapp, E., Crook, A. F., Orizaga, M., Sengar, D. P. S., and Raman, S. 1976. Immunochemotherapy of lung cancer. Ann. NY Acad. Sci., 277:436–466.

Takita, H., Takada, M., Minowada, J., Han, T., and Edgerton, F. 1978. Adjuvant immunotherapy of stage III lung carcinoma. In Terry, W. D., and Windhorst, D. (eds.): Immunotherapy of Cancer: Present Status of Trials in Man. New York, Raven Press, pp. 217–223.

Wright, P. W., Hill, L. D., Anderson, R. P., Hammar, S. P., Bernstein, I. D., and Prentice, R. L. 1977. Immunotherapy of resectable non-small cell cancer of the lung: A prospective comparison of intrapleural BCG + levamisole versus intrapleural BCG versus placebo. In Salmon, S. E., and Jones, S. E. (eds.): Adjuvant Therapy of Cancer. Amsterdam, North-Holland Publishing Co., pp. 217–224.

Yamamura, Y. 1978. Immunotherapy of lung cancer with oil-attached cell-wall skeleton of BCG. In Terry, W. D., and Windhorst, D. (eds.): Immunotherapy of Cancer: Present Status of Trials in Man. New York, Raven Press, pp. 173–179.

Yashphe, D. 1971. Immunological factors in nonspecific stimulation of host resistance to syngeneic tumors: A review. Isr. J. Med. Sci., 8:90–107.

Zbar, B., and Tanaka, T. 1971. Immunotherapy of cancer: Regression of tumors after intralesional injection of living mycobacterium bovis. Science, 172:271–273.

Immunotherapy of Human Cancer,
The University of Texas System Cancer Center
M. D. Anderson Hospital and Tumor Institute.
Raven Press, New York © 1978.

Adjuvant Immunotherapy for Colorectal Cancer

Giora M. Mavligit, M.D., Mary Anne Malahy, Ph.D.,* Nancy Zatopek, B.A., and Evan M. Hersh, M.D.

*Department of Developmental Therapeutics and *the National Large Bowel Cancer Project, The University of Texas System Cancer Center M. D. Anderson Hospital and Tumor Institute, Houston, Texas*

Experimental adjuvant treatment of micrometastases has shown promising results in patients with acute leukemia and a variety of solid tumors, such as melanoma, sarcoma, and breast and lung carcinoma. The natural history of colorectal cancer clearly indicates that, despite the improvement in surgical techniques and diagnostic procedures, overt metastatic disease ultimately develops in a substantial number of patients after potentially curative surgery. This unfavorable development lends ample support to the contention that foci of micrometastases are present in adjacent and distant organs of some patients when the primary lesion is removed.

Because patients with Dukes' class C lesions (tumor penetration through the bowel wall, with involvement of mesenteric lymph nodes and without invasion of adjacent structures or distant organs) are particularly prone to the development of fatal metastatic disease, they were selected for our clinical trial of systemic adjuvant therapy following surgery. With a maximum follow-up of 50 months, the benefits of adjuvant immunotherapy with BCG continue to hold up, while the role of oral 5-fluorouracil (5-FU) in the adjuvant setting is still debatable.

MATERIALS AND METHODS

A total of 121 patients with carcinoma of the large bowel, Dukes' class C, was entered into a clinical trial of adjuvant therapy between 1973 and 1976. Therapy consisted of immunotherapy with bacillus Calmette-Guérin (BCG) by scarification or immunochemotherapy with BCG plus oral 5-FU as previously described (Mavligit *et al.,* 1975). Details of the randomization to treatment groups and the criteria for exclusion from this study have been discussed at length in a previous publication (Mavligit *et al.,* 1975). Treatment evaluation of disease-free interval and overall survival was compared with clinical parameters in a consecutive series of comparable (by the previous definition of Dukes' class C lesions and evaluation of patient characteristics possibly related to prognosis by the Cox regression model) historical control patients with Dukes' class C lesions operated on at M. D. Anderson Hospital between 1963 and 1973. This indicates the lack of a significant change in operative techniques and other unknown factors that might have influenced the surgical management of Dukes' class C patients at M. D. Anderson Hospital. We also found virtually no difference in disease-free interval or overall survival between patients operated on at M. D. Anderson Hospital and those operated on elsewhere. This allowed us to consider in the current study experimental patients who received adjuvant therapy regardless of where surgery was done. All patients were regularly followed up in the outpatient clinic. Their plasma carcinoembryonic antigen (CEA) levels were regularly determined, and the immune status was initially determined by skin tests to recall antigens and subsequently included local graft versus host reaction.

RESULTS AND COMMENTS

The latest analysis, performed in June 1977, shows that preliminary results published earlier continue to hold up. With a maximum follow-up of 50 months, 18 of 52 patients who received BCG alone and 30 of 69 patients who received BCG plus 5-FU have relapsed. The disease-free interval for either treatment group is significantly prolonged when compared with that of the control group ($p = 0.004$, $p = 0.015$). The median disease-free intervals are estimated at 35+ and 34.3 months for the BCG and BCG plus 5-FU groups, respectively, compared with 21.4 months for the controls. It is noteworthy that the difference between BCG and BCG plus 5-FU is not significant ($p = 0.5$).

The overall survival of the patients who received adjuvant therapy was also significantly prolonged, compared to that of the controls. Ten of the 18 patients who received BCG and relapsed and 16 of the 30 who received BCG plus 5-FU and relapsed have died. The median survival for either group has not been reached, but the 75th percentile survival is estimated at 36.5 and 28.3 months for BCG and BCG plus 5-FU, respectively, compared with a 75th percentile survival of 16.6 months for the controls. Again, no significant difference has been noted between BCG and BCG plus 5-FU ($p = 0.5$), although the BCG group has had slightly better results.

In the absence of a significant difference between the two treatment groups, they were combined into one group designated "adjuvant therapy." The combined treatment group was then compared with 143 control patients with Dukes' class B lesions (penetration through the bowel wall into the serosa and/or pericolonic fat, with negative lymph nodes) consecutively operated on at M. D. Anderson Hospital between 1963 and 1973. The median disease-free interval for the adjuvant therapy group was estimated at 35.9 months, compared to 21.4 months for the Dukes' class C controls, but it is still significantly shorter than the median disease-free interval for Dukes' class B controls (86.5 months). This can be considered a modest shift in prognosis as a result of adjuvant therapy; however, the overall survival rates are rather striking. The survival curve for Dukes' class C patients receiving adjuvant therapy almost overlaps the curve for Dukes' class B controls, with 75th percentile figures of 34 and 35 months, respectively ($p = 0.35$), compared with a 75th percentile survival of 16.6 months and a median survival of 39.5 months for Dukes' class C controls ($p = 0.001$). In other words, the administration of adjuvant therapy resulted in a doubling of the 75th percentile survival to a point almost equivalent to the *median* survival time for Dukes' class C controls.

This prolongation of the disease-free interval and particularly the overall survival indicates a clear-cut biologic effect manifested by a marked shift in prognosis of Dukes' class C patients treated with adjuvant therapy. The prolongation of survival has been achieved despite unfavorable prognostic factors resulting in significantly higher hazard ratios ascribed to the adjuvant therapy group by the Cox regression model. Furthermore, the significant prolongation of disease-free interval has been achieved despite (1) the overwhelming effect ostensibly exerted by the absolute number of involved nodes, which may have somewhat masked the effect of adjuvant therapy, and (2) the frequent sequential monitoring of plasma CEA levels in patients receiving adjuvant therapy, which contributed considerably to the early detection of recurrent tumor and therefore had an "unfavorable" (shortening) effect on the disease-free interval. Nevertheless, the prognosis of our historical control patients was demonstrated by the Cox regression model to be comparable to (if not favorable to) that of the patients who received adjuvant therapy. The regression model indicates the importance of the absolute number of involved nodes in the disease-free interval, but when overall survival was considered, it was the percentage rather than the absolute number of involved nodes that determined the prognosis of a given patient. This finding should have an impact on the evaluation of Dukes' class C patients before they are subjected to adjuvant trials. Investigators must secure both the operative and the pathologic reports to accurately assess prognostic factors.

The site of the primary lesion was found by the Cox regression model to be an insignificant factor in disease-free interval and overall survival. However, the model was important in determining the *pattern* of tumor recurrence among patients receiving adjuvant therapy. It became clear that adjuvant therapy, as administered, had no significant effect on the *incidence* of local recurrence in patients with primary lesions arising in the rectum or rectosigmoid portions of the large bowel. This finding has led us to modify our protocol to include postoperative radiotherapy in an attempt to control the tendency of these patients to develop pelvic recurrence. We also have decided to change the administration of 5-FU from the oral to the intravenous route. This decision is based on recent information suggesting that oral administration results in unpredictable absorption, whereas the intravenous route gives more consistent results in plasma drug levels.

The periodic determination of plasma CEA levels was instrumental in the clinical follow-up of patients receiving adjuvant therapy. For a substantial number of patients, the sequential determination has led to a second-look operation at which recurrent tumor was found; in some cases, the tumor was resectable and the patients were saved. However, the elevation in the plasma CEA level correlated with clinical relapse in only 75% of the cases; in the remaining 25%, CEA levels remained low despite the growing tumor. This discrepancy may be related to the degree of differentiation of the various tumors; i.e., differentiated tumors would produce more CEA than would undifferentiated ones. It is important to note that the peak in the CEA level preceded the actual clinical relapse by approximately one to two months in almost all cases.

The immunologic monitoring by skin tests to recall antigens in patients receiving adjuvant therapy was disappointing. No correlation between reactivity to recall antigens prior to administration of adjuvant therapy and subsequent tumor status (no evidence of disease vs. tumor relapse) was observed (Table 1). This lack of correlation was noted also with subsequent changes in skin reactivity to the recall antigens except in the case of Varidase (Table 2). Of 42 patients who were initially anergic to Varidase, 22 remained anergic throughout the administration of adjuvant therapy, and 15 of these ultimately relapsed. Twenty patients experienced conversion to reactivity; of these, only five subsequently relapsed ($p < 0.02$).

Because of this disappointing experience with immunologic monitoring, we recently adopted a new immunobioassay to evaluate the immunocompetence of patients receiving adjuvant therapy. A local graft versus host reaction is elicited by intradermal injection of peripheral blood mononuclear cells (separated by Ficoll-Hypaque density solution centrifugation) into a rat that has been pretreated with cyclophosphamide. Cells from 90 of 91 (99%) normal donors produce a reaction, whereas cells from only 16 of 22 (73%) patients with Dukes' class C lesions and 3 of 10 (30%) patients with Dukes' class D (overt metastatic

Table 1. *Skin Reactivity to Recall Antigens Prior to Adjuvant Therapy:*
Relation to Clinical Outcome

Recall Antigen	No Evidence of Disease	Tumor Recurrence
Dermatophytin		
Negative	19	18
Positive	10	5
Varidase		
Negative	22	20
Positive	7	4
Candida		
Negative	6	4
Positive	23	19
Mumps		
Negative	8	11
Positive	16	11

Table 2. *Changes in Skin Reactivity to Varidase During Adjuvant Therapy: Relation to Clinical Outcome*

Skin Reactivity	Initial Reactivity	
	Negative (n = 42)	Positive (n = 11)
Remained		
Negative	22	...
Positive	...	9
With tumor recurrence	15*	2
Converted		
Negative	...	2
Positive	20	...
With tumor recurrence	5*	2

* $p < 0.02$.

disease) produce a reaction. We hope this new test will be more practical for the sequential evaluation of immunocompetence in patients receiving adjuvant therapy.

ACKNOWLEDGMENTS

This work was supported by Public Health Service grant 1 R26 CA 15458–04 and in part by Hoffmann-LaRoche grant 169196.

Giora Mavligit, M.D., is recipient of Career Development Award CA 1 KO 4 CA 00130–03 from the National Institutes of Health.

REFERENCE

Mavligit, G. M., Gutterman, J. U., Burgess, M. A., Khankhanian, N., Seibert, G. B., Speer, J. F., Reed, R. C., Jubert, A. V., Martin, R. C., McBride, C. M., Copeland, E. M., Gehan, E. A., and Hersh, E. M. 1975. Adjuvant immunotherapy and chemoimmunotherapy in colorectal cancer of the Dukes' C classification. Cancer, 36:2421–2427.

PRINCIPLES AND PROSPECTS FOR IMMUNOTHERAPY

Immunotherapy of Human Cancer,
The University of Texas System Cancer Center
M. D. Anderson Hospital and Tumor Institute.
Raven Press, New York © 1978.

Some New Approaches to Cancer Immunotherapy in Man

Lucien Israël, M.D., Richard Edelstein, M.D., and Raymond Samak, M.D.

Chemotherapy and Immunotherapy Unit, University of Paris XIII, Centre Hospitalier Universitaire de Bobigny, Bobigny, France

The variable results obtained by different groups of chemotherapists no longer surprise anyone, but many oncologists still find this same variability exasperating when encountered in cancer immunotherapy. This is understandable because spontaneous cancer in man, unlike experimental malignant tumors, may be accompanied by immunosuppression related to a wide variety of mechanisms that may occur in a wide variety of combinations and change during the course of the disease. The future of immunotherapy probably lies in identifying individual mechanisms and appropriately correcting them. At present, individual identification and correction is not possible in most cases. However, recent clinical and experimental findings warrant the proposition of new approaches for controlled trials.

We shall confine our considerations to the identification and correction of immunosuppressive states resulting directly or indirectly from the tumor itself. Viewed from this angle, immunosuppression may be considered a series of measures allowing the tumor to protect itself against the host. We shall not discuss the undoubtedly important problem of congenital or acquired immunosuppressive states that may precede or even promote the appearance of certain human tumors.

CONSIDERATIONS OF IMMUNOTHERAPEUTIC APPROACHES IN IMMUNOCOMPETENT PATIENTS

Disease Stage

Some patients with widespread disease do retain a state of immunocompetence, as far as can be assessed, for example, with delayed hypersensitivity skin tests

---

Abbreviations used in this chapter: CCNU—1-(2-chloroethyl)-3-cyclohexyl-1-nitrosourea; EORTC—European Organization for Research on Treatment of Cancer; T-lymphocytes—thymus-dependent lymphocytes; TNM—tumor, node (lymph), metastasis.

and mitogen-induced lymphocyte transformation in vitro. We have reported (Israël, 1973, 1974a) series of lung cancer patients in which similar degrees of immunosuppression were observed in patients with locally confined, operable tumors and those with metastatic disease.

Patients who have retained their immunocompetence have more slowly progressing disease and a better postoperative prognosis (Eilber and Morton, 1970). Our findings in 451 patients with resected lung cancer followed up without treatment confirm this observation (Israël *et al.,* 1973). Longer survival also is associated with an adequate immune status in patients with disseminated disease (Israël and Edelstein, 1975).

Lymph Node Involvement

Irrespective of primary tumor sites, patients with uninvolved lymph nodes have a better postoperative prognosis. This finding has been taken into account in many types of staging more or less derived from the TNM classification. Indeed, we have observed (unpublished data) a close correlation between the delayed hypersensitivity response and lymph node status.

Despite the usual interpretation to the contrary, tumor involvement of lymph nodes should not be considered a phenomenon reflecting or related to the duration of tumor growth. Indeed, the time it would take tumor cells to reach regional lymph nodes from a primary tumor must surely be on the order of a few hours or even days, but certainly not years. Our personal opinion is, therefore, that the absence of lymph node involvement on pathologic examination simply reflects the ability of lymphocytes to kill cancer cells that reach the lymph node and, in fact, reflects the patient's immune status, rather than the tumor's extension in space or time. If, after surgery, lymph nodes succumb to invasion by tumor cells, as is often the case with surgically removed malignant melanoma without radical lymph node dissection, it is probably because cells in regional microscopic foci that have escaped the surgeon's knife eventually suppress regional, and then general, immune reactivity by one of the mechanisms we shall examine later. We feel that this explains the better prognosis associated with cases classified N_0.

Nonspecific Immune Stimulation

We have reported two randomized trials (Israël and Halpern, 1972; Israël, 1974b) comparing chemotherapy alone and chemotherapy combined with *Corynebacterium parvum* for disseminated cancer. These two trials showed that patients who retained their immunocompetence and were treated with immunotherapy did significantly better, in terms of survival, than others.

An interesting, recent study (McKneally *et al.,* 1977) showed that, among patients with resected lung cancer treated postoperatively with intrapleural bacillus Calmette-Guérin (BCG), only those with no lymph node involvement differed from untreated control subjects and derived any benefit from this regional, nonspecific immunostimulation.

In view of the above data, patients who have retained their immunocompetence appear to be good candidates for nonspecific immunostimulation. It is unnecessary to submit these patients to any form of immunorestoration, such as treatment with levamisole or thymosin, nor is it necessary to attempt to remove blocking factors. These patients, from the outset, may be treated with immunotherapy capable of activating (Halpern *et al.,* 1964) and increasing the number of macrophages (Fisher *et al.,* 1975), and enhancing specific antibody secretion (Woodruff *et al.,* 1974). If patients with or without an adequate immune status are submitted indiscriminately to immune stimulation, the results obtained, not surprisingly, will be sometimes perplexing and difficult to interpret. There is also the important question raised by the work of McKneally and his colleagues (1977); i.e., in locally confined tumors, should efforts be directed to regional rather than systemic immune stimulation? At present, only a comparative trial can provide an answer to this question. Our personal experience with prolonged treatment of malignant melanoma of the extremities by regional BCG injections between the primary tumor and draining lymph nodes suggests that regional stimulation is preferable, but does not allow us to reach any definite conclusions.

TUMOR-DEPENDENT IMMUNOSUPPRESSIVE MECHANISMS

Apart from the seemingly few cases in which immunosuppression precedes the appearance of cancer and those in which tumor antigenicity is weak or related to a histocompatibility system, there are many cases, possibly the vast majority, in which immunosuppression is induced directly or indirectly by the tumor itself. We shall not discuss the considerable amount of evidence supporting this, but we shall refer simply to two personal studies (Israël *et al.,* 1968, 1973) in which we observed that, following surgical resection of a tumor, a substantial number of patients whose nonspecific immune reactivity was formerly suppressed once again exhibited an adequate response. A number of clinical and experimental studies have shed light on some of these mechanisms, and we shall briefly describe some of them before discussing the immunotherapeutic approaches to which they may give rise.

Induction of Synthesis of Nonspecific Immunosuppressive and Anti-Inflammatory Factors by the Liver

Numerous reports showing that some acute-phase reactants attain elevated levels in tumor-bearing animals and cancer patients have been published (Greenspan *et al.,* 1951; Greenspan, 1955; Sarcione, 1967; Zacharia and Pollard, 1969; Snyder and Ashwell, 1971; Ablin *et al.,* 1971, 1973; Lilley *et al.,* 1974; Harris *et al.,* 1974; Cooper *et al.,* 1976; Krolikowski *et al.,* 1976; Latner *et al.,* 1976). Our own studies (Israël *et al.,* 1976b, 1977; Israël and Edelstein, 1978) have shown that this is a general, though unequally distributed, phenomenon among cancer patients and that there is a correlation between the serum levels of acute-phase reactants and extent of disease such that these proteins may, to some extent, be considered markers of tumor growth. We also have observed (Israël and Edelstein, 1978) that some of these proteins can inhibit phytohemagglutinin (PHA) blastogenesis in vitro, particularly when their concentration in the medium is higher than that found in normal subjects and approximates the levels found in cancer patients. Therefore, the presence of a tumor triggers hepatic synthesis of globulins, essentially those migrating in the α_1 and α_2 regions, endowed with immunosuppressant properties. These glycoproteins are all rich in sialic acid, by which they might be able to mask receptor sites on lymphocytes and macrophages. Our hypothesis, then, is that these proteins work as nonspecific blocking factors with regard to immunocytes and provide a partial explanation for the negativity of various tests of delayed hypersensitivity, the suppressed lymphocyte response to mitogens, and the reduction or suppression of specific cytotoxicity. Moreover, sera from cancer patients can inhibit PHA blastogenesis in vitro, and in vitro washing of these lymphocytes improves responsiveness to PHA (Mannick *et al.,* 1977).

Secretion of Nonspecific Immunosuppressive Substances by Tumor Cells

It has been shown also that tumor cells secrete and tumor cell membranes bear immunosuppressive glycoproteins and polypeptides (Graham and Graham, 1975; Mongini and Rosenberg, 1975; Reznik and Winzler, 1975; Bhavanandan and Davidson, 1976; Wang *et al.,* 1977) and that tumor cells also can secrete substances that repel macrophages (Fauve *et al.,* 1974). Therefore, in addition to the previously described secretion of nonspecific blocking factors by the host in response to a signal from the tumor, nonspecific blocking factors are produced also by the tumor itself and contribute very early to its protection against immune surveillance and destruction mechanisms.

Depletion of Nonspecific Immunostimulant Substances

Normal persons possess various immunostimulant compounds that exert non-specific effects (Badger *et al.,* 1976; Chapman and Hibbs, 1977). One of these is a nonspecific opsonin that migrates with the α_2-globulins (DiLuzio *et al.,* 1972; Saba, 1975; Blumenstock *et al.,* 1976). This nonspecific opsonin has been shown to diminish rapidly in the sera of animals bearing experimentally induced tumors, and its reinjection results in an increase in activated macrophage-mediated tumor cell killing. Humoral control of reticuloendothelial function probably plays an important role. The challenge resulting from the introduction of a sufficiently large number of tumor cells conceivably might lead to disturbance and weakening of this control mechanism through a reduction of available opsonizing factors.

Specific Blocking Factors Produced by Tumor and by Host-Tumor Interaction

The phenomenon of specific blocking of antitumor immunity described by the Hellströms and colleagues (1971) initially was ascribed to antitumor antibodies that, by binding to membrane antigens of tumor cells, were believed to protect the latter against cellular mechanisms mediated by lymphocytes and macrophages. It was soon recognized that specific blocking was due, in fact, either to immune complexes formed by soluble antigen and antibody or to circulating tumor-associated antigen itself (Sjögren *et al.*, 1971; Currie and Basham, 1972; Grosser and Thompson, 1976; Friedman *et al.*, 1976). Tumor cells produce and shed soluble antigen (Bystryn, 1977; Nordquist *et al.*, 1977) that can block receptor sites on lymphocytes and macrophages. Circulating immune complexes bind to immunocytes in the presence of excess antigen and to target cell membranes in the presence of excess antibody. The role of these immune complexes in inhibiting specific immune reactions appears to be well established.

Effects of Immunosuppressive Phenomena on Antitumor Immunity

Ideally, one day we will be able to determine for each patient and for each period in the development of a tumor how the described factors interact, as this would allow individualized immunotherapy. Today we already can appreciate the overall effects of these phenomena on antitumor immunity: (1) Certain nonspecific blocking factors inhibit inflammation, i.e., chemotaxis, vasodilatation, and release of biogenic amines in the tumor's immediate environment (Bernstein *et al.*, 1972; Franchi *et al.*, 1972; Hirata-Hibi and Murray, 1974; Fauve *et al.*, 1974; Boetcher and Leonard, 1974; Snyderman and Pike, 1976; McVie *et al.*, 1977; Normann and Sorkin, 1977). (2) The absence of nonspecific stimulant factors inhibits phagocytosis and the contact between nonspecifically activated macrophages and tumor cells. (3) Nonspecific recognition by macrophages (Hibbs, 1973) is inhibited by glycoproteins, which mask binding sites on immunologically competent cells. (4) Specific recognition by macrophages and lymphocytes is inhibited by circulating immune complexes and circulating, soluble tumor-associated antigen. (5) Secretion of lymphokines and other products showing lymphocyte tropism secreted by macrophages, which normally occurs when the immunocytes come in contact with target cell membranes, does not take place.

When these various phenomena are combined, one can easily see why the prognosis for initially immunosuppressed patients is poor and why attempts at immunostimulation, both specific and nonspecific, meet with such poor results. For immunosuppressed patients, there is a need for new immunotherapeutic procedures capable, if possible, of reversing or overcoming the above-described situations.

PROPOSALS FOR NEW IMMUNOTHERAPEUTIC PROCEDURES

Removal of Circulating Blocking Factors

It may be hypothesized that all the described circulating factors, both specific and nonspecific, bind to macrophages and lymphocytes as they are produced in the bone marrow, rendering them nonoperational as soon as they enter the circulation. For this reason, we have begun treating patients with disseminated disease by repeated plasmapheresis (Israël *et al.,* 1976a,c, 1977; Israël and Edelstein, 1978). The procedure consists of two 5-liter plasma exchanges weekly with replacement using fresh frozen plasma from normal donors, washing and reinjection of leukocytes, and reinjection of red cells and platelets. The total number of plasma exchange sessions varies from six to 12. Among 23 evaluable patients with metastatic disease, we have observed eight partial responses. We observed a transient decrease in all the acute-phase reactants, as well as other plasma proteins, including the gamma globulins (IgG and IgM, but not IgA) and transferrin. These preliminary investigations did not include assays for circulating immune complexes. A study currently in progress (Israël *et al.,* unpublished data) has shown that, following a single plasmapheresis, levels of acute-phase reactants return to their base line within 48 hours; hence, the ideal schedule for plasma exchange would be three times rather than twice a week.

Plasmapheresis is an entirely empirical procedure and probably could be improved upon. Also, we do not know what effect it has on levels of nonspecific factors of tumor origin or specific blocking factors. Nevertheless, the fact that we have observed objective responses in patients with widely disseminated tumors is highly encouraging. It also emphasizes the fact that the immune system stands ready to fulfill its function as soon as inhibiting factors are removed, even temporarily; this supports our hypothesis that protective mechanisms triggered by the tumor against the host may play a major role in the host-tumor relationship. Our observations do not exclude the possibility that the fresh frozen plasma used as replacement fluid may contain immunostimulant factors, such as aspecific opsonins, which may contribute to the phenomena observed.

Removal of Membrane-Bound Blocking Factors

Removal of circulating blocking factors is most often insufficient for obtaining the desired immunotherapeutic effect; then it is necessary to remove blocking factors bound to the membranes of lymphocytes and macrophages. This may be achieved by successive washings, as we have performed and as Mannick and co-workers (1977) have shown to be effective in vitro. More complete elimination probably would be achieved by incubating patients' leukocytes with an enzyme at the end of each plasma exchange session before reinjecting them, and this technique is about to be initiated in our unit. Neuraminidase is probably the most adequate enzyme in this respect, in view of the high sialic acid content of glycoproteins belonging to the group of acute-phase reactants. Other enzymes probably would have to be used to detach other types of specific or nonspecific blocking factors from immunocyte membranes.

Compensation of Exhaustible Factors

To the best of our knowledge, no clinical trials have been undertaken with the previously described humoral recognition factor reported by Saba (1975) and DiLuzio *et al.* (1972). This α-globulin would be a good candidate for clinical trials in man in situations in which blocking factors are absent or have been removed.

Immunocytes themselves may be considered, in some respect, exhaustible factors because lymphocytes and macrophages are often found in abnormally small numbers in cancer patients and this is associated with poor prognosis. This reduction in lymphocyte and macrophage numbers may be due to the higher proliferation rate of tumor cells and hence to "consumption" of immunocytes. The solution, then, would be to reinject isogenic cells previously obtained and stocked for this purpose, and it might well be that in the future, all types of surgery on cancer patients will include obtaining bone marrow tissue to be stocked for future use.

Reduction in the number of immunocytes, of course, also may be due to chemotherapy. It has been shown that nonspecific immunostimulants may induce proliferation of macrophage precursors in bone marrow (Fisher *et al.,* 1975; Dimitrov *et al.,* 1975). Numerous reports have shown also that, in man, the addition of immunotherapy to chemotherapy prolongs the duration of response (Israël, 1975, 1976). These reports recently have been confirmed by the preliminary results of the EORTC study of patients with resected lung cancer (Israël *et al.,* unpublished data). This study showed that, following surgery, disease-free intervals differed little among patients followed up with systemic immunotherapy with BCG; chemotherapy with cyclophosphamide, CCNU, and methotrexate; and no treatment. In contrast, a combination of the same chemotherapy and the same immunotherapy gave significantly better results at two and three years.

Restoration of Reticuloendothelial System and Lymphocyte Functions

It has been shown that levamisole (Amery, 1976; Schmidt and Douglas, 1976) and thymosin (Constanzi *et al.,* 1977) can restore altered immune function after prolonged malfunction. Here again it seems that these agents should be given clinical trials in immunoincompetent patients after removal of blocking factors.

Direct Injection of Lymphokines

Lymphokines secreted by immunocytes stimulated in vitro have been used with some immediate, positive effects in cancer patients (Djerassi, personal communication). In situations in which lymphokines are no longer secreted, owing to a recognition and stimulation defect, reinjection of such material into cancer patients could help restore some immune mechanisms of tumor cell killing.

IDEAL SEQUENCES, TIMING, AND SITUATIONS FOR NEW IMMUNOTHERAPEUTIC APPROACHES

We have mentioned that the turnover of blocking factors is rapid. In this respect, it is evident that plasmapheresis cannot be of lasting benefit; yet during the 24 hours that follow each plasma exchange session (with reinjection of lymphocytes that have been washed and, ideally, treated with neuraminidase), there is a propitious situation for maximum immune stimulation. This period is theoretically the most satisfactory for replacing the depleted pool of nonspecific opsonins and for restoring the functional capacity of T-lymphocytes and macrophages with thymosin or levamisole. Also during this period, nonspecific immune stimulation might be expected to produce its best results. We have undertaken a trial to compare successive plasmapheresis alone and plasmapheresis immediately followed by an intravenous injection of *C. parvum,* which we consider one of the most effective, clinically practicable immunostimulants (Israël *et al.,* 1975).

Circulating tumor antigen increases considerably following massive tumor destruction, regardless of whether this is achieved by radiotherapy or chemotherapy. It would seem logical, therefore, to undertake plasmapheresis immediately following such therapy to avoid immunologic blocking, which interferes with complete control of tumor growth. Serum assays for circulating immune complexes and tumor antigen prior to and following radiotherapy and chemotherapy would be essential and should precede clinical trials designed to compare these treatment modalities alone and in alternation with plasma exchange. The relatively high incidence of nephrotic syndromes supervening during chemotherapy may be relevant in this respect.

The highest levels of nonspecific blocking factors are observed before treatment, when a large tumor burden is present. Thus, extensive, rapidly growing tumors are good indications for plasmapheresis. However, in practice, plasmapheresis may prove difficult to perform before and after chemotherapy or radiotherapy. The most satisfactory approach, therefore, seems to be that described above, i.e., conventional treatment by physical or chemical agents, followed by adequate restoration of conditions for proper immunologic function. In such cases, an objective tumor response cannot be expected from immunotherapy because the tumor already will have responded to chemotherapy or radiotherapy.

However, this is a problem to which conventional therapists will have to become accustomed. The efficacy of these procedures will have to be assessed by end results and survival rates, rather than response rates.

The fact remains that, for both immunotherapy and more conventional treatment modalities, the ideal situation is that in which tumor cells are as few as possible.

If the procedures described prove feasible and safe, we would like to see them undertaken after surgery. We explained earlier why there is no point undertaking such procedures in patients with stage I disease. In contrast, completely excised stage II disease with lymph node involvement is a highly satisfactory indication. It is in this direction that we plan to develop our future studies. A trial with various stage II cancers comparing no treatment and plasmapheresis, or chemotherapy and chemotherapy preceded by plasmapheresis as postoperative follow-up presently appears the most appropriate design to elucidate the role these new immunotherapeutic approaches may play in the coming years.

CONCLUSIONS

The ideas developed in this paper confirm that immunotherapy has an important role in oncology, a role that is in keeping with the importance and complexity of the immunologic phenomena involved in tumor growth and that is only beginning to be taken into account.

Among the numerous phenomena involved, we have emphasized particularly those that depend on the tumor itself because we believe they are decisive, and we have attempted to describe them so that they may serve as a guideline for future immunotherapeutic attempts. The following facts emerge from this description: (1) The various modalities of immunostimulation currently in use should be applied only to patients who have retained an adequate immune status, whereby they can respond to these modalities. (2) Immunoincompetence probably is due, to a large extent, to the conjunction of specific and nonspecific blocking factors secreted by the host or the tumor, or to host-tumor interaction. Immunoincompetent patients, therefore, cannot be expected to respond to immunostimulation or immunorestoration until such factors have been removed as completely as possible. For this reason, we have suggested, on an empirical basis, repeated plasmapheresis, which in our experience has proved capable of inducing objective tumor regression. Our studies of plasmapheresis are being pursued and currently are directed to deriving the maximum efficacy from this procedure and to combining it with traditional therapeutic methods under optimal conditions. These attempts have been made in patients with widespread disease; as with chemotherapy, however, it is in patients with less extensive disease, such as postoperative stage II cases, that the future of these modalities lies.

REFERENCES

Ablin, R. J., Soanes, W. A., Bronson, P. M., and Gonder, M. J. 1971. Serum proteins in patients with benign and malignant diseases of the prostate. Neoplasma, 18:271–276.

Ablin, R. J., Gonder, M. J., and Soanes, W. A. 1973. Serum proteins in prostatic cancer. I. Relationship between clinical stage and level. J. Urol., 110:238–241.

Amery, W. K. 1976. Double-blind levamisole trial in resectable lung cancer. Ann. NY Acad. Sci., 277:260–268.

Badger, A. M., Merluzzi, V. H., and Cooperband, S. R. 1976. Immunostimulatory and immunosuppressive factors in human cancer ascites fluids: Effect on the primary plaque forming response in vitro. Cell. Immunol., 27:126–130.

Bernstein, I. D., Zbar, B., and Rapp, H. J. 1972. Impaired inflammatory response in tumor-bearing guinea pigs. J. Natl. Cancer Inst., 49:1641–1647.

Bhavanandan, V. P., and Davidson, E. A. 1976. Characteristics of a mucin type sialoglycopeptide produced by B16 mouse melanoma cells. Biochem. Biophys. Res. Commun., 70:139–145.

Blumenstock, F., Saba, T. M., Weber, P., and Cho, E. 1976. Purification and biochemical characterisation of a macrophage stimulating alpha-2-globulin opsonic protein. J. Reticuloendothel. Soc., 19:157–172.

Boetcher, D. A., and Leonard, E. J. 1974. Abnormal monocyte chemotactic response in cancer patients. J. Natl. Cancer Inst., 52:1091–1099.

Bystryn, J. C. 1977. Release of cell-surface tumor-associated antigens by viable melanoma cells from humans. J. Natl. Cancer Inst., 59:325–328.

Chapman, H. A., Jr., and Hibbs, J. B., Jr. 1977. Modulation of macrophage tumoricidal capability by components of normal serum: A central role for lipid. Science, 97:282–285.

Constanzi, J. J., Gagliano, R. G., Delarey, F., Harris, N., Thurman, G. B., Sakai, H., Goldstein, A. L., Loukas, D., Cohen, G. B., and Thomson, P. D. 1977. The effect of thymosin on patients with disseminated malignancies. A phase I study. Cancer, 40:14–19.

Cooper, E. H., Turner, R., Geekie, A., Munro-Neville, A., Goligher, J. C., Graham, N. G., Giles, G. R., Hall, R., and MacAdam, W. A. F. 1976. Alpha-globulins in the surveillance of colorectal carcinoma. Biomedicine, 24:171–178.

Currie, G. A., and Basham, C. 1972. Serum mediated inhibition of the immunological reactions of the patient to his own tumor: A possible role for circulating antigen. Br. J. Cancer, 26:426–438.

DiLuzio, N. R., McNamee, R., Olcay, I., Kitahama, A., and Miller, R. H. 1972. Alterations in plasma recognition factor activity in experimental leukemia. J. Reticuloendothel. Soc., 11:186–197.

Dimitrov, N. V., Andre, S., Eliopoulos, G., and Halpern, B. 1975. Effect of Corynebacterium parvum on bone marrow cell cultures. Proc. Soc. Exp. Biol. Med., 148:440–442.

Eilber, F. R., and Morton D. L. 1970. Impaired immunologic reactivity and recurrence following cancer surgery. Cancer, 25:362–367.

Fauve, R. M., Hevin, B., Jacob, H., Gaillard, J. A., and Jacob, F. 1974. Antiinflammatory effects of murine malignant cells. Proc. Natl. Acad. Sci. USA, 71:4052–4056.

Fisher, B., Wolmark, N., and Fisher, E. R. 1975. Results of investigations with Corynebacterium parvum in an experimental animal system. In Halpern, B. (ed.): *Corynebacterium parvum.* Applications in Clinical and Experimental Oncology. New York, Plenum Press, pp. 218–243.

Franchi, G., Reyers-Degli Innocenti, I., Standen, S., and Garattini, S. 1972. The inhibitory effect of cancer cell dissemination on the phagocytic activity of the reticuloendothelial system in tumor-bearing mice. J. Reticuloendothel. Soc., 12:618–628.

Friedman, H., Specter, S., Kamo, I., and Kateley, J. 1976. Tumor associated immunosuppressive factors. Ann. NY Acad. Sci., 276:417–430.

Graham, R. M., and Graham, M. M. 1975. Immunosuppressive peptides in patients with cancer (Letter to the Editor). N. Engl. J. Med., 292:701.

Greenspan, E. M. 1955. Clinical significance of serum mucoproteins. In Dock, W., and Snapper, I. (eds.): Advances in Internal Medicine. Chicago, Year Book Medical Publishers Inc., vol. 7, pp. 101–123.

Greenspan, E. M., Lehman, I., Graff, M. M., and Schoenbach, E. B. 1951. A comparative study of the serum glycoproteins in patients with parenchymatous hepatic disease or metastatic neoplasia. Cancer, 4:972–983.

Grosser, N., and Thompson, D. M. P. 1976. Tube leukocyte (monocyte) adherence inhibition assay for the detection of anti-tumour immunity. III. "Blockade" of monocyte reactivity by excess free antigen and immune complexes in advanced cancer patients. Int. J. Cancer, 18:58–66.

Halpern, B., Prévot, A. R., Biozzi, G., Stiffel, C., Mouton, D., Morard, J. C., Bouthillier, Y., and Decreusefond, C. 1964. Stimulation de l'activité du système réticuloendothélial provoquée par Corynebacterium parvum. J. Reticuloendothel. Soc., 1:77–96.

Harris, C. C., Primack, A., and Cohen, M. H. 1974. Elevated alpha-1-antitrypsin serum levels in lung cancer patients. Cancer, 34:280–281.

Hellström, I., Sjögren, H. O., Warner, G., and Hellström, K. E. 1971. Blocking of cell mediated tumor immunity by sera from patients with growing neoplasma. Int. J. Cancer, 7:226–237.

Hibbs, J. B., Jr. 1973. Macrophage non-immunologic recognition: Target cell factors related to contact inhibition. Science, 180:868–870.

Hirata-Hibi, M., and Murray, I. M. 1974. Acute inflammation as a prerequisite for the immune response. J. Reticuloendothel. Soc., 16:69–74.

Israël, L. 1973. Cell-mediated immunity in lung cancer patients: Data, problems and propositions. Cancer Chemother. Rep., 4:279–281.

Israël, L. 1974a. Non-specific immunostimulation in bronchogenic cancer. Scand. J. Resp. Dis., 89:95–105.

Israël, L. 1974b. A randomized study of chemotherapy versus chemotherapy and immune therapy with Corynebacterium parvum in advanced breast cancer (Abstract). In: Abstracts, XIth International Cancer Congress, Florence. Geneva, UICC, vol. 1, pp. 222–223.

Israël, L. 1975. Report on 414 cases of human tumors treated with Corynebacteria. In Halpern, B. (ed.): *Corynebacterium parvum.* Applications in Clinical and Experimental Oncology. New York, Plenum Press, pp. 389–401.

Israël, L. 1976. Immunochemotherapy with Corynebacterium parvum in disseminated cancer. Ann. NY Acad. Sci., 277:241–251.

Israël, L., Bouvrain, A., Cros-Decam, J., and Mugica, J. 1968. Contribution à l'étude des phénomènes d'immunité cellulaire chez les cancéreux pulmonaires avant traitement. Poumon Coeur, 24:339–344.

Israël, L., and Edelstein, R. 1975. Nonspecific immunostimulation with *Corynebacterium parvum* in human cancer. In: Immunological Aspects of Neoplasia (The University of Texas System Cancer Center M. D. Anderson Hospital and Tumor Institute 26th Annual Symposium on Fundamental Cancer Research, 1973). Baltimore, The Williams & Wilkins Company, pp. 485–504.

Israël, L., and Edelstein, R. 1978. In vivo and in vitro studies on non-specific blocking factors of host origin in cancer patients: Role of plasma exchange as an immunotherapeutic modality. Isr. J. Med. Sci., 14:105–130.

Israël, L., Edelstein, R., Depierre, A., and Dimitrov, N. V. 1975. Daily intravenous infusions of Corynebacterium parvum in twenty patients with disseminated cancer: A preliminary report of clinical and biological findings. J. Natl. Cancer Inst., 55:29–33.

Israël, L., Edelstein, R., Mannoni, P., and Radot, E. 1976a. Plasmapheresis and immunological control of cancer (Letter to the Editor). Lancet, 2:642–643.

Israël, L., Edelstein, R., Mannoni, P., Radot, E., and Greenspan, E. M. 1977. Plasmapheresis in patients with disseminated cancer: Clinical results and correlation with changes in serum proteins. The concept of non-specific blocking factors. Cancer, 40:3146–3154.

Israël, L., Greenspan, E. M., and Rousselet, F. 1976b. Distribution and significance of acute phase reactants in cancer patients at various stages and correlation with skin tests (Abstract). Proc. Am. Assoc. Cancer Res., 17:17.

Israël, L., and Halpern, B. 1972. Le Corynebacterium parvum dans les cancers avancés. Nouv. Presse Med., 1:19–23.

Israël, L., Mannoni, P., Radot, E., and Greenspan, E. M. 1976c. Réactions immunitaires et tumorales à l'échange de plasma dans les cancers avancés (Letter to the Editor). Nouv. Presse Med., 5:433.

Israël, L., Mugica, J., and Chahinian, P. 1973. Prognosis of early bronchogenic carcinoma. Survival curves of 451 patients after resection of lung cancer in relation to the results of the preoperative tuberculin skin test. Biomedicine, 19:68–72.

Krolikowski, F. J., Reuter, K., Waalkes, T. P., Sieber, S. M., and Adamson, R. H. 1976. Serum sialic acid levels in lung cancer patients. Pharmacology, 14:47–51.

Latner, A. L., Turner, G. A., and Lawin, M. M. 1976. Plasma alpha-1-antitrypsin levels in early and late carcinoma of the cervix. Oncology, 33:12–14.

Lilley, D. P., Burger, D. R., and Vetto, R. M. 1974. Tumor growth in the guinea pig: Alpha-globulin changes associated with lymphocyte suppression. J. Natl. Cancer Inst., 53:701–709.

Mannick, J. A., Constantian, M., Pardridge, E., Saporoschetz, L., and Badger, A. 1977. Improvement of phytohemagglutinin responsiveness of lymphocytes from cancer patients after washing in vitro. Cancer Res., 37:3066–3070.

McKneally, M. F., Maver, C. M., and Kausel, H. W. 1977. Intrapleural BCG immunostimulation in lung cancer (Letter to the Editor). Lancet, 1:593.

McVie, J. G., Logan, E. C. M., and Kay, A. B. 1977. Monocyte function in cancer patients Eur. J. Cancer, 13:351–353.

Mongini, P. K., and Rosenberg, L. T. 1975. Inhibition of lymphocyte trapping by cell free ascitic fluid cultivated in syngeneic mice. J. Immunol., 114:650–654.

Nordquist, R. E., Anglin, J. H., and Lerner, M. P. 1977. Antibody-induced antigen redistribution and shedding from human breast cancer cells. Science, 197:366–367.

Normann, S. J., and Sorkin, E. 1977. Inhibition of macrophage chemotaxis by neoplastic and other rapidly proliferating cells in vitro. Cancer Res., 37:705–711.

Reznik, A. Z., and Winzler, R. J. 1975. Glycoproteins from ascitic fluid of Ehrlich ascites tumor. Isolation and chemical characterization. Biochim. Biophys. Acta, 404:268–273.

Saba, T. M. 1975. Aspecific opsonins. In Neter, E., and Milgrom, F. (eds.): The Immune System and Infectious Diseases. Basel, S. Karger, pp. 489–504.

Sarcione, E. J. 1967. Hepatic synthesis and secretory release of plasma alpha-2 (acute-phase)-globulin appearing in malignancy. Cancer Res., 27:2025–2033.

Schmidt, M. E., and Douglas, S. D. 1976. Effects of levamisole on human monocyte function and immunoprotein receptors. Clin. Immunol. Immunopathol. 6:299–305.

Sjögren, H. O., Hellström, I., Bansal, S. C., and Hellström, K. E. 1971. Suggestive evidence that the blocking antibodies of tumor-bearing individuals may be antigen-antibody complexes. Proc. Natl. Acad. Sci. USA, 68:1372–1375.

Snyder, S., and Ashwell, G. 1971. Quantitation of specific serum glycoproteins in malignancy. Clin. Chim. Acta, 34:449–455.

Snyderman, R., and Pike, M. C. 1976. An inhibitor of macrophage chemotaxis produced by neoplasms. Science, 192:370–372.

Wang, B. S., Badger, A. M., Nimberg, R. R., Cooperband, S. R., Schmid, K., and Mannick, J. A. 1977. Suppression of tumor-specific cell-mediated cytotoxicity by immunoregulatory alpha-globulin and by immunoregulatory alpha-globulin-like peptides from cancer patients. Cancer Res., 37:3022–3025.

Woodruff, M. F. A., McBride, W. H., and Dunbar, N. 1974. Tumour growth, phagocytic activity and antibody response in Corynebacterium parvum-treated mice. Clin. Exp. Immunol., 17:509–518.

Zacharia, T. P., and Pollard, M. 1969. Elevated levels of alpha-globulins in sera from germ-free rats with methylcholanthrene-induced tumors. J. Natl. Cancer Inst., 42:35–38.

Immunotherapy of Human Cancer,
The University of Texas System Cancer Center
M. D. Anderson Hospital and Tumor Institute.
Raven Press, New York © 1978.

Limitations, Obstacles, and Controversies in the Optimal Development of Immunotherapy

Michael J. Mastrangelo, M.D., David Berd, M.D., and Robert E. Bellet, M.D.

Melanoma Unit, The Fox Chase Cancer Center, Philadelphia, Pennsylvania

The first decade of the modern age of human tumor immunotherapy is coming to a close. The great enthusiasm with which this period began was based on the exciting results achieved by Morton (1971) in malignant melanoma, Klein *et al.* (1973) in cutaneous neoplasms, van Scott and Winters (1970) in mycosis fungoides, and Mathé *et al.* (1969) in acute lymphoblastic leukemia. However, subsequent advances have been modest. The early promise of human tumor immunotherapy still awaits fulfillment. Our hypothesis is that if tumor immunotherapy can be effective, this will be most readily demonstrable in animal models. In the paragraphs that follow, we will attempt to define and analyze the obstacles and limitations in human tumor immunotherapy by comparing the progress made in this area with the results achieved in animal tumor immunotherapy. Controversies, which are usually man-made, will be considered separately from obstacles and limitations, which are generally naturally occurring phenomena.

OBSTACLES AND LIMITATIONS

Animal Tumor Immunotherapy

Immunotherapy for animal tumors is reviewed in detail by Basombrio (1973); thus, only highlights and more recent developments will be presented.

Demonstration of Animal Tumor Antigens

By the end of the 19th century, investigators had succeeded in adapting spontaneously arising mouse tumors to grow in allogeneic hosts. The celebrated work of Pasteur with infectious diseases undoubtedly stimulated attempts at tumor immunotherapy. Ehrlich (1907) was probably the first to demonstrate that mice could be immunized against these allogeneic tumors. He observed that animals in which low-virulence tumors had grown and regressed were resistant to subsequent inoculations of more virulent tumors. Similar observations were made by others. Bashford *et al.* (1908), in studies of the growth of a mouse tumor in rats, showed that the initial mouse tumor transplant survived eight to nine days in the rat; however, a second mouse tumor transplant was destroyed in three to four days. The investigators erroneously postulated that this accelerated tumor destruction represented the development of antitumor immunity in the rat. It soon became clear that not only cancer tissues, but also normal tissues could immunize against tumor grafts (Bridre, 1907). Further, it was observed that there was an essential difference between primary and transplanted tumors in that primary tumors seldom regressed and an animal could not be made resistant to its own primary tumor.

The discovery of histocompatibility antigens provided an explanation for these observations. The immunity that developed against transplantable tumors was directed, at least in part, against normal histocompatibility antigens, those antigens normally present in all tissues of an individual and that differ from individual to individual (except between identical twins) within a species.

The inability with then available techniques to distinguish between tumor-specific and transplantation immunity led to a decline in interest in tumor immunology. Of the possible solutions to this problem, two are apparent. Ideally, techniques could have been developed to isolate, purify, and characterize tumor-specific antigens. Such antigens would have been powerful tools in the study of both animal and human tumor immunology. Instead, the influence of histocompatibility antigens was eliminated through the development of syngeneic strains of animals. The availability of syngeneic animals provided a stimulus to the study of animal tumor immunology, but unfortunately, this approach is not applicable to the study of human tumor immunology.

The definitive demonstration of tumor-specific transplantation antigens was reported by Prehn and Main (1957). These investigators demonstrated that syngeneic mice could be immunized (with the growth and excision technique) against a chemically induced tumor and yet accept a skin graft from the animal in which the tumor had arisen. The antigens involved were unique to the tumor tissue and not shared by normal tissue. Since these initial studies, tumor-specific transplantation antigens have been demonstrated to be present in some spontaneous animal tumors, as well as in most tumors induced by chemical agents, viruses, and physical agents. The antigens present on chemically induced tumors were originally thought to be unique to individual tumors; however, newer in vitro techniques suggest some cross-reactivity.

Accomplishments in Animal Tumor Immunotherapy

Tumor antigens have been conclusively demonstrated in a large number of animal tumors. Both outbred and syngeneic animals are available in relative abundance. Their manipulation is not hampered by ethical considerations. If tumor immunotherapy can be effective, this should be most readily demonstrable in animal models.

Immunoprophylaxis by Active-Specific Immunization

It is possible to immunize a variety of animals against the induction of viral cancers and leukemias. This has been achieved with rabbit fibromas (Allison, 1966) and papillomas (Shope, 1937), and with a variety of viral sarcomas, carcinomas, and lymphoid neoplasms of chickens, hamsters, and mice (Burmester, 1955; Friend, 1966; Larson *et al.,* 1967; Biggs *et al.,* 1970). In most of these experiments, the oncogenic virus was applied after vaccination. However, in the more relevant case of a virus that is already present in the animal at the time of vaccination, it has been possible, in a few situations, to achieve measurable immunization. For example, the incidence of spontaneous lymphomas can be reduced in AKR mice inoculated with irradiated extracts of syngeneic leukemias (Latarjet, 1964).

The immunologic prevention of chemically induced tumors is complicated by the theoretical problem that the specific antigen needed for vaccination may not be available until the tumor appears. It is thus important to know whether the antigenic determinants on chemically induced tumors are unique, or at least partially cross-reactive or limited in diversity to a reasonable total number, in which case vaccination with pools of several tumors might expose the animal to all the possible antigenic determinants that any tumor might develop. This issue has not been resolved, and at present, the prevention of chemically induced tumors has not been achieved by specific immunization. However, syngeneic animals can be immunized against transplanted, chemically induced tumors. This, of course, is not a clinically relevant experiment.

Immunoprophylaxis by Nonspecific Immunostimulation

The injection of substances and organisms, such as bacillus Calmette-Guérin (BCG) and *Corynebacterium parvum,* that stimulate the reticuloendothelial system can prevent the appearance or retard the growth of tumors in the autochthonous or syngeneic host (Laucius *et al.,* 1974; Berd, 1978). However, these successes may not be based on stimulation of tumor-specific immunity, but on activation of a nonspecific killer mechanism.

Immunoprophylaxis by Passive or Adoptive Transfer of Immunity

Some success has been achieved with passive and adoptive immunoprophylaxis in animal tumor systems. Many investigators have demonstrated that immune lymphocytes administered to animals prior to challenge with tumor cells are capable of preventing the subsequent outgrowth of tumor. This work has been reviewed extensively (Old and Boyse, 1964; Klein, 1966). The effects of immune serum are less dramatic. Gorer and Amos (1956) raised antibody to EL-4 lymphoma in allogeneic mice and noted that this antibody could protect against tumor growth if given prior to EL-4 injection. This approach to immunoprophylaxis requires that the immune-effector elements be given in close proximity to the oncogenic stimulus and thus is not clinically applicable.

Treatment of Established Tumors by Specific Immunization

Attempts have been made to immunize the host animal against a tumor that is already growing by reinjecting tumor cells away from the primary growth. The rationale is that the in situ growing tumor may not be eliciting the maximum or optimal immune response, and reexposure of tumor cells at a different site might do so. The literature is replete with failures. The few positive trials warrant brief mention. The added immunotherapeutic procedure of reinjecting irradiated autologous tumor tissue in rats bearing primary methylcholanthrene-induced sarcomas improved the therapeutic effect of partial excision and irradiation of the tumor (Alexander, 1968). Mathé et al. (1969b) were able to substantially prolong the survival of mice transplanted with L1210 leukemia cells by immunotherapy with BCG plus irradiated L1210 cells. The effect was indirectly related to the number of living L1210 cells transplanted. By reinjecting tumor cells incubated with *Vibrio cholerae* neuraminidase into mice bearing a transplanted methylcholanthrene-induced sarcoma, Rios and Simmons (1972) achieved remarkable therapeutic results. The growth of most tumors was retarded, and some regressed completely. Likhite (1976a) specifically conjugated *Bordetella pertussis* to T1699 tumor cells using toluidine-2-4-diisocyanate and used this conjugate to treat DBA/2 mice with established (seven-day-old) subcutaneous tumors. After a period of tumor growth, all tumors regressed, some completely.

Treatment of Established Tumors with Nonspecific Immunostimulants

The striking therapeutic successes with nonspecific immunostimulants have been in their intralesional application in the guinea pig hepatoma model. Working with an inbred strain of guinea pigs and a transplantable hepatocarcinoma, Zbar et al. (1971) demonstrated that intralesional BCG can induce regression of established, dermal tumor transplants as well as stimulate tumor-specific cell-mediated immunity. They found that tumor regression requires an intact immune system and direct contact between BCG and tumor cells. The therapeutic efficacy of intralesional therapy has been extended to an ocular cancer in cattle (Rapp et al., 1976).

There are many other animal tumor models in which therapeutic success has been achieved with nonspecific immune modulators. The therapy trials with BCG (Laucius et al., 1974), *C. parvum* (Berd, 1978), and levamisole (Symoens and Rosenthal, 1977) have been reviewed. In general, the therapeutic effect has been modest, that is, retardation of tumor growth rather than tumor regression and cure. Further, success has been achieved under such strictly defined conditions that duplication of results in other laboratories is often difficult and extension to other species almost impossible. For example, the results achieved by Likhite (1974) and Purnell *et al.* (1975) with intralesional *B. pertussis* in the CAD$_2$ mammary adenocarcinoma system varied widely. The frequency of this inconsistency may result from the facts that the models in studies reported in the literature are carefully chosen from a larger number of negative systems and thus represent only a small fraction of the models tested, that the therapeutic effects are meager, and that test conditions are critical. Attempts to extrapolate these models to the clinic, therefore, would be hopeless. The guinea pig hepatoma model differs in that tumor regression is achieved routinely, the results are readily reproducible, and the technique has been successfully extended to other species, including man.

Treatment of Established Tumors by Adoptive or Passive Transfer of Immunity

This subject has been extensively reviewed by Rosenberg and Terry (1977), who concluded that the passive administration of immune serum has yielded disappointing results. Therapeutic benefit is largely limited to those situations in which immune serum is administered almost simultaneously with tumor challenge. The two exceptions are the studies of sarcomas induced by Moloney sarcoma virus (Hellström and Hellström, 1970) and tumors induced by polyoma virus (Bansal and Sjögren, 1971). The high immunogenicity of the Moloney sarcoma (as evidenced by its spontaneous regression when induced in adult mice) may have facilitated the immunotherapeutic success of immune serum. The prolongation of survival of rats bearing polyoma virus-induced tumors required the administration of large quantities of immune serum (almost five times the rat's blood volume).

The adoptive administration of immune cells has met with somewhat more success as therapy for established animal tumors. Several workers have induced regression of both autochthonous and transplanted tumors in animals by the administration of immunized cells (Delorme and Alexander, 1964; Fefer, 1969; Borberg *et al.,* 1972). Large numbers of cells were required. In some studies, allogeneic or heterologous cells were effective, although not as effective as syngeneic cells.

Summary

The data clearly indicate that many animal tumors have tumor-associated antigens demonstrable by postimmunization challenge-rejection techniques. The presence of these antigens has been successfully exploited in an array of immunoprophylaxis experiments. Success with active-specific or active-nonspecific immunotherapy in tumor-bearing animals has been minimal. Of the examples cited, only one has been repeatedly confirmed and successfully extended to other animals: intralesional therapy in the guinea pig hepatoma model. By comparison to the volume of research in active immunotherapy, passive and adoptive approaches have been virtually ignored. Nonetheless, regression of established tumors has been reported in several systems. Adoptive and passive modes of therapy could be utilized to augment the immunity generated by irrevocably impaired or already maximally responding, normally functioning immune systems. Further, they may be logically combined with immunosuppressive chemotherapy.

Human Tumor Immunotherapy

Demonstration of Human Tumor Antigens

The sine qua non for successful immunotherapy is the demonstration that human tumors, like animal tumors, possess tumor-specific antigens not present (qualitatively or quantitatively) in normal tissue. The presence of tumor-specific antigens in or on human neoplasms is suggested by two clinical observations, which indicate a possible host immune response to these antigens. First, spontaneous and sometimes dramatic regressions of metastatic malignancies have been reported (Everson and Cole, 1966). The spontaneous regression of cancer well may be a result of host immunity, but other factors, such as hormonally induced regression or spontaneous maturation to a benign form, cannot be excluded. A second line of clinical evidence for the existence of tumor-specific antigens in human tumors and a host response against these antigens is the relatively favorable prognosis that is associated with tumors that are infiltrated by lymphocytes (Thomas, 1973).

The convincing demonstration of tumor-specific antigens in animal tumors relied heavily on transplantation techniques in syngeneic hosts, a technique poorly suited to use in humans. Such studies must be limited to autotransplants in patients with incurable malignant disease. A number of investigators have studied human cancer with this methodology. The most extensive of these studies were conducted by Southam and Beunschwig (1961). Using cells from fresh tumor specimens, these investigators demonstrated that inocula of 10^8 cells would almost always grow, whereas only 50% takes were noted with inocula of 10^6 cells and no growth was noted with inocula of 10^4 tumor cells. These studies probably demonstrated some measure of host resistance, even in patients with incurable, progressive disease. Despite these results, the autotransplantation techniques are of limited usefulness in the detection of tumor-specific antigens.

In vitro assays have been developed in an effort to demonstrate tumor-specific antigen. The tumor most extensively studied with these techniques has been malignant melanoma. The data from these assays have been extensively reviewed in an attempt to determine if they supported the existence of tumor antigens and a host immune response to these antigens (Clark *et al.,* 1977). Although the data were often conflicting, controls absent or inappropriate, and the design inadequate to distinguish tumor-associated from other antigens, the conclusions were that there probably are melanoma-associated antigens and a host immune response to these antigens. Subsequent to that report, Shiku *et al.* (1976), using the immune adherence assay, tested sera from 18 melanoma patients on autologous melanoma cell lines. Autologous serum reactivity was demonstrated in ten patients. No reactivity was seen with autologous fibroblasts. Sera from two patients that were most strongly and consistently reactive against autologous melanoma cells were studied in detail. The serum from one patient reacted against no other autologous, allogeneic, or xenogeneic cell type and thus represented a reaction against an individually distinct (private) melanoma antigen. Serum from the other patient reacted against 4/11 allogeneic melanoma cell lines but none of the other normal or neoplastic cells tested; this reaction was against a common, but not universal, melanoma antigen. Similar results were achieved with the mixed hemadsorption assay (Carey *et al.,* 1976). These studies provide the most compelling evidence for the existence of human tumor-specific antigens. They are limited, however, to a single tumor type, and only a modest number of cases were studied. Data supporting the existence of tumor-specific antigens in other tumors are decidedly more limited.

Is this an adequate data base from which to launch an array of immunotherapy trials? With the question considered in isolation, the answer is no. However, other factors also must be weighed. First, a large body of data demonstrates the presence of tumor-specific antigens in a variety of animal tumors; it is likely that at least some human tumors will have similar antigens. The failure to demonstrate these antigens to date probably results from the lack of appropriate technology rather than the antigens' nonexistence; the transplantation rejection technique relied on in animal systems is not applicable in man. Secondly, even if human tumor-specific antigens do not exist, "immunotherapy" might still be effective; e.g., Hibbs *et al.* (1972) have demonstrated that activated macrophages kill tumor cells nonspecifically. Thirdly, the current modalities of therapy for patients who are no longer candidates for potentially curative surgery or irradiation are usually inadequate because only short-term palliation is provided. Faced with this reality, the clinician feels an urgency to try new therapeutic approaches if he is convinced that the risk to the patient is reasonable. Indeed, many approaches to "immunotherapy" have been "tested" in cancer patients.

Accomplishments in Human Tumor Immunotherapy

The current status of human tumor immunotherapy has been reviewed recently (Mastrangelo *et al.,* 1976; Terry and Windhorst, 1978). These presentations will not be repeated. Rather, we will attempt to determine if the successes noted in animal tumor immunotherapy have been duplicated in human trials. It seems unreasonable to expect or demand greater success in man.

Immunoprophylaxis

In animals, immunotherapy has been most effective in the tumor prophylaxis setting. In man, there have been no randomized, prospective trials of tumor immunoprophylaxis. Such trials would require the inclusion of large numbers of patients followed over decades. In view of the current status of human tumor immunology, such trials cannot be justified. There has been as yet no clear demonstration of the presence of tumor-specific antigens in a reasonable variety of tumors. The cross-reactivity and diversity of these alleged tumor-specific antigens have not been defined, and the antigens are unavailable for active immunization or for the generation of immune-effector elements for passive or adoptive use. Several retrospective attempts to assess the prevalence of a variety of malignancies (primarily leukemias) in persons who received BCG (a nonspecific immunostimulant) to effect tuberculosis prophylaxis in infancy have yielded conflicting results. These studies have been analyzed in detail (Mastrangelo *et al.,* 1976). No conclusions can be drawn because of serious faults in study design. Further, it must be remembered that BCG was administered to these persons to effect tuberculosis prophylaxis, and not in a way specifically designed to reduce the subsequent appearance of malignancy. A prospective attempt to achieve immunoprophylaxis is not indicated at present. We have not yet determined the most effective dose, schedule, or route of administration of these materials. Further, there is the theoretical problem of inducing autoimmune diseases.

Treatment with Active-Specific Immunotherapy

Success with active-specific immunotherapy in tumor-bearing animals has been limited. Nonetheless, several exceptions are noted. Have similar types of therapy been tested in man and have they been successful? Mathé *et al.* (1969b) extended their study of BCG and/or tumor cells in the L1210 leukemia system to a maintenance therapy trial for human acute lymphoblastic leukemia (Mathé *et al.,* 1969a). Remissions maintained by immunotherapy (BCG and/or irradiated allogeneic leukemia cells) were significantly longer than unmaintained remissions. The results of this trial as well as improvements in chemotherapy made confirmative trials with unmaintained control subjects unethical. However, the European Organization for Research on Treatment of Cancer has compared maintenance chemotherapy (6-mercaptopurine plus methotrexate) with maintenance immunotherapy (BCG plus irradiated allogeneic tumor cells) and could demonstrate no difference (Stryckmans and Otten, 1976). This, then, is an example of the adaptation of a successful animal immunotherapy trial to clinical practice.

The results achieved by Likhite (1976a) with a tumor cell–*B. pertussis* conjugate in an established animal tumor system are striking. An attempt at confirmation is required, however. Likhite (1976b) has treated patients with far-advanced solid tumors with autologous tumor cells conjugated to *B. pertussis.* To date, these have been reported only in anecdotal fashion. Eight of 15 colon cancer patients, 2/2 esophageal cancer patients, and 1/1 melanoma patient are alleged to have had objective remissions. A further assessment of this approach must await a more detailed report as well as attempts at corroboration.

Surprisingly, attempts to extend the use of *V. cholerae* neuraminidase-treated tumor cells to the clinical setting have been modest. This may be related to the difficulty encountered in reproducing the animal data. Rosato *et al.* (1976) have employed autologous, *V. cholerae* neuraminidase-treated tumor cells on a postsurgical adjuvant basis in a small number of patients with a wide variety of tumors. The lack of a control population makes these studies difficult to interpret. Holland (1978) is comparing chemotherapy alone versus chemotherapy plus *V. cholerae* neuraminidase-treated tumor cells in the maintenance of remission in acute myelogenous leukemia; preliminary data suggest a benefit in favor of chemoimmunotherapy. The use of neuraminidase-treated tumor cells in patients with clinically evident residual tumors has not been reported. Likewise, attempts to combine systemic, active-specific immunotherapy with conventional approaches to treatment of the primary lesion in a fashion similar to that reported by Alexander (1968) have not been reported.

Treatment with Active-Nonspecific Immunotherapy

The systemic use of active-nonspecific immunotherapy in animal models has been ineffective except in a few instances. Similarly, this approach has been minimally effective in humans. Moertel *et al.* (1975) reported three objective responses in 26 patients with advanced gastrointestinal cancer treated with methanol extraction residue of BCG (MER). There of seven melanoma patients experienced objective remissions when treated with oral BCG (Falk *et al.,* 1973). Objective responses were noted in 8 of 20 patients with a variety of advanced cancers treated with intravenous *C. parvum* (Israël *et al.,*1975). Although confirmation of these observations has not yet been reported, they are encouraging.

Substantial and reproducible therapeutic results in animals have been achieved with intralesional BCG treatment of established cutaneous tumor transplants. Injected lesions regress, and microscopic regional lymph node metastases are eradicated. Similarly striking and equally reproducible results have been achieved in the treatment of intradermal melanoma metastases. Regression of injected as well as uninjected lesions has been well documented (for review, see Mastrangelo *et al.,* 1976). Although the therapeutic effects are undeniable, the concept that an immunologic mechanism is responsible for these regressions has been disputed. The controversy arises because regression of uninjected lesions is seen most often when the dermal metastases are confined to an extremity and the uninjected lesions are in close proximity to injected lesions. It has been postulated that regression of uninjected lesions is simply a result of the nonspecific activation of macrophages at sites in close proximity to BCG injection. There are insufficient data to resolve this question. Nonetheless, the results achieved in animals and man are strikingly similar.

Treatment by Passive or Adoptive Means

Again, results with passive and adoptive immunotherapy have been reviewed by Rosenberg and Terry (1977). They report that there is no convincing evidence that immune serum from any source has had a beneficial effect on the course of human malignant disease. Positive reports on the use of allogeneic serum from cured patients, such as that of Ngu (1967), are not well documented and have not been corroborated (Fass *et al.,* 1970). The successes claimed with the use of immune, heterologous sera are poorly detailed and have not been confirmed by others (Murray, 1958; DeCarvalho, 1963). Nevertheless, the latter studies should not be ignored; the area is deserving of further study.

Success with the passive administration of immune cells also has been meager. Attempts to utilize cell transfer immunotherapy in humans are hampered by the unavailability of suitable immune cells. The cross-immunization of cancer patients with subsequent transfer of immune cells was best studied by Nadler and Moore (1966, 1969), who provided evidence that immune cell transfer is capable of affecting the growth of tumors in humans. Of 118 patients with advanced cancer, 23 had objective responses. However, documentation of many responses was not presented. These studies and similar attempts by Humphrey *et al.* (1971) demonstrated that at least small therapeutic effects are achievable in some patients with advanced cancer.

Summary

What has been accomplished in human tumor immunotherapy, and how do these accomplishments compare with the results achieved with animal tumor immunotherapy? The area in which the greatest successes have been achieved in animals, immunoprophylaxis, has not been pursued in humans. In tumor-bearing hosts, success has been modest but comparable in animal and human tumor systems. Overall, immunotherapy as presently practiced seems to be a relatively ineffective way of treating both animal and human tumors.

Future Directions

In what direction(s) should human tumor immunotherapy proceed? Based on past experience in the control of infectious diseases and the animal data demonstrating successful tumor immunoprophylaxis, one could argue that clinical trials should cease until an adequate data base and appropriate technology with which to pursue human tumor immunoprophylaxis are available. Unfortunately, attainment of successful human tumor immunoprophylaxis is not a certainty awaiting only the technology to provide the vaccine. Some tumors may be devoid of tumor-specific antigens. The tumor-specific antigens associated with chemically induced tumors indeed may be individually unique and infinitely diverse. Oncogenic viruses may be present during gestation and throughout life, thus making immunoprophylaxis more difficult. Work in this area must continue. Immunoprophylaxis is our most desired goal; success is far from certain, however.

If immunoprophylaxis is not now technically feasible and if the treatment of patients with more advanced disease is of limited value, should our efforts be concentrated on patients with micrometastases? Results of animal studies indicate that tumor burden is a major factor limiting the effectiveness of immunotherapy. Further, the most encouraging clinical data are being generated in this area. In addition to the previously cited success of Mathé *et al.* (1969a) in acute lymphoblastic leukemia, McKneally *et al.* (1976) have had success with intrapleural BCG as a postsurgical adjuvant for stage I lung cancer (non-oat cell type), and Rojas *et al.* (1976) have improved survival rates with levamisole following irradiation for patients with stage III breast cancer.

Adjuvant studies are, by nature, of protracted duration, they require a large number of patients (including a conventionally treated or untreated control group), and unavoidably include a significant number of disease-free persons. All of these factors necessitate the selection of a rational therapy with known toxicity and a reasonable expectation of success. Appropriate animal models (that is, minimum residual metastatic disease following treatment of the primary lesion) are being developed, and their utility remains to be determined. Several of the current adjuvant trials evolved from animal models. In other trials, therapy was selected to correct real or postulated problems: Levamisole was used to restore naturally or iatrogenically suppressed immune function in breast and lung cancer patients; BCG has been employed similarly in patients with Hodgkin's disease and other lymphomas. When using this approach to the design of lengthy and potentially dangerous (especially to the disease-free subjects) trials, one must be certain to confirm the presence of the postulated problem and to demonstrate that the proposed therapy addresses the problem. For example, if serum blocking activity is shown to correlate with a poor prognosis in clinically disease-free persons and if the addition of substance X to the assay abrogates this blocking, one must demonstrate before initiating a therapeutic trial that administering substance X to the patient will also abrogate the serum blocking effect. Surprisingly, such simple procedures frequently are overlooked.

Active-specific (or nonspecific) immunotherapy has been used to further heighten the response of a normally functioning immune system to tumor cells that, because of their number, location, or immunogenicity, may not be eliciting a maximum immune response. Whether the currently available nonspecific immune modulators and tumor antigen preparations can heighten tumor-specific immunity and whether this heightened immunity will be therapeutically effective can be determined only through well-designed clinical trials. The success with intralesional therapy in the guinea pig hepatoma and dermal melanoma metastases has been seemingly rationally extended to the adjuvant setting. Trials are under way in malignant melanoma and lung, bladder, and gastric cancer to test the therapeutic efficacy of injecting the primary lesion with a nonspecific immune modulator prior to definitive surgical therapy.

Another consideration is the nature of and the need for clinically relevant animal models. Tumor immunoprophylaxis studies have been termed clinically irrelevant because clinical circumstances necessitate treatment of patients with cancer. These trials are not irrelevant, but simply not presently applicable in the clinic. Models then were developed in tumor-bearing animals. A variety of immunologic treatments were found to be of limited therapeutic value in carefully chosen animal systems. These results were achieved in single species and under strict laboratory conditions not easily duplicated in the clinic. Toxicity has not been a major concern. Reproducibility is a common problem, and extension to other animal species, in general, has not been successful. It is not surprising that extrapolation of these data to man has been difficult. Further, these animal tumor models have been labeled irrelevant in that the tumors do not metastasize beyond the site of placement or the regional nodes, whereas human cancer is a systemic disease. Thus, newer, more widely metastasizing models are being developed. These also will be subjected to a variety of criticisms. If, for example, the model employs a transplantable, chemically induced tumor in syngeneic animals, a criticism will be that this single, chemically induced tumor extrapolates to represent only a single patient with a chemically induced tumor irrespective of the number of syngeneic animals into which it is transplanted.

What, then, is the ideal animal tumor system? It is a tumor that arises spontaneously in an outbred strain at about the same frequency as similar tumors in humans and that evolves over a time interval proportional to the human counterpart. Of course, it should disseminate widely. Further, the animals must be readily available in large numbers at a uniform stage of disease for testing purposes. The larger, outbred domestic animals, such as dogs, horses, and cattle, in which tumors arise spontaneously seem suitable. However, supply is likely to be a problem and costs may be prohibitive. The development of new models undoubtedly will lead to refinement of clinical immunotherapy, but is unlikely to pave the way for major clinical progress. We respectfully submit that we have an abundance of animal models. What we need are useful approaches to therapy.

What is to be done with cancer patients during the next quarter-century while approaches to immunoprophylaxis and adjuvant therapy are being perfected? The major thrust of our therapeutic approach has rested on the concept that the immune system of cancer patients is not functioning maximally, either because it is suppressed or because it is being inadequately stimulated. We can agree that terminally ill patients generally are immunosuppressed. At the time of initial diagnosis and treatment, the situation is variable and appears dependent on the tumor type: melanoma patients are minimally immunosuppressed, if at all (Camacho *et al.,* 1977), whereas patients with squamous carcinoma of the head and neck appear to be substantially immunosuppressed (Browder and Chretien, 1977). The immunologic status of patients at the inception of the malignant process is unknown but is unlikely to be impaired as determined by currently available techniques. Whether detected levels of immunosuppression are of clinical consequence remains to be determined; nonetheless, it seems reasonable to treat patients who are unable to adequately perform a specific immunologic function with a material known to correct that defect. Ideally, the immunologic function measured should reflect the patient's ability to respond to his own tumor and should also correlate with prognosis. In the interim, while appropriate assays are being developed, it is not unreasonable to rely on immunologic assays not directly related to tumor-specific immunity. Whether nonspecific stimulation of a normally functioning immune system will be therapeutically beneficial in cancer patients can be determined only through clinical trials. However, results of animal studies indicate that substantial benefit is unlikely.

With respect to treatment, we presently rely on bacteria and bacterial products that nonspecifically activate the reticuloendothelial system. (We will not consider the question of whether this nonspecific stimulation of the reticuloendothelial system is, in fact, immunotherapy.) The magnitude of the therapeutic effect achieved with these materials generally has been modest. Improvements of log magnitude are required to have a substantial impact on the clinical course of cancer. Whether this can be accomplished by fractionating these materials, identifying the active components, and then modifying them remains to be determined. If investigators are successful, a new spectrum of toxicity—namely, autoimmune disease—may be opened. Uveitis and vitiligo have already been associated with BCG treatment (Donaldson *et al.,* 1974).

It is our belief that the aforementioned approaches to immunotherapy are unlikely to have a significant impact on the clinical course of cancer patients. The emphasis in immunotherapy must change from an approach predicated on increasing the magnitude of the host response to attempts to render escape mechanisms ineffective. There are data consistent with the view that tumors that metastasize (the major clinical problem) and grow progressively develop the capacity to bypass host reactions directed against tumor-specific antigens on their surfaces (in much the same way as many bacterial infections persist in the presence of an active immune response). In animal models, Alexander (1974) found that tumors that were able to release antigens in a soluble form into the host environment were able to escape immune destruction in vivo. Moreover, he noted that when tumors were passaged, they frequently changed from a nonmetastasizing to a metastasizing form. This progression was not necessarily associated with the loss of tumor-specific antigens, but occurred because antigens were more rapidly shed.

Other observations are similarly of interest. The established lines of allogeneic transplantable mouse tumors (for example, Ehrlich's ascites) are not rejected by their hosts, despite theoretical incompatibility. Effective immunity against these lines can be induced by immunization with irradiated or chemically treated tumor cells. Apffel *et al.* (1966) demonstrated that nonimmunized animals could recover from a lethal inoculation of various ascites tumors (EL-4 leukemia, S-37 sarcoma, Krebs-2 tumor) if subjected to paracentesis daily beginning 12 to 14 days after inoculation. Following recovery, the animals were able to reject challenge doses of tumor. The paracenteses did not significantly reduce tumor burden, as only a small number of cells were removed. Reinjection of the cell-free supernatant from the paracentetic fluid completely abrogated the influence of the paracentesis. This cell-free supernatant was nontoxic to normal mice and was effective in immunizing mice against challenge with the various ascites tumors. This latter observation suggests that the cell-free supernatant contained tumor-related antigens. This observation again suggests that free tumor antigen can abrogate an immune response that otherwise might be therapeutically effective.

These and other observations serve to highlight the need to reassess our approach to tumor-bearing patients. There is a need to document the escape mechanisms that are operative so that techniques can be devised to circumvent them.

CONTROVERSIES

The ultimate objective of clinical research in human tumor immunotherapy is to ascertain if a given treatment is effective. The results of several hundred trials have been reported, and hundreds more trials are in progress. Despite this wealth of data, definite conclusions are relatively infrequent. The controversies that have erupted generally center around selection of treatments and their dose and schedule of administration, selection of treated and control populations, and interpretation of results.

Selection of Treatments and Dose and Schedule of Administration

In the bulk of immunotherapy, nonspecific immune modulators, such as BCG, *C. parvum,* or levamisole, are employed. These materials have been placed into clinical trial largely on the basis of results of animal tumor immunoprophylaxis studies or their ability to nonspecifically improve immunocompetence. Evidence of their efficacy in animals with established tumors, however, has not been convincing. As the early chemotherapists hoped for more effective drugs, we, too, hope for more effective immune modulators. We have two alternatives: First, we can terminate clinical trials until materials with more convincing antitumor activity are found. This is unacceptable in view of the currently desperate plight of cancer patients. The second and only reasonable solution is to continue our trials but to conduct them in such a fashion as to yield reliable data with the minimum expenditure of patients, personnel, and monies.

Clinical trials are being initiated with little, if any, of the traditional phase

I work required for chemotherapy. This has resulted not so much from our lack of awareness of the need for phase I trials, but from the difficulty in designing and conducting useful ones. Phase I studies of immunotherapeutic agents differ substantially from traditional phase I chemotherapy trials. In the latter, the maximum tolerated dose is assumed to be the dose most likely to demonstrate antitumor effect, and dose-limiting toxicity is usually hematologic. The dose-limiting toxicities of immune modulators are not so obvious; levamisole is an example. In addition, the maximum tolerated dose well may not be the most efficient dose for stimulation of immunity. For BCG (Chee and Bodurtha, 1974), *C. parvum* (Berd and Mitchell, 1976), and levamisole (Sampson *et al.,* 1977), variations in dose can enhance animal tumor growth. This is not a problem solely related to nonspecific immune modulators. As early as 1907, Flexner and Jobling showed that prior immunization may facilitate the growth of an allogeneic tumor.

Although several cancer centers currently are conducting phase I trials of immune modulators, there remains considerable controversy over the general format of these trials. Of particular concern is the best method of assessing immune modulation. We have no ready answers. It would seem most desirable to measure antitumor immunity, but the in vitro assays of cellular immunity have been disappointing because they have correlated with neither clinical course nor response to therapy (Clark *et al.,* 1977). Serologic assays have not been extensively studied; we hope they will be more useful. A number of non-tumor-directed parameters of immunity have been measured in patients receiving non-specific immune modulators, but with few exceptions (Biran *et al.,* 1976), are not consistently affected by immunomodulating agents.

Several other categories of tests might be useful but have not been employed yet for the evaluation of immunomodulating agents in patients. Reticuloendothelial clearance is augmented in mice treated with macrophage-stimulating agents (Halpern *et al.,* 1964). Reticuloendothelial clearance can be measured in man. The technique is safe and seems to produce reliable results (Biozzi *et al.,* 1958). Immunostimulants might act as adjuvants to the production of antibody in humans, as they do in experimental animals. Finally, immune modulators also might act as adjuvants to primary delayed hypersensitivity responses.

The question of schedule also must be considered, especially if we are to continue combining potentially immunosuppressive chemotherapy with immune modulators. With the use of materials such as BCG, which persists for long periods, this may not be a critical issue. However, newer immune modulators, such as levamisole, may have a much shorter duration of action, thus making scheduling a crucial factor.

Selection of Treatment and Control Populations

In the early history of chemotherapy, phase II trials included tumors of diverse histologic types and infrequently included sufficient numbers of patients with any one kind of tumor to allow a conclusion regarding the merits of the drug. This was likewise the case in many of the earlier immunotherapy trials. As with chemotherapy, certain tumors are more likely to be responsive to immunotherapy than are others. For example, immunocompetence, which is probably a significant factor in determining responsiveness to immunotherapy, varies not only by tumor type but by stage of disease as well. The study populations must be as homogeneous as is clinically practical.

The choice of an appropriate control is also of vital importance. The greatest difficulty is encountered in adjuvant trials in which the conventionally treated control subjects receive no additional treatment. We and others have found it difficult to convince truly informed patients, that is, patients who are aware that they are at significant risk for tumor recurrence and that we are testing a therapy that we hope will improve prognosis, to accept control status. There are also ethical and legal factors to be considered in denying patients a treatment that may be beneficial and is not known to be significantly toxic. The alternative is to use a historical control. However, it then becomes virtually impossible to demonstrate the comparability of the historical control and the current treatment groups in regard to known and unknown prognostic variables. Partial compensation might be achieved by using larger numbers of patients and selecting as controls patients seen at the same institution and who were accrued over a relatively brief interval preceding accrual of the current treatment group. Nonetheless, acceptance of a treatment as being of clinical benefit is of major significance when one considers the costs and toxicities (both known and unknown) of the treatment. Such decisions must be based on the most reliable data, and these are generated by randomized, prospective trials.

Interpretation of Results

The application of life table methods of data analysis to immunotherapy trials, particularly adjuvant trials, has allowed projection of results prior to completion of patient accrual and follow-up. The early analysis of data not infrequently yields survival curves that are widely disparate although not significantly different statistically. The interpretation of these data causes little difficulty for the experienced clinical investigator; however, presentation to less experienced primary care physicians can produce problems, including the widespread use of an unproven therapy and the reluctance of physicians to refer patients for control treatment.

The "sifting" of data from negative trials can identify subsets of patients who appear to have benefited from therapy. Although these findings are a valid basis on which to formulate new hypotheses to be tested in future trials, they are not valid conclusions to be drawn from the initial trial. Again, the interpretation of these data is no problem for the experienced investigator. Presentation of these findings to less experienced primary care physicians can create the same problems cited in the preceding paragraph.

Finally, when should a trial be terminated? Matters of toxicity aside, a therapy trial should be terminated when either a significant difference has been shown or a clinically significant benefit has been excluded. The common conclusion of negative trials is that treatment A was not demonstrated to be better than B. This does not mean that treatment A is, in fact, no better than B; it indicates only that a benefit, which may or may not exist, was not demonstrated. The exclusion of a small but clinically significant benefit often necessitates accrual of large numbers of patients and continuation of the trial long beyond the interests of the investigator and referral physician. The least that should be provided is a statistical statement regarding the magnitude of clinical benefit that was excluded with reasonable certainty.

In summary, the reader may conclude erroneously that we are advocating that something that is not worth doing is worth doing well. Rather, we have taken the position that the current plight of the cancer patient is such that trials designed to clearly identify a modestly effective treatment are worthwhile.

ACKNOWLEDGMENT

This work was supported in part by Public Health Service grants CA-13456, CA-06927, and RR-05539 from the National Institutes of Health, Department of Health, Education and Welfare; and by an appropriation from the Commonwealth of Pennsylvania.

REFERENCES

Alexander, P. 1968. Immunotherapy of cancer: Experiments with primary tumors and syngeneic tumor grafts. Prog. Exp. Tumor Res., 10:23–71.

Alexander, P. 1974. Escape from immune destruction by the host through shedding of surface antigens: Is this a characteristic shared by malignant and embryonic cells? Cancer Res., 34:2077–2082.

Allison, A. C. 1966. Immune responses to Shope fibroma virus in adult and newborn rabbits. J. Natl. Cancer Inst., 36:869–876.

Apffel, C. A., Arnason, B. G., Twinam, C. W., and Harris, C. A. 1966. Recovery with immunity after serial tapping of transplantable mouse ascites tumors. Br. J. Cancer, 20:122–126.

Bansal, S. C., and Sjögren, H. O. 1971. "Unblocking" serum activity *in vitro* in the polyoma system may correlate with antitumor effects of antiserum *in vivo*. Nature [New Biol.], 233:76–78.

Bashford, E. F., Murray, J. A., and Haaland, M. 1908. Resistance and susceptibility to inoculated cancer. In: Third Scientific Report of the Cancer Research Fund, p. 359.

Basombrio, M. A. 1973. The immunology of cancer. J. Oral Pathol., 2:231–253.

Berd, D. 1978. Effects of *Corynebacterium parvum* in immunity. Pharmacol. Ther. [A], 2:373–395.

Berd, D. A., and Mitchell, M. S. 1976. Immunological enhancement of leukemia L1210 by *Corynebacterium parvum* in allogeneic mice. Cancer Res., 36:4119–4124.

Biggs, P. M., Payne, L. N., Milne, B. S., Churchill, A. E., Chubb, R. C., Powell, R. C., and Harris, A. H. 1970. Field trials with an attenuated cell-associated vaccine for Marek's disease. Vet. Rec., 87:704–709.

Biozzi, G., Benaceraff, B., Halpern, B. N., Stiffel, C., EsSc, L., and Hillemand, B. 1958. Exploration of the phagocytic function of the reticuloendothelial system with heat denatured human serum albumin labeled with I^{131} and application to the measurement of liver blood flow in normal man and in some pathological conditions. J. Lab. Clin. Med., 51:230–239.

Biran, H., Moake, J. L., Reed, R. C., Gutterman, J. U., Hersh, E. M., Freireich, E. J, and Mavligit, G. M. 1976. Complement activation *in vivo* in cancer patients receiving *Corynebacterium parvum* immunotherapy. Br. J. Cancer, 34:493–499.

Borberg, H., Oettgen, H. F., Choudy, K., and Beattie, E. J., Jr. 1972. Inhibition of established transplants of chemically induced sarcomas in syngeneic mice by lymphocytes from immunized donors. Int. J. Cancer, 10:539–547.

Bridre, J. 1907. Recherches sur le cancer des souris. Ann. Inst. Pasteur, 21:760–776.

Browder, J. P., and Chretien, P. B. 1977. Immune reactivity in head and neck squamous carcinoma and relevance to the design of immunotherapy trials. Semin. Oncol., 4:431–439.

Burmester, B. R. 1955. Immunity to visceral lymphomatosis in chickens following injection of virus into dams. Proc. Soc. Exp. Biol. Med., 88:153–155.

Camacho, E. S., Pinsky, C. M., Wanebo, H. J., Mike, V., Golbey, R. B., Fortner, J. G., and Oettgen, H. F. 1977. DNCB reactivity and prognosis in 358 patients with malignant melanoma (Abstract). Proc. Am. Assoc. Cancer Res., 18:226.

Carey, T. E., Takahashi, T., Resnick, L. A., Oettgen, H. F., and Old, L. J. 1976. Cell surface antigen of human malignant melanoma: Mixed hemadsorption assays for humoral immunity to cultured autologous melanoma cells. Proc. Natl. Acad. Sci. USA, 73:3278–3282.

Chee, D. O., and Bodurtha, A. J. 1974. Facilitation and inhibition of B16 melanoma *in vivo* and by lymphoid cells from BCG-treated mice *in vitro*. Int. J. Cancer, 14:137–143.

Clark, W. H., Jr., Mastrangelo, M. J., Ainsworth, A. M., Berd, D., Bellet, R. E., and Bernardino, E. A. 1977. Current concepts of the biology of human cutaneous malignant melanoma. Adv. Cancer Res., 24:267–338.

DeCarvalho, S. 1963. Preliminary experimentation with specific immunotherapy of neoplastic disease in man. I. Immediate effects of equine immune gamma globulin. Cancer, 16:306–330.

Delorme, E. J., and Alexander, P. 1964. Treatment of primary fibrosarcomata in the rat with immune lymphocytes. Lancet, 2:117–120.

Donaldson, R. C., Canaan, S. A., Jr., McLean, R. B., and Ackerman, L. V. 1974. Uveitis and vitiligo associated with BCG treatment of malignant melanoma. Surgery, 76:771–778.

Ehrlich, P. 1907. Experimentelle studies an mausetumoren. Z. Krebsforsch., 5:59–81.

Everson, T. C., and Cole, W. H. 1966. Spontaneous Regression of Cancer. Philadelphia, W. B. Saunders.

Falk, R. E., Mann, P., and Langen, B. 1973. Cell mediated immunity to human tumors. Arch. Surg., 107:261–266.

Fass, L., Herberman, R. B., Ziegler, J., and Morrow, R. H., Jr. 1970. Evaluation of the effect of remission plasma on untreated patients with Burkitt's lymphoma. J. Natl. Cancer Inst., 44:145–149.

Fefer, A. 1969. Immunotherapy and chemotherapy of Moloney sarcoma virus-induced tumors in mice. Cancer Res., 29:2177–2183.

Flexner, S., and Jobling, W. 1907. Restraint and promotion of tumor growth. Proc. Soc. Exp. Biol. Med., 5:16–18.

Friend, C. 1966. Immunological relationship among some of the murine leukemia viruses. In Burdette, W. J. (ed.): Viruses Inducing Cancer. Salt Lake City, University of Utah Press, pp. 51–60.

Gorer, P. A., and Amos, D. B. 1956. Passive immunity of mice against C57B1 leukosis EL4 by means of isoimmune serum. Cancer Res., 16:338–343.

Halpern, B. N., Prevot, A. R., Biozzi, G., Stiffel, C., Mouton, D., Morard, J. C., Bouthillier, Y., and Decreusefond, C. 1964. Stimulation de l'activite phagocytaire du systeme reticuloendothelial provoquee par *Corynebacterium parvum*. J. Reticuloendothel. Soc., 1:77–96.

Hellström, I., and Hellström, K. E. 1970. Colony inhibition studies on blocking and non-blocking effects on cellular immunity to Moloney sarcomas. Int. J. Cancer, 5:195–201.

Hibbs, J. B., Jr., Lambert, L. H., Jr., and Remington, J. S. 1972. Control of carcinogenesis: A possible role for the activated macrophage. Science, 177:998–1000.

Holland, J. F. 1978. Comparison of chemotherapy to chemotherapy plus VCN-treated cells in acute myelogenous leukemia. In Terry, W. D., and Windhorst, D. (eds.): Immunotherapy of Cancer: Present Status of Trials in Man. New York, Raven Press, p. 347.

Humphrey, L. J., Jewell, W. R., Murray, D. R., and Griffen, W. O. 1971. Immunotherapy for the patient with cancer. Ann. Surg., 173:47–54.

Israël, L., Edelstein, R., Depierre, A., and Dimitrov, N. 1975. Daily intravenous infusions of *Corynebacterium parvum* in twenty patients with disseminated cancer: A preliminary report of clinical and biological findings. J. Natl. Cancer Inst., 55:29–33.

Klein, E., Holtermann, O. A., Papermaster, B., Milgrom, H., Rosner, D., Klein, L., Walker, M. J., and Zbar, B. 1973. Immunologic approaches to various types of cancer with the use of BCG and purified protein derivatives. Natl. Cancer Inst. Monogr., 39:229–239.

Klein, G. 1966. Tumor antigens. Annu. Rev. Microbiol., 20:223–252.

Larson, V. M., Raupp, W. G., and Hilleman, M. R. 1967. Prevention of SV40 virus tumorigenesis in newborn hamsters by maternal immunization. Proc. Soc. Exp. Biol. Med., 126:674–677.

Latarjet, R. 1964. Action inhibitrice des extraits leucemiques isologues irradiés sur la leucemogenese spontanee de la souris AKR. Ann. Inst. Pasteur, 106:1–26.

Laucius, J. F., Bodurtha, A. J., Mastrangelo, M. J., and Creech, R. H. 1974. Bacillus Calmette-Guerin in the treatment of neoplastic disease. J. Reticuloendothel. Soc., 16:347–373.

Likhite, V. V. 1974. Rejection of mammary adenocarcinoma cell tumors and the prevention of progressive growth of incipient metastases following intratumor permeation with killed *Bordetella pertussis*. Cancer Res., 34:2790–2794.

Likhite, V. V. 1976a. Rejection of growing tumors in mice following immunotherapy with killed *Bordetella pertussis*-ICTD-tumor cell conjugates. ICRS Med. Sci., 4:565.

Likhite, V. V. 1976b. Clinical cancer immunotherapy. In Martin, M., and Dionne, L. (eds.): Immuno-cancerology in Solid Tumors. New York, Stratton Intercontinental Medical Book Corporation, pp. 135–154.

Mastrangelo, M. J., Berd, D., and Bellet, R. E. 1976. Critical review of previously reported clinical trials of cancer immunotherapy with non-specific immunostimulants. Ann. NY Acad. Sci., 277:94–123.

Mathé, G., Amiel, J. L., Schwarzenberg, L., Schneider, M., Cattan, A., Schlumberger, J. R., Hayat, M., and DeVassal, F. 1969a. Active immunotherapy for acute lymphoblastic leukemia. Lancet, 1:697–699.

Mathé, G., Pouillart, P., and Lapeyraque, F. 1969b. Active immunotherapy of L1210 leukemia applied after the graft of tumor cells. Br. J. Cancer, 23:814–824.

McKneally, M. F., Maver, C., and Kausel, H. W. 1976. Regional immunotherapy of lung cancer with intrapleural BCG. Lancet, 1:377–379.

Moertel, C. G., Ritts, R. E., Jr., Schutt, A. J., and Hahn, R. G. 1975. Clinical studies of methanol extraction residue fraction of *Bacillus Calmette-Guerin* as an immunostimulant in patients with advanced cancer. Cancer Res., 35:3075–3083.

Morton, D. L. 1971. Immunological studies with human neoplasms. J. Reticuloendothel. Soc., 10:137–160.

Murray, G. 1958. Experiments in immunity in cancer. Can. Med. Assoc. J., 79:249–259.

Nadler, S. H., and Moore, G. E. 1966. Clinical immunologic study of malignant disease: Response to tumor transplants and transfer of leukocytes. Ann. Surg., 164:482–490.

Nadler, S. H., and Moore, G. E. 1969. Immunotherapy of malignant disease. Arch. Surg., 99:376–381.

Ngu, V. A. 1967. Host defenses in Burkitt tumor. Br. Med. J., 1:345–347.

Old, L. J., and Boyse, E. A. 1964. Immunology of experimental tumors. Annu. Rev. Med., 15:167–186.

Prehn, R. T., and Main, J. M. 1957. Immunity to methylcholanthrene induced sarcomas. J. Natl. Cancer Inst., 18:769–778.

Purnell, D. M., Kreider, J. W., and Bartlett, G. L. 1975. Evaluation of antitumor activity of *Bordetella pertussis* in two murine tumor models. J. Natl. Cancer Inst., 55:123–128.

Rapp, H. J., Kleinschuster, S. J., Lueker, D. C., and Kainer, R. A. 1976. Immunotherapy of experimental cancer as a guide to the treatment of human cancer. Ann. NY Acad. Sci., 276:550–556.

Rios, A., and Simmons, R. L. 1972. Comparative effect of Mycobacterium bovis and neuraminidase-treated tumor cells on the growth of established methylcholanthrene-fibrosarcomas in syngeneic mice. Cancer Res., 32:16–21.

Rojas, A. F., Mickiewicz, E., Feierstein, J. N., Glait, H., and Olivari, A. J. 1976. Levamisole in advanced human breast cancer. Lancet, 1:211–215.

Rosato, F. E., Miller, E., Rosato, E. F., Brown, A., Wallack, M. K., Johnson, J., and Moskowitz, A. 1976. Active specific immunotherapy in solid tumors. Ann. NY Acad. Sci., 277:332–338.

Rosenberg, S. A., and Terry, W. D. 1977. Passive immunotherapy of cancer in animals and man. Adv. Cancer Res., 25:233–288.

Sampson, D., Peters, T. G., Lewis, J. D., Metzig, J., and Kurtz, B. E. 1977. Dose dependence of immunopotentiation and tumor regression induced by levamisole. Cancer Res., 37:3526–3529.

Shiku, H., Takahashi, T., Oettgen, H. F., and Old, L. J. 1976. Cell surface antigens of human malignant melanoma. II. Serologic typing with immune adherence assays and definition of two new surface antigens. J. Exp. Med., 144:873–881.

Shope, R. E. 1937. Immunization of rabbits to infectious papillomatosis. J. Exp. Med., 65:219–231.

Southam, C. M., and Beunschwig, A. 1961. Quantitative studies of autotransplantation of human cancer. Cancer, 14:971–978.

Stryckmans, P. A., and Otten, J. 1976. Immunotherapy in acute lymphoblastic leukemia (Abstract). Proc. Am. Assoc. Cancer Res., 17:217.

Symoens, J., and Rosenthal, M. 1977. Levamisole in the modulation of the immune response: The current experimental and clinical state. J. Reticuloendothel. Soc., 21:175–221.

Terry, W. D., and Windhorst, D. (eds.) 1978. Immunotherapy of Cancer: Present Status of Trials in Man. New York, Raven Press, 696 pp.

Thomas, E. 1973. Current thoughts on factors that influence prognosis of gastric cancer. Med. J. Aust., 2:821–824.

van Scott, E. J., and Winters, P. L. 1970. Response of mycosis fungoides to intensive external treatment with nitrogen mustard. Arch. Dermatol., 102:507–514.

Zbar, B., Bernstein, I. D., and Rapp, H. J. 1971. Suppression of tumor growth at the site of injection with living Bacillus Calmette-Guerin. J. Natl. Cancer Inst., 46:831–839.

Immunotherapy of Human Cancer,
The University of Texas System Cancer Center
M. D. Anderson Hospital and Tumor Institute.
Raven Press, New York © 1978.

Prospects for the Future of Immunotherapy: The Need for Individualism

Jordan U. Gutterman, M.D.

*Department of Developmental Therapeutics, The University of Texas System Cancer Center
M. D. Anderson Hospital and Tumor Institute, Houston, Texas*

I have been given the challenge to project the future of immunotherapy for human cancer. At first, this appeared to be an unenviable task; however, after a great deal of thought, I consider this an exciting and important challenge. I am reminded of the new member of the House of Commons who asked the eminent British politician Disraeli if he should participate actively in debates. After a quick appraisal, Disraeli replied, "No, I think not. It would be better for people to wonder why you did not speak rather than why you did." I hope my remarks do not encourage a similar response.

It has been more than 100 years since the control of cancer by immunologic methods was suggested by physicians who observed that cancer partially or totally regressed after acute bacterial infections. William B. Coley (1911) pioneered the study of mixed bacterial vaccines or their products, and there is no doubt that these vaccines were effective in many cases. During the last ten years, there has been an explosion of knowledge in basic tumor immunology. I feel that we are on the verge of making great progress with a new form of cancer treatment. It is crucial that we examine where we are and consider the long-range future prospects.

Four and a half years ago, we held a basic tumor immunology symposium here at M. D. Anderson Hospital. Many distinguished speakers attended and participated in that exciting meeting. Nearly 1,000 people attended every session. There was tremendous excitement in the air at that time, in 1973. Since then, there has been a precipitous decline in enthusiasm for tumor immunology and immunotherapy. I feel the pendulum has swung in the negative direction. Our more sophisticated knowledge of the immune system, however, should make us more courageous. As clinical investigators, we have two alternatives. We can say that the immune system is too complicated and in too delicate a balance, and thus, immunotherapy will not become a major factor in cancer treatment. With that attitude, which is prominent among some circles, a self-fulfilling prophecy will occur and immunotherapy will fail to flourish. We have only one choice:

to hypothesize that immunotherapy can work and that it will play a major role in the control or prevention of cancer. With this choice, we can succeed or we can fail; nothing is foolproof. No great accomplishments have ever been made with certainty prior to their discovery.

It is often said that if we do not learn from history, we will be compelled to relive it. Similarly, if we do not manipulate the future, we shall be compelled to endure it, and that could be worse. It may be surprising to many of you that the word "futurist" has come to be used commonly in the social sciences and other scientific spheres of today. Before we prophesy the future of immunotherapy, I think it is useful to see how others have fared scientific predictions. Arthur C. Clarke (1972) has described two failures of predictions in science: the failure of nerve and the failure of imagination.

Failure of nerve occurs when, given all the relevant facts, the prophet cannot see the point of an inescapable conclusion. "They said it could not be done" is a phrase used throughout the history of discoveries and inventions. It is often impossible to recall the attitudinal climate that existed, for example, when the first locomotives were being built. Many critics asserted that speeds greater than 30 miles per hour were impossible. It was only 80 years ago that the idea of a domestic light was thought impossible by many experts, with the exception of Thomas Edison. Scientists often stated that flight was impossible. Many of the things that have happened in the last 50 years indeed have been fantastic. It is only by assuming that great developments will continue that we have any hope of planning and anticipating a future. To predict the future, therefore, we need logic, but we also need faith (Clarke, 1972).

The above-described failures in predicting the future were made in the face of all the facts. The critics did not assume the courage that their scientific convictions had offered them. They could not believe the truth, even when it had been spelled out before them. The second type of failure according to Clarke, which is more interesting, occurs when all the available facts are appreciated but the vital link is still undiscovered and the possibility of its existence is not admitted. This is lack of imagination. An example of this type of failure is that of Lord Rutherford, who, more than any other man, bared the internal structure of the atom; however, he frequently made fun of those who suggested that one day we would be able to harness the energy locked up in matter. Only five years after his death, in 1937, the first nuclear chain reaction was started in Chicago. Despite his insight, Rutherford had failed to take into account that a nuclear reaction that would release more energy than that required to start it might be discovered. There are numerous accomplishments in science that seemed impossible with the existing techniques but proved to be of ease with subsequent scientific breakthroughs. These breakthroughs never can be totally anticipated.

We have heard elegant discussions of the accomplishments made and problems, limitations, and obstacles of the further development of immunotherapy for cancer. I will consider the aspects on which, I think, our nerve and imagination should be spent, because these aspects are critically important for the future of cancer immunotherapy.

PHILOSOPHY

One of the largest problems we face is how to incorporate a new modality in the treatment strategy for the cancer patient. This problem is certainly not easy to resolve because often incorporated in the practice of immunotherapy in the clinic are modalities that are new and therefore foreign, strange, and somewhat frightening. Clinical oncologists, in some ways, are confined by paradigms, which are a shared set of assumptions, a model, or a pattern (Smith, 1975). We are trained to treat the cancer patient in a certain way, and it is difficult to imagine any other way or pattern of treatment. All of us share assumptions; a new idea that does not fit the paradigm makes us feel uncomfortable and sounds bizarre. Also, the establishment always has invested in the old paradigms, so new ones often do not get adopted even though they are neater and work better than the old ones. Thus, paradigms do not change easily.

In his famous book *The Ascent of Man,* Bronowski (1973) shows that the progress of man depends on ascent, on new ideas. Every great movement needed leadership, however, such as that of Mendell, Darwin, and Einstein. As Bronowski reminds us, the ascent of man can be halting at times. There have been many great civilizations, all of which failed by limiting the freedom of the imagination of the young. They became static—static because the son did what the father did and the father what the grandfather did—and minority cultures set in. In the Middle Ages, the ladder of promotion was through the Church. At the end of the ladder, there was always the icon of the Godhead that said, "Now you have reached the last commandment: Thou shalt not question." We must not allow clinical and basic cancer research to reach this level. Every new program encounters massive resistance at first, even if only the resistance of inertia and indifference. History is full of struggles such as this. For example, in 1607, Colonel Lancaster noted that with fresh fruits, his crew had no scurvy on journeys to India but the crews of the other ships in the same squadron were all helpless with the disease. Despite the work of Lind years later, it was 192 years before lemons and limes were included in the daily ration of the British Navy.

Most of you are familar with the fascinating stories of smallpox research (Langer, 1976). Years before Edward Jenner began to apply vaccinations, there were many pilot "clinical trials" of smallpox vaccination. In this country, in 1718, Reverend Cotton Mather learned of African natives who recognized that the scars of smallpox meant that one would never have the disease again. They even occasionally gave each other the disease on purpose. Mather convinced a man in Boston by the name of Boylston, who was the son of a doctor, to do some clinical experiments. After being convinced by Mather that inoculation would protect against smallpox, Boylston started with his own child. The boy developed what his father called a discrete case: He was sick for a few days and got well. Boylston went on to give many other people the inoculation, which was with the virus of smallpox, not cowpox. The early results suggested that those people inoculated had a lower incidence of smallpox. This experiment was carried out with little background and the most primitive of knowledge, and paved the way for protection against epidemic smallpox. Boylston was ridiculed and scorned but lived to receive honor and vindication both here and abroad. He paved the way for acceptance in the United States of Jenner's great contribution of cowpox vaccination in England. He was persuaded to undertake his experiment with no preliminary animal work. It was based largely on the observation that if you had the scar, you had the "badge of immunity."

How often we make observations that could be put into clinical practice. An example for us is the fact that patients with spontaneous bacterial infections can undergo complete, permanent regression of cancer. Yet there is still great reluctance, even today, to introduce bacteria in the strategy of treatment of cancer patients. As we think about the future of immunotherapy, all of us—clinical investigators, clinical practitioners, and our colleagues in basic science—must struggle constantly to try new ideas in the clinic, not to supplant but to improve the current, partially successful treatment of cancer.

INVESTIGATOR

A critical person for the future of immunotherapy is the clinical investigator, the pivotal point around which the future takes place. To assure a great future, it is imperative that the investigator have the freedom to maintain and investigate his or her own ideas. Individualism is crucial to continued discovery. The Renaissance taught us to respect the individual, and the result was a surge of individual achievement. Remember the father's description of the camel's gait to his young son, when he said, "A camel walks as though it has been put together by a committee." This is not to say that large groups of individuals working together will not achieve more than the individual—far from it. Multidisciplinary departments and groups have produced extraordinary results in clinical oncology, but once again, we must respect the ability of the individual investigator to express his or her ideas.

Some of the greatest discoveries have evolved from chance, a belief, an inspiration. The inspiration, the "eureka" phenomenon, emphasized by Van Potter (1975), must not be squelched. Imagination, logic, and enthusiasm have constituted the backbone of many discoveries. Enthusiasm, unfortunately, is frequently criticized today, but there is great merit in the childlike curiosity and enthusiasm for discoveries. Bronowski (1973) said that the creative scientist is more primitive, more cultured, more destructive, more constructive, and crazier than the average person. How often we have heard this of great, creative persons, that they are indeed a little crazy. The investigator must not be forced into a posture to produce new results every month or perhaps every year. We are all impatient;

needless to say, patients are dying every day, but the clinical oncologist must not be programmed to the extent that he cannot investigate imaginative ideas.

Lewis Thomas (1974), in his important book *Lives of a Cell*, states something that I cannot agree with: ". . . what distinguishes applied from basic science is the element of surprise." He says that in basic research, at the outset, a high degree of uncertainty is important; otherwise, the problem is not likely to be an important one. "You plan experiments on the basis of probability or possibility rather than certainty. If an experiment turns out as predicted this can be nice, but only a great event if it is a surprise." This I agree with. He, however, goes on to state that "clinical research or applied research is when you are organized to apply knowledge, set up targets, produce a useable product requiring a high degree of certainty from the outset. All the facts on which you base protocols must be reasonably hard facts with unambiguous meaning. The challenge is to plan the work and organize the workers so that it will come out precisely as predicted. For this you need centralized authority, elaborately detailed time schedules and some sort of reward system based on speed and perfection. But most of all you need the intelligible basic facts to begin with and these must come from basic research. There is no other source." I agree that part of applied research should be organized in this way. Unfortunately, applied research is going too much in this direction. Certainly, large-scale organized trials are important, but what is missing in clinical research today is the same approach that Thomas talks about in basic research: empirical eureka phenomena, starting with an incomplete roster of facts and resulting in the unexpected. Certainly, the history of smallpox vaccination is one example. Therefore, the clinician is truly a scientist and should not be so organized that he will produce only predictable results.

I see increasing frustration of many young investigators with the bureaucratic organizations that tend to control research. I am not going to discuss governmental activities or social structures of today, but as a clinical investigator, I think it is imperative for all of us to be thinking about and discussing the maintenance of freedom from regimentation. Men can become so entrapped in a bureaucratic organization that only rage and frustration result. We should be aware that the powers of governmental organization can be so overwhelming that counter-productivity results. A river kept within its bounds is both beautiful and powerful; however, when the river overflows its banks, it becomes impetuous and can be destructive.

An extension of the clinical investigator is the clinical trial. Despite tremendous amounts of discussion, there is still uncertainty about how to carry out the ideal or the best clinical trial and how to best incorporate immunotherapy in the treatment of human cancer, and reasonably so, because the precise role of immunotherapy has not been defined. However, I think the future depends on much more insight in our thinking and planning. Most trials, at best, seem to be random, and immunotherapy is merely tagged on to some standard protocol, with little thought of such factors as interactions. How do we incorporate phases

I, II, and III immunotherapy with phases I, II, and III chemotherapy? There is certainly no need for a tug-of-war between the chemotherapy and immunotherapy investigators. More planning is needed in terms of how we can bring immunotherapy and drug development together with, not opposed to, chemotherapy.

In many respects, the father of both chemotherapy and tumor immunology is Paul Ehrlich. Certainly, we immunologists frequently refer to Ehrlich as our founding father; he was one of the first to suggest the presence of tumor-associated antigens and that the immune system may be necessary not only to reject foreign parasites but also to reject tumor cells. That same person, Paul Ehrlich, was one of the founders of pharmacology and chemotherapy. In today's world, it is difficult to find a Paul Ehrlich, but it is not impossible. In other words, a leader of chemotherapy and immunotherapy could be the same person.

Little attention has been paid to the important interactions of chemotherapy and immunotherapy. For example, the pharmacology and pharmacokinetics of drugs may be altered substantially by these materials. Chemotherapeutic drugs have tremendously different effects on the immune system. Some are immunosuppressive, but some of these may suppress aspects of the immune system that may weaken a tumor-host relationship. What is important is that immunotherapy be incorporated in chemotherapy protocols only with careful thought. I often wonder, is it in the patients' and clinical oncologists' best interests to continue to investigate in the same patient one phase I chemotherapeutic drug after another when the patient is immunologically so suppressed? Could we not work out a strategy in the development of chemotherapeutic and immunotherapeutic agents whereby the two are given sequentially in some fashion so that we can understand and learn about both modalities? For example, after exclusion of a phase I chemotherapeutic modality, it would seem logical in programs in which both chemotherapy and immunotherapy are being investigated that a patient be given phase I immunotherapy in an attempt to reconstitute or restore deficient immune response. Certainly, the possibility for response to a new chemotherapeutic agent after immunologic restoration would be greater.

I think it is time that drug development at the national level be better organized. There is an urgent and persuasive need for a unified development program for cancer immunostimulants. Since there is essentially no adequate preclinical pharmacology, screening, and toxicology program with immunotherapy, a "catch-22" situation develops. The materials are crude and poorly evaluated in many cases. The exciting developments, for example, with microbial purification products are important, but these products should be subjected to preclinical screening in many models with and without chemotherapy. In reviewing the drug development program for chemotherapy, it is worthwhile to recall that Shear was one of the first to organize a screening program to test and isolate microbial polysaccharides that primarily evoked a Shwartzman reaction. By the 1940s, this program was extended to evaluate chemotherapeutic drugs. In the enactment of the National Cancer Institute Act in 1937, a committee stated that in any program for cancer research, patience in the adoption of a long-term point of view is absolutely essential. I am not sure that this attitude has been assumed in the development of immunotherapeutic agents. Other questions come to mind in planning clinical trials. For example, what is an adequate trial for immunostimulants? The same ground rules established for chemotherapeutic agents may not necessarily be applicable for the evaluation of immunotherapy. What is a course of immunotherapy? In evaluation of data, it will be crucial to evaluate patients and treatment for varying lengths of time with not only clinical but immunologic responses.

As Weiss has pointed out, we have to be aware of the "double-edged sword" effects of immunomodulating agents. That is, we can immunostimulate as well as immunosuppress patients. Thus, continuous use of the same immunomodulating agent may not be in the best interest of the patient. Witness the immunologic consequences of chronic parasitic infections. It may be more logical to rotate different immunostimulants for short periods rather than administering the same immunoadjuvant on a long-term basis. Thus, we must ask ourselves: When during long-term immunotherapy should we stop treating? We also have a unique opportunity to do immunoprophylaxis in clinical trials. Chemotherapy is capable of curing 50% to 70% of patients with certain tumors, including Hodgkin's disease, childhood lymphocytic leukemia, and histiocytic lymphoma. Thus, the potential role for immunotherapy in these situations would be to decrease the secondary complications of chemotherapy, including the development of secondary neoplasms. This, indeed, is immunoprophylaxis and can be evaluated immediately.

Thus, empirical trials will continue to play an important role for the future of immunotherapy. Excellent correlations have been observed between the development of postoperative empyemas in patients and subsequent prognosis, and led to the important trial of intrapleural BCG, as described by McKneally. Many accomplishments in science were empirical, for example, those of Jenner. Although there is still controversy regarding the true role of immunotherapy today, we know that, if given properly, it is safe and that potentiation of tumor growth is a clinical rarity. We must move toward earlier application of immunotherapy. Although live BCG has been the prototype, we should initiate the use of partially purified fractions of microorganisms, as pioneered by Ribi, as well as other workers, including Lederer and Yamamura.

BASIC RESEARCH

We have a tremendous amount of work to do to elucidate the basic immunologic mechanisms underlying tumor-host control. The foundation of immunotherapy is the presence of tumor antigens. I see in the future continued increase in our understanding of both nonspecific as well as specific mechanisms for the killing of tumor cells. Little is still known about how the immune system allows for the regression of tumors. It will be crucial to purify as well as possible tumor-specific or at least tumor-associated antigens. Methods to increase immunogenicity of tumor cells have been encouraging, as illustrated by the trial of neuraminidase-treated cells for acute myeloid leukemia. The use of haptens has been disappointing, but important leads with the use of viruses infecting tumor cells, at least in animal models, are encouraging. Although viral vaccinations have been successful in at least one tumor model, we must await definition of human oncornaviruses and the study of horizontal transmission before attempting this in man.

The use of sensitized lymphocytes or subcellular fractions of lymphocytes has not been greatly successful. However, there seems little doubt that fractions removed from lymphocytes can have powerful biologic activity, and I sense that further progress along these lines will be made. The use of lymphocytes sensitized in vitro against tumor cells is an important experimental lead that must be followed up.

Long neglected clinically because of logistical problems is the use of serum or plasma to deliver antibody, which can kill directly with complement or via lymphocytes. Clear-cut antitumor responses can be seen in animals and occasionally in man. As Israël has pointed out, removal of unwanted factors, presumably antigen-antibody complexes and other inhibitory materials, not only can cause significant antitumor effects but, we hope, will potentiate other therapeutic endeavors. We must look more closely at defects, such as complement deficiencies, in the serum.

Of course, the greatest clinical effort thus far has been in the application of microbial vaccines and, more recently, mediators released by these nonspecific approaches. What are the molecular mechanisms responsible for macrophage selectivity in the recognition of tumor cell membranes? Our increasing understanding of the molecular definitions of subfractions of BCG and other microorganisms responsible for killing tumor cells is encouraging. I see in the future further application of the use of synthetic materials that can simulate directly microbial materials. Equally important will be the study of molecules that appear to inhibit proliferation of the tumor cells and kill tumor cells directly. In other words, mediators of the immune response will be important. Their characterization and purification will allow a fine tuning of the use of nonspecific immunotherapy and, we hope, will allow the development of a true immunopharmacology.

It is going to be important to distinguish between tumors in which there is evidence of antigens inducing tumor rejection and in which the malfunctioning of the effector mechanisms may have contributed to the original development of the tumor. In systems in which the tumor cells are not recognized immunologically in the first place, immunotherapeutic approaches obviously will vary considerably. In the latter case, the problem is not how to strengthen and establish response or how to counteract blocking or enhancing factors, but how to render response in genetically unresponsive patients to a given tumor antigen.

The concept of immune surveillance has come under sharp attack during the past several years. The concept, first proposed by Ehrlich and later extended by Thomas and Burnett (1970), is more complicated than once conceived. Prehn suggested that spontaneous tumors may be stimulated by an immune reaction. Does this mean there is little hope for immunologic control of cancer? I think not. Both in vitro and in vivo evidence of host reaction to tumor is unequivocal. Virus-induced neoplasms give the most convincing evidence for tumor immunogenicity and surveillance (Klein and Klein, 1977). Unfortunately, we do not know if human tumors, with occasional exceptions, fit in this category. In terms of spontaneous tumors that we see clinically, we must recall the work Foulds published more than 20 years ago when he described the model of tumor progression (1958). Multiple changes are responsible for the development of most naturally occurring tumors. Many concepts of immunotherapy are based on the notion that tumors are rejectable in the autologous host and that tumor growth is a failure of the rejection response. This may be an important weakness in our current thinking. The poor rejectability of spontaneous tumors may have several causes. Antigenic modulation and the shedding of antigens are other ways tumor cells escape the immune response. These antigens flood the body and inhibit lymphocytes and macrophages. Tolerance, therefore, may play a critical role in the lack of recognition. We must deal with these escape mechanisms much more carefully.

I foresee an important increase in our understanding of the aging process and how it relates to the immune response and to cancer. One of the greatest potentials for immunologic intervention will be in the aged population. In addition, work on tumor immunology and immunotherapy has profound implications not only for cancer but for other diseases associated with aging, including autoimmune phenomena, arthritis, and neurologic diseases. Thus, the spin-off of research in the immunotherapy of cancer will be tremendous.

Immunodeficiency associated with aging in certain strains of mice can be altered dramatically by diet; reduced dietary protein intake in mice from the time of weaning is associated with decreased weight gain in both male and female mice and increased longevity, which, in turn, is associated with more vigorous antibody and cellular response. Deficiencies of essential amino acids also may influence the immune system. Although there are conflicting data, there is a suggestion that high-cholesterol environments may be inimical to the ability of macrophages to kill tumor cells. There is increasing evidence of the importance of heavy metals on the aging process and the immune response. Deficiencies of certain metals play an important role in interfering with materials such as interferon. Zinc deficiency can lead to immunosuppression. Because the incidence of some cancers, such as colon and breast cancer, is higher in western cultures, we need to better understand the relationship between diet and the immune system. Therefore, dietary manipulation may be an important aspect of immune modulation or immune engineering, and may be crucial in true immunoprophylaxis.

Another influence on the immune system is stress. Possibly, emotional stress could play a part in causing a lymphocyte breakdown. It will be difficult to study prolonged periods of anxiety and frustration, but we know that certain personality types have a higher incidence of cancer, and I think this needs further evaluation.

FINANCIAL SUPPORT

How will all this work get done? Until the beginning of the 20th century, research was largely confined to the university. Then, industry began to see the advantage of creating its own research laboratories, and finally, around World War II, the US government became an active participant in research, particularly through contracts and grants. In addition to industry and the federal government, the private sector has played an increasingly important role in the support of biomedical research. I think it is going to be crucial during the coming years that the private sector contribute to our progress. However, the modern research laboratories of the pharmaceutical industry may be one of the only places where the search for new and better drugs can take place. Only industry is so organized with capable scientists directed toward the search for better drugs and has the essentials for further advancement.

It seems to me that the pharmaceutical industry, the university, as well as the federal government must work more closely together. One of the problems with drug development is the long, expensive ordeal to clear various agencies of the government. Investigators tend to give up early because of the tedious time it takes to develop new drugs. We should recall the agonizing time from Fleming's original discovery of the bacteriostatic activity of mold until Florey and Chain's effort to isolate and produce penicillin. As Chain has stressed recently, granting bodies seem reluctant to provide funds for the large-scale production of biologically active substances occurring in the natural source in trace amounts. Thus, it has frequently fallen on the private research organizations to provide funds for this activity.

ETHICS

The cancer patient is also crucial for the future of immunotherapy. We must constantly try to help the patient without doing harm. The patient has the legal as well as moral right to be properly informed of potential, new therapy. What is important is that the physician be humble in his responsibilities of administering new treatments. We must deal with patients as we would ourselves or our own family members.

In 1950, the French author Vercours wrote a story entitled "You Shall Know Them," in which a group of missing links was found to resemble humans. They were gentle, tractable, and highly educable. Soon, they were used widely to do all sorts of labor. The hero of the story, who believed the creatures to be human, becomes upset by the exploitation and decides to kill a young one to settle the issue of whether the creatures were human. If the hero wins the issue, he will be convicted of murder. If he loses, his protégés will be destined for exploitation forever. The resolution was that the creatures were indeed human. However, the judge points out that the hero really slaughtered an animal because the only criterion for humanness is acceptance by other humans, and until that was done by killing one of the creatures, they were not actually human.

Requesting informed consent of patients being submitted for clinical investigation not only informs the patient but also says to the physician, "This is a human being like yourself." This should be a reminder and a caution, for we have a spectrum of ideas of humanness. We often perceive those persons different from us as a little less human. Informed consent should have its greatest meaning to the investigator, therefore, when the subject seems a little different. To many, the sick person, in a sense, is different, weaker, thus also a little less human; clinical investigators constantly must be aware of this.

CONCLUSION

What will the scientific historians think of our era? Will they describe it as a period of pessimism, despair, and cynicism, or will it be a period of enlightenment, a Renaissance? I think the latter will be true, but we must be careful to avoid despair and pessimism. It would be tragic if tumor immunology failed to flourish. We cannot actually see where the future is going, but we must remember that primitive man shivered and froze on the site of what are now the great coal mines.

Too many of us are afraid of driving anything but the latest model automobile and insist on the most modern gadgets in our homes, only to manifest an obsolete or even Victorian philosophy regarding new ideas and research. After the second World War, a novel, *The Tin Drum,* was written by Gunther Grass. It was about a boy who, at three years of age, decided that he was never going to grow up. There are countless people in our world who have decided at one time or another that they were not going to grow up. They had their little drum, their favorite tantrums, and they made out very well by staying as they were. As someone said, "In this kind of world, we need only to fear the small scale individual whose very littleness will bring the larger world down around our heads."

We must open our minds and grow with the times. We must be creative, innovative, and open to new possibilities. Many of our ideas will become reality and many will not. What is important is that we try to develop better treatment, not to replace, but to supplement our current approaches. Thus, we must be willing to brave the disapproval of our colleagues. This is the one essential quality for those who seek to change the way cancer patients now live. It is easy to follow the familiar paths, but the future does not belong to those who are content with today or apathetic toward the problems that exist. We must have a vision that we can shape a better future for the cancer patient. Robert Kennedy was fond of saying that it is the individual who makes the difference.

"Each time a man stands up for an ideal or acts to improve the lot of others or strikes out against injustice, he sends forth a tiny ripple of hope and crossing each other from a million different centers of energy and daring these ripples build a current which can sweep down the mightiest walls of oppression and resistance."

I would like to close with a story. Two jealous, cynical disciples decided to discredit their Rabbi for their own ends. To test the Rabbi, they caught a small bird. If the Rabbi said it was alive, they planned to crush and kill it. If the Rabbi said the bird was dead, they planned to permit it to fly off dramatically before the multitude. With one holding the bird behind him, the other asked the Rabbi which of them had the bird. "The one who is silent." The silent one then asked, "Is the bird alive or dead?" The Rabbi looked him straight in the eye and said, "That depends on you." Indeed, I think the future of immunotherapy depends on all of us. Whether it lives or dies depends on our attitudes, our cooperation, our leadership, and our enthusiasm.

Let this be our call to arms. Let us return to our labs and clinics working as individuals and together. I am confident that if we can keep in mind some of the principles that I have reviewed, we will develop a new form of therapy that will become uniquely important for the cancer patient of today and of the future.

REFERENCES

Bronowski, J. 1973. Ascent of Man. Boston, Little Brown.

Burnett, F. M. 1970. The concept of immunological surveillance. Prog. Exp. Tumor Res., 13:1–27.

Clarke, A. 1972. In Toffler, A. (ed.): The Futurists. New York, Random House, pp. 133–150.

Coley, W. B. 1911. A report of recent cases of inoperable sarcomas successfully treated with mixed toxins of erysipelas and bacillus prodigiosus. Surg. Gynecol. Obstet., 13:174.

Foulds, L. 1958. The natural history of cancer. J. Chron. Dis., 8:2–37.

Klein, G., and Klein, E. 1977. Immune surveillance against virus induced tumors and nonrejectability of spontaneous tumors: Contrasting consequences of host versus tumor evolution. Proc. Natl. Acad. Sci. USA, 74:2121–2125.

Langer, W. L. 1976. Immunization against smallpox before Jenner. Sci. Am., Jan:112–117.

Smith, A. 1975. Power of Mind. New York, Random House.

Thomas, L. 1974. The Lives of a Cell; Notes of a Biology Watcher. New York, Viking Press, p. 153.

Van Potter, R. 1975. Humility with responsibility: A bioethic for oncologists. Presidential address. Cancer Res., 35:2297–2306.

Author Index[*]

A
Amery, William K., 181-195
Amiel, Jean-Louis, 245-256
Azuma, Ichiro, 131-154

B
Bartold, Shelley L., 257-265
Bekesi, J. George, 237-244
Bellet, Robert E., 375-394
Belpomme, Dominique, 245-256
Benjamin, Robert S., 257-265
Berd, David, 375-394
Blumenschein, G. R., 321-345
Bottino, Joseph C., 83-97
Brehmer, Werner, 131-154
Burgess, Michael A., 257-265
Buzdar, A. U., 321-345

C
Cantrell, John L., 131-154
Cattan, Albert, 245-256
Chirigos, Michael A., 181-195
Clark, R. Lee, *ix-xi*
Cuttner, Janet, 237-244

D
Delgado, Miguel, 245-256
de Vassal, Francoise, 245-256

E
Edelstein, Richard, 363-374
Eidinger, David, 289-301
Ezaki, Khoji, 83-97

F
Fahey, J. L., 31-39
Farquhar, David, 83-97
Fidler, Isaiah, J., 63-81

G
Gall, Stanley A., 303-319
Gehan, Edmund A., 257-265
Gil, Marianne, 245-256
Goldstein, Allan L., 83-97, 173-179
Granatek, Christine H., 83-97
Gutterman, Jordan U., 83-97, 257-265, 321-345, 395-406

H
Hanna, M. G., Jr., 111-129
Hayat, Maurice, 245-256
Hersh, Evan M., *ix-xi,* 83-97, 257-265, 321-345, 355-359
Hickey, Robert C., *ix-xi,* 3-4
Holland, James F., 237-244
Hollinshead, Ariel C., 213-233
Hortobagyi, G. N., 321-345
Hwang, Kou M., 131-154

I
Israël, Lucien, 363-374

J
Jasmin, Claude, 245-256

K
Kennedy, Anne, 257-265

---

[*]*See also* List of Contributors, pp. *xiii-xix.*

407

L

Lawrence, H. Sherwood, 197-211

M

Machover, David, 245-256
Malahy, Mary Anne, 355-359
Marshall, Gailen D., Jr., 173-179
Mastrangelo, Michael J., 375-394
Mathé, Georges, 5-27, 245-256
Mavligit, Giora M., 83-97, 257-265,
  355-359
McBride, Charles M., 257-265
McKneally, Martin F., 347-353
McLaughlin, Charles A., 131-154
McMurtrey, Marion J., 267-288
Misset, Jean-Louis, 245-256
Morris, Dexter, 83-97
Musset, Marina, 245-256

P

Papadopoulos, Nicholas, 267-288
Patt, Yehuda Z., 83-97
Pena-Angulo, Juan, 245-256
Peters, Leona C., 111-129
Peters, Lester J., 155-172
Pico, José-Luis, 245-256
Plager, Carl, 267-288
Pouillart, Pierre, 245-256

R

Ribaud, Patricia, 245-256
Ribi, Edgar, 131-154

Richman, Stephen P., 83-97, 257-265,
  321-345
Rios, Adan, 83-97
Rivera, Ernesto, 83-97
Romero, Jimmy J., 267-288
Romsdahl, Marvin M., 267-288
Rosenfeld, Claude, 245-256
Rossen, Roger D., 83-97
Rossio, Jeffrey L., 173-179

S

Samak, Raymond, 363-374
Schneider, Maurice, 245-256
Schwarzenberg, Léon, 245-256
Sinkovics, Joseph G., 267-288
Strain, S. Michael, 131-154

T

Toubiana, Raoul, 131-154

W

Waldinger, Ruth, 267-288
Weiner, Roy, 245-256
Weiss, David W., 41-61, 101-109
Wiseman, C., 321-345

Y

Yamamura, Yuichi, 131-154

Z

Zatopek, Nancy, 355-359

Subject Index

A

N-Acetylmuramyldipeptide, 144-146
Actinomycin D, 275, 277, 308
  in malignant melanoma, 258, 261-264
Adenocarcinoma of endometrium, 305
Adrenergic hormones, 77
Adriamycin (doxorubicin), 165, 277, 279, 308, 317, 324
  in breast cancer, 327-338
Aging process, 403
Alkylating agents, 305
ALL, see Leukemia, acute lymphoblastic
Allogeneic
  cells, 37
  mice, 75-76
AML, see Leukemia, acute myelocytic
AMP, cyclic, levamisole and, 192
Amplification mechanisms, impaired, 34-35
Anergy, 199-200, 323
Animal models, 63-64, 101-109, 385, 386
  for BCG immunotherapy, 111-128
  domestic, 108-109
  ideal, 386
  of metastases, 71-76
Antibody, blocking, 33
Antigen
  administration, intralymphatic, 37
  -antibody complexes, 33
  lack, 36
Antigenic conversion, 273
Antigenicity
  relative, 66-69
  tumor, minimal hypothesis of, 42
Antigens
  animal tumor, 375-376
  cancer cell membrane, 216
  carcinoembryonic, see Carcinoembryonic antigen
  cell surface, 83-84
  complement-fixing, see Complement-fixing antigen
  diffuse cytoplasmic, see Diffuse cytoplasmic antigen
  doses of, 33

granular cytoplasmic, see Granular cytoplasmic antigen
  sarcoma-specific, 273-276
  T cell responses to, 31-32
  tumor-associated, see Tumor-associated antigens
  tumor-specific, see Tumor-specific antigens
Antilymphocyte serum, 69
Antipyrine half-time, 86
  Corynebacterium parvum and, 93-94
Antithymocyte serum, 12
Arabinose mycolate, 140
Arabinosylcytosine, 247
Arlacel A, 227
L-Asparaginase, 69, 246-247
Azathioprine, 191-192

B

B cells, 34
  immune deficiency diseases of, 32
B16 melanoma, 65-66
  BCG and, 7, 9
  immunogenicity and, 66-69
Bacillus Calmette-Guérin (BCG), ix-x
  adjuvant immunotherapy, 292-298
  in ALL, 245-251
  ascitic tumor cells and, 13
  in B16 melanoma, 7, 9
  in bladder cancer, 291, 292-297, 298-299
  in breast cancer, 326-328
  cell wall (CW), 132-137
  colony-forming units and, 14
  in colorectal cancer, 355-356
  contralateral challenge and, 116
  cyclophosphamide and, 7-8, 15-18
  dermatophytin and, 91
  dosage, 389
  in genitourinary cancer, 290-299
  in gynecologic malignancies, 308-309
  hepatic microsomal enzymes and, 93
  immunotherapy, 111-128
  -induced septicemia, 9

Bacillus Calmette-Guérin (BCG) *(contd.)*
 intralesional, 114-119, 378
 L1210 leukemia and, 7-8
 Lewis tumor and, 7-11
 in lung cancer, 347-350
 lymphoid stem cells and, 14
 in malignant melanoma, 257-264
 Mathé, Dr. Georges, and, 3-4
 into melanoma nodules, 279
 in metastatic renal cell tumors, 297-298,
  299
 methanol extraction residue of, 239-244;
   see also Methanol extraction residue
 purified protein derivative and, 122
 reactions to, 131
 RFCNU and, 17-18
 in sarcomas, 276
 thymosin and, 94
 transfer factor and, 204
 -tumor cell vaccine
  micrometastases and, 119-124
  after surgery, 124-125
 tumor growth and, 12, 116
 vaccine preparation, 113-114
 viral oncolysates and, 280
BCG, *see* Bacillus Calmette-Guérin
BCNU, 165
 levamisole and, 182, 188-189
Bisdiazobenzidine, 337
Bladder cancer, 291, 292-297, 298-299
Blocking antibody, 33
Blocking factors, 33, 218, 366, 367
 circulating, 95
  removal of, 368
  removal of membrane-bound, 368-369
Boosting, immunologic, 90-93
Bordetella pertussis, 382-383
Breast cancer, 200-201, 321-340
Brucella abortus, 23, 24

C

C1q binding activity, 89, 90
Calmette-Guérin bacillus, *see* Bacillus
  Calmette-Guérin
Candida, 87-88
 in colorectal cancer, 358
Carcinoembryonic antigen (CEA), 89, 304
 in colorectal cancer, 356-358
CCNU, 240
 methyl CCNU, 182, 238
CEA, *see* Carcinoembryonic antigen
Cell
 -mediated immunity, 55-56, 198-199
  transfer factor and, 199-200
 recognition systems, 36-37
 surface antigens, 83-84
 surfaces, tumor, 213
 wall (CW)

BCG, 132-137
 skeleton (CWS), 132-137, 148
Cervical cancer, tumor immunity in, 87
CFU, *see* colony-forming units
Chemoimmunotherapy, 11-18; *see also*
  Chemotherapy
 for ALL, 245-254
 for AML, 237-244
 for breast cancer, 321-340
  micrometastases, 335-337
Chemotaxis, monocyte, 34
Chemotherapy, 84
 Corynebacterium parvum interactions
  with, 164-166
 immunotherapy versus, 382
 interactions with immunotherapy, 95-96
  400
 intermittent, 11-18
 interrelationship with immunotherapy,
  228-231
 levamisole and, 189-190
 transfer factor and, 202-203
Chloramphenicol, 164
Coley, Dr. William B., 267-269
Colony-forming units, (CFU)
 assay, 85-86
 BCG and, 14
Colorectal cancer, 355-359
Complement-fixing (S3) antigen, 275
Concanavalin A (ConA), 24, 44, 45, 85, 88
 levamisole and, 184
 in sarcomas, 269
Contralateral challenge, 121
 BCG and, 116
Cord factor, purified, *see* Trehalose
  dimycolate
Corticosteroids, 156, 165-166, 324
Cortisone acetate, 165-166
Corynebacterium, 21-23
 granulosum, 23, 248
 parvum, 21, 91-92, 155-157
  antipyrine half-time and, 93-94
  in breast cancer, 326-327, 331-333
  chemotherapy and, 164-166
  cyclophosphamide and, 164-165
  in disseminated cancer, 364
  in experimental tumors, 155-168
  in genitourinary cancer, 290-291
  in gynecologic malignancies, 307,
   309-313
  heat and, 166-167
  immunoprophylaxis with, 157
  in malignant melanoma, 258-264
  radiation and, 162-164
  in sarcomas, 276
  T cells and, 161-162
  thymosin fraction 5 and, 162
  tumor-specific immune responses and,
   161-162

Corynomycolic acid, 145
Coxiella burnetii, 141
CW, *see* Cell wall
CWS, *see* Cell wall skeleton
Cyclic
    AMP, *see* AMP, cyclic
    GMP, *see* GMP, cyclic
Cyclophosphamide, 240, 277, 317
    in ALL, 246-248
    BCG and, 7-8, 15-18
    in breast cancer, 327-328
    Corynebacterium parvum and, 164-165
    effector cells and, 49
Cytosine arabinoside, 240-243
Cytotoxicity assays, lymphocyte-mediated,
        270-272

D
Daunorubicin, 240-242
Dedifferentiation, 197
Defense mechanism, host, *see* Host defense
        mechanism
Dermatophytin, 87-88
    BCG and, 91
    in colorectal cancer, 358
    levamisole and, 92-93
Dexamethasone, 243
Dextran sulfate, 24, 44, 45
Diffuse cytoplasmic antigen (S2), 275
Dimethyl triazeno imidazole carboxamide
        (DTIC), 277
    chemotherapy, 91
    demethylase, 93
    in malignant melanoma, 257-264
Dinitrochlorobenzene (DNCB), 269, 306
    in breast cancer, 323, 326-327
    in vaginal cancer, 309
Dinitrofluorobenzene (DNFB), 306-307
DNCB, *see* Dinitrochlorobenzene
DNFB, *see* Dinitrofluorobenzene
Doxorubicin, *see* Adriamycin
DTIC, *see* Dimethyl triazeno imidiazole car-
        boxamide
Dukes' class B lesions, 356-357
Dukes' class C lesions, 355-359

E
EAE, *see* Encephalomyelitis, experimental
        "allergic"
Effector cells, 47-52, 307
    deficiency of, 89-90
    kinetics of development of, 51
Electrophoresis, *see under* Polyacrylamide
        gel
Embolus formation, 77
Encephalomyelitis, experimental "allergic"
        (EAE), 228
Endometrium, adenocarcinoma of, 305

Endotoxin, 135-136, 267-269, 282
    antitumor properties of, 141-143
    effects in man, 268
Environmental determinants, 106-107
Epodyl (triethylene glycol diglycidyl ether),
        293
Epstein-Barr (E-B) virus-immune transfer
        factor, 205
Erysipelas, 267
Escherichia coli, 135, 141
Estrogens
Ewing's sarcoma, 272, 275-276

F
Fc receptors, 307
α-Fetoprotein, 304
Fibrosarcomas, 272
5-Fluorouracil (5-FU), 58
    in breast cancer, 327-338
    in colorectal cancer, 355-357
Freund's adjuvant, 226-228, 350
5-FU, *see* 5-Fluorouracil

G
Genital cancer, *see* Gynecologic malignancies
Genitourinary cancer, 289-299
Glucan, 326-327
Glycolipids, Re, *see* Re glycolipids
Glycoproteins on tumor cells, 217, 281
GMP, cyclic, levamisole and, 192
Granular cytoplasmic antigen (S1), 275
Gynecologic
    cancer patient, immune status of, 306-
        308
    malignancies, 303-317
        experimental immunotherapy for
            clinical, 308-317
        features of, 304-306

H
Heat and *Corynebacterium parvum,* 166-167
Heath Memorial Award
    lecture, 5-25
    recipient, introduction of, 3-4
Helper cells, 281
Hemocyanin, keyhole limpet (KLH), 24, 290
Hepatic microsomal enzymes and BCG, 93
Hepatocarcinoma, line 10, 111-112
Hepatoma isografts and MER, 55
Histiocytoma, 283
Histiocytosis, sinus, 322
Hodgkin's disease, transfer factor and, 207
Host
    defense mechanism, 65
    and environment interactions in neo-
        plasia, 106-107
    immune
        responses, evidence for, 321-322

Host
  immune *(contd.)*
    status, tumor cell growth and, 72-76
  immunity, metastasis and, 69-71
  -tumor interaction, 76-77
Humoral recognition factor, 369
Hydrocortisone, 166
Hypernephroma, 297-298, 299
Hypernephroma-specific transfer factor, 205
Hypersensitivity
  Jones-Mote, 218
  reactions, delayed, 31, 91-93, 306-307
    in malignant melanoma, 87-88
Hyperthermia, 156
Hysterectomy, total abdominal, 310-311

I

Immune
  assessment of patients with sarcoma,
    269-272
  complexes, 367
  deficiency diseases of B cells, 32
  monitoring, 224
  paralysis, 33
  resistance, failure of, 32-36
  response to tumor, 31-32
  responses, tumor-specific, 161-162
  status of gynecologic cancer patient,
    306-308
  system
    influence of therapeutic maneuvers
      on, 323-324
    stress and, 403-404
    tumor isolation from, 35
Immunity
  cell-mediated, *see* Cell-mediated immunity
  endocrine thymus and, 174
  host, *see* Host immunity
  sarcoma-directed, 270-272
  transfer of, 377-378, 379
Immunization, *see also* Immunotherapy
  active-specific, 377
  sarcoma-specific, 276
  specific, 378
Immunobiology, tumor, *x*
Immunocompetence, 84, 363-364, 390
  prognosis and, 322-323
  thymosin dose and, 94
Immunocytes, 43, 369
Immunodeficiency, progressive, 84
Immunogenicity
  B16 melanoma lines and, 66-69
  low, 36
Immunogens, delayed hypersensitivity, 31
Immunoglobulin deficiencies, 32
Immunologic
  boosting, 90-93
  concomitants of tumor initiation, 197-198

consequences of tumor growth, 198
Immunology, immunotherapy and, 104
  principles of, 31-38
Immunomodulation with MER, 44-59
Immunoprophylaxis, 377-378, 382, 384-
    386, 401
  with *Corynebacterium parvum,* 157
Immunoresistance, 12
Immunosuppressive
  mechanisms, tumor-dependent, 365-367
  phenomena, 323, 363, 367
  serum factors, 88-89
  treatment modalities, 324
Immunosurveillance, 32, 42, 402-403
Immunotherapy, *see also* Immunization
  accomplishments in, 381-384
  active, 5-25
    development of clinical trial, 20-25
    for minimal residual disease, 5-11
  active-nonspecific, 290-291, 383-384
    for breast cancer, 326-327
  active-specific, 213-231, 382-383, 385
    for breast cancer, 337-339
    for genitourinary cancer, 289-290
    for gynecologic malignancies, 308-
      309
  adjuvant, for colorectal cancer, 355-359
  adoptive, 95, 292, 384
    for animal tumors, 379
    -passive specific, 48
  animal
    models of, 101-109
    tumor, 375-380
  approaches to, 93-233
  basic research in, 401-404
  with BCG, *see* Bacillus Calmette-Guérin
  for breast cancer, 321-340
    micrometastases, 335-337
  chemotherapy and, *see* Chemoimmuno-
    therapy, chemotherapy
  clinical, 235-359
    foundations of, *ix-x*
    rationale for, 83-96
  controls in, 390
  controversies about, 388-391
  with *Corynebacterium parvum,* 158-159
  detrimental effects of, 93-95
  for established micrometastases, 119-
    124
  ethics in, 404-405
  experimental, for clinical gynecologic
    cancer, 308-317
  experimental basis of, 63-78; *see also*
    Animal models
  financial support for, 404
  future of, 384-388, 395-406
  for genitourinary cancer, 289-299
  goals of, 325

Immunotherapy *(contd.)*
  for gynecologic malignancies, 303-317
  immunologic and clinical basis of, 29-97
  immunology and, 104, 279-283
  intralymphatic, 35, 37
  introduction to, *ix-xi*
  investigators in, 398-401
    with levamisole, *see* Levamisole
  limitations and obstacles in, 375-388
  for line 10 tumors, 148-149
  local, 20, 325-326
  for lung cancer, 226-231
  for malignant melanoma, 203-205, 257-
    264
  with MER, *see* Methanol extraction
    residue
  with microbial constituents, 131-150
  for micrometastases, 63
  new approaches to, 363-371
  nonspecific
    for animal tumors, 378-379
    for lung cancer, 347-351
    for ovarian carcinoma, 309-317
    tumor growth and, 41-59
    for vaginal cancer, 309
  objectives of, 95
  before other cancer treatments, 18-19
  passive, 384
    for animal tumors, 379
    for breast cancer, 339
  passive-nonspecific, 292
  passive-specific, 291-292
  philosophy of, 397-398
  principles
    of immunology and, 31-38
    and prospects for, 361-406
  procedures, new, 368-371
  regional, 19-20
  results, interpretation of, 390
  for sarcomas, 267-283
  scheduling of, 35-36
  side effects of, 108
  termination of, 391
  with thymosin, *see* Thymosin
  with transfer factor, 197-209
Individualism, need for, 395-406
Inflammatory response capability, 34
Interferon, 278, 334
Isoniazid, 348
Isotachophoresis, 218-219

J
Jones-Mote hypersensitivity, 218

K
K cells, 43
Kaposi's sarcoma, 269
  cells, 275

Keyhole limpet hemocyanin, *see* Hemocyanin,
  keyhole limpet
Killer cells, 173, 280-281
  natural (NK), 43, 50
  spontaneous (SK), 32
KLH, *see* Hemocyanin, keyhole limpet

L
L1210 leukemia, 237-238
  BCG and, 7-8
  cells, survival times with, 6-7
Lethality, 141-143
Leukemia
  acute lymphoblastic
    chemotherapy-immunotherapy
      protocols for, 245-254
    transfer factor and, 207
  acute myelocytic (AML), 92, 237-244
  AKR, 20, 237-238
  EAKR, 20
  L1210, *see* L1210 leukemia
  transfer factor and, 207
Leukocyte migration inhibition
  assay, 85
  levamisole and, 190
Levamisole, 181, 369, 385
  AMP and, 192
  BCNU and, 182, 188-189
  chemical structure of, 182
  chemotherapy and, 189-190
  dermatophytin and, 92-93
  dosage, 389
  dose effect of, 186-187
  GMP and, 192
  in human breast cancer, 333, 334
  immunologic profile of, 190-192
  leukocyte migration inhibition and, 190
  in lung cancer, 349-351
  lymphocyte cytotoxicity and responsive-
    ness and, 191
  metastasis and, 187
  mitogens and, 184
  neutrophils and, 190
  therapy, combined, 181-192
Lewis tumor, BCG and, 7-11
Lipid composition of mycobacteria, 138-139
Lipopeptides, 144
Lipopolysaccharide (LPS), 24, 25, 44, 45
  bacterial, 282; see also Endotoxin
Liposarcoma, 283
LPS, *see* Lipopolysaccharide
Lung Cancer
  immunotherapy trials, 226-231
  nonspecific immunotherapy for, 347-
    351
Lymph node
  involvement, 364
  metastases, 257

Lymphoblastogenesis inhibitory factor, 217
Lymphocyte
  blastogenic response to mitogens, 85,
    88, 269
  count, 323
  cytotoxicity, levamisole and, 191
  infiltration, 322
  -mediated cytotoxicity assays, 270-272
  mitogen, polyclonal, 44-46
  products, 278-279
  responsiveness, levamisole and, 191
  transfer, 277-278
  : tumor cell clumping, 68-69
Lymphocytes
  sensitized, 402
  syngeneic, 67
  thymus-dependent, *see* T cells
  "trephocytic" function of, 69
Lymphoid stem cells and BCG, 14
Lymphokine generation assay, 86
Lymphokines, 34
  injection of, 370
Lymphoma, cytotoxic, 281

M

Macrophage
  activation, 155-156, 282
  activities, MER stimulation of, 52-54
  depletion, 47
Macrophages, 31, 269
  syngeneic, 67
Mammary tumor D7T4S, 57-58
Mathé, Dr. Georges, 3-4
Megestrol, 291
Melanoma
  B16, *see* B16 melanoma
  malignant
    immunodeficiency and, 87-88
    immunotherapy for, 203-205, 257-
     264
  nodules, BCG into, 279
  radioimmunoassay, 223-225
  -specific transfer factor, 204
  tumor-associated antigens, 219-224
Melphalan, 308, 310-313
MER, *see* Methanol extraction residue
6-Mercaptopurine in ALL, 246-248
Metastases, tumor
  artificial, 117-118
  BCG and, 111-128
  cryptic distant, 349
  development of, 64-65
  extent of, 66-69
  host immunity and, 69-71
  levamisole and, 187
  low versus high, 66-69
  lymph node, 257
  micrometastases, *see* Micrometastases

organ-specific, 77
  pulmonary, 118
  radiation and, 164
  transfer factor and, 204
  tumor cell properties and, 65-66
Metastatic
  potential, 77-78
  renal cell tumors, 297-298, 299
Methanol extraction residue (MER) of BCG,
  21-22, 239-244
  hepatoma isografts and, 55
  immunomodulation with, 44-59
  immunotherapy with, 55-59
  mammary tumor D7T4S and, 57-58
  Rous sarcoma virus and, 56
  stimulation
    of macrophage activities, 52-54
    of T cell functions, 47-52
Methotrexate, 228-229, 279, 308, 324
  in ALL, 246-248
  in breast cancer, 329-338
Methyl CCNU, 182, 238
Microbial constituents, immunotherapy with,
  131-150
Micrometastases, *see also* Metastases, tumor
  formation of, 74
  breast cancer, 335-337
  immunotherapy for, 63
    established, 119-124
Migration inhibitory factor (MIF), 197
Mithramycin, 275
Mitogen
  lymphocyte blastogenic response to, 85,
    88, 269
  pokeweed, *see* Pokeweed mitogen
  polyclonal lymphocyte, 44-46
Mitomycin C, 147-148
Moloney sarcoma virus, 379
Monocyte chemotaxis, 34
Mortality, *see* Survival times
Mycobacterial
  cell walls, 132-137
  lipid composition, 138-139
Mycobacterium
  bovis, 291
  smegmatis, 22
Mycolic acid, 138-140, 145

N

Nandrolone decanoate, 333
Nasopharyngeal cancer, transfer factor for,
  205
Necrosis factor, tumor, 269
Neuraminidase, 369
  Vibrio cholerae, 237
Neutrophils and levamisole, 190
NK, *see* Killer cells, natural
Nocardomycolic acid, 145

Null cells, 280-281

O

Omentectomy, 310-311
Oncolysates, viral
 allogeneic sarcoma, 277
 BCG and, 280
Oncornavirus, 273-275
Oncovin, *see* Vincristine
Opsonin, nonspecific, 366
Osteoclasts, 272
Osteosarcoma, 201-203, 269, 283
 cells, 272
 transfer factor, 201-203
Ovarian carcinoma, 304-305, 307
 histologic types of, 312
 nonspecific immunotherapy for, 309-317

P

P3, *see* Trehalose dimycolate
PAGE, *see* Polyacrylamide gel electrophoresis
Paget's osteitis deformans, 275
L-PAM, *see* L-Phenylalanine mustard
Papillomatosis of larynx, transfer factor for,
 206
Paralysis, immune, 33
PGPE, *see* Polyacrylamide gel preparative
 electrophoresis
PHA, *see* Phytohemagglutinin
L-Phenylalanine mustard (L-PAM), 336
Phytohemagglutinin (PHA), 24, 44, 45, 85,
 184, 242, 269
 blastogenesis, 366
Plasmapheresis, *x*, 95, 368, 370
Pokeweed mitogen (PWM), 85, 88, 184, 242
Polyacrylamide gel
 electrophoresis (PAGE), 215, 217, 218
 preparative electrophoresis (PGPE), 218
Polyoma virus, 379
Polypeptides, nomenclature for thymosin,
 174-176
PPD, *see* Protein derivative, purified
Prednisone, 246-248, 336, 338
Procarbazine, 165
Prognosis, immunocompetence and, 322-323
Propionibacterium, 155
Protein derivative, purified (PPD), 44, 45,
 200
 BCG and, 122
 in bladder cancer, 293, 298
 in breast cancer, 326-327
Pseudomonas aeruginosa, 23-25
Pseudomonas vaccine, 333
PWM, *see* Pokeweed mitogen
Pyrogenicity, 141-143

R

Radiation, 324

Corynebacterium parvum interactions
 with, 162-164
 metastases and, 164
Radioimmunoassay, melanoma, 223-225
Radiotherapy, 83, 84
Randomization procedures, 282
Re glycolipids, 135, 137-150
 CWS and, 148
 P3 and, 146-147
 tumor regression and, 140
Red blood cells, sheep (SRBC), 24
 MER and, 46
Regression, tumor, *x*, 143-144
 Re glycolipid and, 140
 spontaneous, 111, 303
Renal cell tumors, 297-298, 299
 transfer factor for, 205-206
Residual disease, treatment of, 5-11
Retabolil, 333
Reticuloendothelial
 clearance, 389
 system activation, 69, 89, 95
RFCNU and BCG, 17-18
Rhabdomyosarcoma, 283
Rous sarcoma virus (RSV), MER and, 56

S

S1, *see* Granular cytoplasmic antigen
S2, *see* Diffuse cytoplasmic antigen
S3, *see* Complement-fixing antigen
Salmonella, 141-142
 enteritidis, 141-142
 minnesota, 141
 typhimurium, 135, 137, 141-142
Salpingo-oophorectomy, bilateral, 310-311
Sarcoma, 267-283
 -directed immunity, 270-272
 immune assessment of patients with,
  269-272
 osteogenic, *see* Osteosarcoma
 -specific
  antigens, 273-276
  immunization, 276
Second signal hypothesis, 36
Septicemia induced by BCG, 9
Serratia marcescens, 267
Serum factors, immunosuppressive, 88-89
Sézary syndrome, 281
Side effects of immunotherapy, 108
SK-SD, *see* Streptokinase-streptodornase
SRBC, *see* Red blood cells, sheep
Staphylococcus albus, 52-53
Stilbestrol, 324
Streptokinase-streptodornase (SK-SD), 200
Streptolysin O, 85
Stress, immune system and, 403-404
Suppressor cells, 34, 281
 thymosin and, 177

Survival times
  with acute lymphoid leukemia, 251-254
  with breast cancer, 328-337
  with L1210 leukemia cells, 6-7
  with line 10 hepatocarcinoma, 120-125
  with ovarian carcinoma, 312-317
Syngeneic
  lymphocytes, 67
  preference, 36-37

T

T cell
  depression, 324
  functions, MER stimulation of, 47-52
  immune reactions, 31
  measurement, 85
  responses to antigen, 31-32
T cells
  Corynebacterium parvum and, 161-162
  pre-, 177
  suppressor, 34
TAA, *see* Tumor-associated antigens
Terminal deoxynucleotidyl transferase (TdT), 177
Thioguanine, 240, 243
Thiotepa (triethylenethiophosphoramide), 293
Thrombocytopenia, 76-77
Thymectomy, 70, 177
Thymidine, tritiated, 52-53
Thymosin, 93, 369
  BCG and, 94
  dose and immunocompetence, 94
  fraction 5
    action, postulated, 176-178
    basic properties of, 173-176
    Corynebacterium parvum and, 162
    therapy, 173-178
  immunoreconstitution and, 176
  polypeptides, nomenclature for, 174-176
  suppressor cells and, 177
Thymus, endocrine, immunity and, 174
Thymus-dependent lymphocytes, *see* T cells
Transfer factor, 199
  BCG and, 204
  bovine, 209
  breast-tumor-specific, 201
  cell-mediated immunity and, 199-200
  chemotherapy and, 202-203
  Epstein-Barr virus-immune, 205
  in Hodgkin's disease, 207
  hypernephroma-specific, 205
  immunotherapy and, 197-209
  in leukemia, 207
  melanoma-specific, 204
  metastases and, 204
  in nasopharyngeal cancer, 205
  in osteosarcoma, 201-203

  in papillomatosis of larynx, 206
  pooled, "nonspecific," 200-201
  in renal cell carcinoma, 205-206
  in sarcomas, 278-279
  varicella-immune, 207
  zoster-immune, 207
Trehalose
  dibehenylbehenate, 144
  dimycolate (P3), 132-139
    Re glycolipid and, 146-147
    trimethylsilylated, 138-139
  dipalmitate, 144
Triethylene glycol diglycidyl ether (Epodyl), 293
Triethylenethiophosphoramide (thiotepa), 293
Trinitrophenol, 47
Trophoblastic tumors, 305-306
Tumor
  antigenicity, *see* Antigenicity, tumor
  -associated antigens (TAA), 20-25, 106, 213-214, 303-304, 322
    identification and isolation of, 214-216
    identification of inhibitory components of, 216-228
    melanoma, 219-224
    production of, 218-224
  cell
    adhesion, 65-66
    clumping, lymphocyte:, 68-69
    growth, *see* Tumor growth
    lines, 105
    properties, metastasis and, 65-69
    surfaces, 213
  cells, glycoproteins on, 217
  -dependent immunosuppressive mechanisms, 365-367
  growth, 71-72
    BCG and, 116
    curves, BCG and, 12
    host immune status and, 72-76
    immunologic consequences of, 198
    nonspecific immunotherapy and, 41-59
    suppression, 143
  immunity
    in cervical cancer, 87
    systemic tumor burden and, 118
  immunobiology, *x*
  immunology, 279-283
  immunotherapy, *see* Immunotherapy
  initiation, immunologic concomitants of, 197-198
  interaction, host-, 76-77
  isolation from immune systems, 35
  metastases, *see* Metastases, tumor
  necrosis factor, 269
  regression, *see* Regression, tumor

Tumor *(contd.)*
  -specific
    antigens, 280, 376, 380-381
    immune responses, *Corynebacterium
      parvum* interactions with, 161-162
    immunity, 161
  systems, experimental, 101-233; *see also*
    Animal models

U
Ultrasonication, 135

V
Vaccine
  adjuvant, 226-228
  BCG-tumor cell, micrometastases and,
    119-124

preparation, BCG, 113-114
Vaginal cancer, 309
Varicella-immune transfer factor, 207
Varidase, 87-88, 358-359
Vasospasm, pulmonary, 77
Vibrio cholerae, 237, 383
Vincristine (Oncovin), 243, 246-248, 277,
    279
  in breast cancer, 329-338

W
Winn test, 48-49, 51-52

Z
Zoster-immune transfer factor, 207
Zymosan, 334